T0294594

Esophageal Cancer

Editors

JONATHAN C. YEUNG
ELENA ELIMOVA

THORACIC SURGERY CLINICS

www.thoracic.theclinics.com

Consulting Editor
VIRGINIA R. LITLE

November 2022 • Volume 32 • Number 4

ELSEVIER

1600 John F. Kennedy Boulevard ● Suite 1800 ● Philadelphia, Pennsylvania, 19103-2899

http://www.thoracic.theclinics.com

THORACIC SURGERY CLINICS Volume 32, Number 4
November 2022 ISSN 1547-4127, ISBN-13: 978-0-323-84989-0

Editor: John Vassallo (j.vassallo@elsevier.com)
Developmental Editor: Jessica Nicole B. Cañaberal

Thoracic Surgery Clinics (ISSN 1547-4127) is published quarterly by Elsevier Inc., 360 Park Avenue South, New York, NY 10010-1710. Months of publication are February, May, August, and November. Business and editorial offices: 1600 John F. Kennedy Boulevard, Suite 1800, Philadelphia, PA 19103-2899. Periodicals postage paid at New York, NY, and additional mailing offices. Subscription prices are $405.00 per year (US individuals), $875.00 per year (US institutions), $100.00 per year (US students), $473.00 per year (Canadian individuals), $893.00 per year (Canadian institutions), $100.00 per year (Canadian students), $225.00 per year (international students), $494.00 per year (international individuals), and $893.00 per year (international institutions). Foreign air speed delivery is included in all Clinics' subscription prices. All prices are subject to change without notice. **POSTMASTER:** Send address changes to Thoracic Surgery Clinics, Elsevier Health Sciences Division, Subscription Customer Service, 3251 Riverport Lane, Maryland Heights, MO 63043. **Customer Service (orders, claims, online, change of address): Telephone: 1-800-654-2452 (U.S. and Canada); 314-447-8871 (outside U.S. and Canada). Fax: 314-447-8029. E-mail: journalscustomerservice-usa@elsevier.com (for print support); journalsonlinesupport-usa@elsevier.com (for online support).**

Reprints. For copies of 100 or more, of articles in this publication, please contact Commercial Rights Department, Elsevier Inc., 360 Park Avenue South, New York, NY 10010-1710. Tel: 212-633-3874; Fax: 212-633-3820; E-mail: reprints@elsevier.com.

Thoracic Surgery Clinics is covered in *MEDLINE/PubMed (Index Medicus), EMBASE/Excerpta Medica, Science Citation Index Expanded (SciSearch®), Journal Citation Reports/Science Edition,* and *Current Contents®/Clinical Medicine.*

Contributors

CONSULTING EDITOR

VIRGINIA R. LITLE, MD
Section Chief of Thoracic Surgery, Medical
Director of Thoracic Surgery, Intermountain
Healthcare, Murray, Utah, USA

EDITORS

JONATHAN C. YEUNG, MD, PhD, FRCSC
Assistant Professor, Department of Surgery,
University of Toronto, Toronto General
Hospital, Toronto, Ontario, Canada

ELENA ELIMOVA, MD, MSc, FRCPC
Assistant Professor, Department of Medicine,
University of Toronto, Toronto, Ontario,
Canada

AUTHORS

AHMED ABDELHAKEEM, MD
Department of Internal Medicine, Baptist
Hospitals of Southeast Texas, Beaumont,
Texas, USA

EVAN T. ALICUBEN, MD
Independent Fellow, Department of
Cardiothoracic Surgery, University of
Pittsburgh Medical Center, University of
Pittsburgh School of Medicine, UPMC
Presbyterian, Pittsburgh, Pennsylvania,
USA

FATEH BAZERBACHI, MD
Director of Interventional Endoscopy,
CentraCare, Interventional Endoscopy
Program, St Cloud Hospital, Cloud, Minnesota,
USA

SHANDA H. BLACKMON, MD, MPH
Department of Surgery, Division of Thoracic
Surgery, Mayo Clinic, Rochester, Minnesota,
USA

MARIELA BLUM MURPHY, MD
Department of Gastrointestinal Medical
Oncology, The University of Texas MD
Anderson Cancer Center, Houston, Texas,
USA

SIDRA N. BONNER, MD, MPH, MSc
General Surgery Resident, Department of
Surgery, University of Michigan Medicine,
University of Michigan, Ann Arbor, Michigan,
USA

PAUL CARROLL, MB, BCh, MD, FRCSI
Consultant Upper GI and General Surgeon,
Galway University Hospital, Honorary Senior
Lecturer, School of Medicine, University of
Galway, Galway, Ireland

LIN-CHI CHUANG, BS
Department of Nursing, Taipei Veterans
General Hospital, Taipei, Taiwan

NICOLAS DEVAUD, MD
GI and HPB Surgical Oncology Attending,
Instituto Oncológico Fundación Arturo López
Pérez (FALP), Associate Professor,
Universidad de Los Andes, Santiago, Chile

AKIRA DOBASHI, MD, PhD
Department of Endoscopy, The Jikei University
School of Medicine, Minato City, Tokyo, Japan

DAFFOLYN RACHAEL FELS ELLIOTT, MD, PhD, FRCPC
Clinical Assistant Professor, Department of
Pathology and Laboratory Medicine, University

of Kansas Medical Center, Kansas City, Kansas, USA

PO-KUEI HSU, MD, PhD
Division of Thoracic Surgery, Department of Surgery, Taipei Veterans General Hospital and School of Medicine, National Yang Ming Chiao Tung University, Taipei, Taiwan

AUDREY JAJOSKY, MD, PhD
Assistant Professor, Department of Pathology and Laboratory Medicine, University of Rochester Medical Center, West Henrietta, New York, USA

YELENA Y. JANJIGIAN, MD
Associate Attending, Chief of Gastrointestinal Oncology Service, Department of Medicine, Memorial Sloan Kettering Cancer Center, Department of Medicine, Weill Cornell Medical College, New York, New York, USA

SANGEETHA N. KALIMUTHU, MD FRCPath, FRCPC
Department of Laboratory Medicine and Pathobiology, University of Toronto, University Health Network, Toronto, Ontario, Canada

YI-YING LEE, MD
Division of Thoracic Surgery, Department of Surgery, Taipei Veterans General Hospital and School of Medicine, National Yang Ming Chiao Tung University, Taipei, Taiwan

SHIRLEY LEWIS, MD, DNB, FRCR
Radiation Oncology Fellow, Radiation Medicine Program, Princess Margaret Cancer Centre, University Health Network, Department of Radiation Oncology, University of Toronto, Toronto, Ontario, Canada; Associate Professor, Department of Radiotherapy and Oncology, Manipal Comprehensive Cancer Care Centre, Kasturba Medical College, Manipal Academy of Higher Education, Manipal, India

DARRICK K. LI, MD, PhD
Department of Medicine, Section of Digestive Diseases, Yale School of Medicine, New Haven, Connecticut, USA

JAMES D. LUKETICH, MD
Henry T. Bahnson Professor and Chair, Chief, Division of Thoracic and Foregut Surgery, Department of Cardiothoracic Surgery,

University of Pittsburgh Medical Center, University of Pittsburgh School of Medicine, UPMC Presbyterian, Pittsburgh, Pennsylvania, USA

JELENA LUKOVIC, MD, FRCPC, MPH
Assistant Professor, Department of Radiation Oncology, University of Toronto, Radiation Oncologist, Radiation Medicine Program, Princess Margaret Cancer Centre, University Health Network, Toronto, Ontario, Canada

GAD MAROM, MD, MSc
Department of General Surgery, Hadassah-Hebrew University Medical Center, Faculty of Medicine, Hebrew University of Jerusalem, Jerusalem, Israel

GEORGIOS MAVROGENIS, MD
Division of Hybrid Interventional Endoscopy, Department of Gastroenterology, Mediterraneo Hospital, Glyfada, Athens, Greece

ANITA T. MOHAN, MBBS, PhD
Division of Plastic Surgery, Rochester, Minnesota, USA

RYAN REBERNICK, BA
Medical Student, University of Michigan Medical School, University of Michigan, Ann Arbor, Michigan, USA

SAMIR MARDINI, MD
Division of Plastic Surgery, Rochester, Minnesota, USA

MANUEL VILLA SANCHEZ, MD
Chief of Thoracic Surgery, Staten Island University Hospital, Northwell Health Physician Partners, Staten Island, New York, USA

INDERPAL S. SARKARIA, MD, MBA
Associate Professor of Cardiothoracic Surgery, Chair in Minimally Invasive Surgery, Vice Chair, Clinical Affairs, University of Pittsburgh Medical Center, University of Pittsburgh School of Medicine, Pittsburgh, Pennsylvania, USA

KAVEL H. VISRODIA, MD
Division of Digestive and Liver Diseases, Department of Medicine, Columbia University Irving Medical Center, New York, New York, USA

ELLIOT WAKEAM, MD, MPH
Assistant Professor of Surgery, Section of
Thoracic Surgery, Assistant Professor, Section of
Thoracic Surgery, Department of Surgery,
University of Michigan, Ann Arbor, Michigan, USA

YU-CHUNG WU, MD
Division of Thoracic Surgery, Department of
Surgery, Taipei Medical University Hospital,
Department of Surgery, College of Medicine,
Taipei Medical University, Taipei, Taiwan

JESSICA YANG, MD
Assistant Attending, Gastrointestinal Oncology
Service, Department of Medicine, Memorial
Sloan Kettering Cancer Center, Department of
Medicine, Weill Cornell Medical College, New
York, New York, USA

ROMAN E. ZYLA, MD
Department of Laboratory Medicine and
Pathobiology, University of Toronto, Toronto,
Ontario, Canada

Contents

Esophageal adenocarcinoma (EAC) is increasing in prevalence. Barrett's esophagus (BE) has long been recognized as the putative precursor lesion for EAC, but much is still unknown regarding its cell of origin and what molecular factors influence its neoplastic progression. Accurate pathologic assessment of BE biopsies is important for identifying patients most at risk of progressing to EAC, whereas pathologic assessment of EAC specimens plays a major role in influencing therapeutic decision-making.

Comprehensive genomic profiling has advanced our understanding of the molecular basis of esophageal cancer. Marked genomic heterogeneity between individual patients and the 2 major histologic subtypes of esophageal cancer likely contributes to the poor survival and lack of universally effective therapies. Esophageal adenocarcinoma and squamous cell carcinoma are molecularly and biologically distinct entities, with unique risk factors and geographic distributions, that may benefit from individualized treatment strategies. Molecular characterization of tumors enables personalized care by providing prognostic information and identifying those most likely to benefit from targeted therapy and/or immunotherapy.

Accurate staging is imperative in the management of esophageal cancer Over the years, different treatment modalities have evolved, ranging from endoscopic resection to traditional surgical resection and multimodal approaches, including the addition of chemotherapy, with or without radiation. In this article, we discuss the different stage groups, which guide the clinician in determining staging for esophageal cancer, and subsequent guidance in appropriate treatment modalities for each patient. These groups are based on tumor, node, and metastasis (TNM) staging and have recently been refined into clinical (cTNM) pathologic (pTNM), and post-neoadjuvant (ypTNM).

Locally advanced esophageal cancer has a dismal prognosis. Surgery remains the cornerstone treatment with 5-year survival rates of approximately 12–39%. Rates of local failure and distant metastases are high following surgical resection of locally advanced tumors. Neoadjuvant therapy (either radiation therapy, chemotherapy, or a combination) prior to surgery carries the advantage of tackling micrometastases and improving complete resection rates. Neoadjuvant concurrent chemotherapy and radiotherapy are a favored approach with evidence for improved pathologic complete response (pCR) rates and improved survival compared with surgery alone. Randomized trials of the optimal neoadjuvant approach are ongoing.

Ahmed Abdelhakeem and Mariela Blum Murphy

Esophageal cancer is the sixth most common cause of cancer mortality worldwide and is considered a major worldwide health challenge. Most patients diagnosed with esophageal cancer require extensive workup and management strategies. Multiple clinical trials have been conducted to evaluate the role of chemotherapy, chemoradiotherapy, and recently immunotherapy before or after surgery in the setting of localized esophageal cancer. Trimodality approaches, including preoperative chemoradiation followed by surgery or perioperative chemotherapy, have been widely accepted for treating localized esophageal cancer. However, the addition of immunotherapy to the current trimodality approach produced an advantage in disease-free survival. Our review will focus on the existing data on adjuvant therapies for locally advanced esophageal and gastroesophageal adenocarcinomas and squamous cell carcinomas.

Jessica Yang and Yelena Y. Janjigian

Advanced esophageal cancer has one of the lowest 5-year survival rates. Historically, treatment options have been limited to cytotoxic chemotherapy but recent trials have established a key role for immune checkpoint inhibitors. Chemotherapy plus nivolumab or pembrolizumab now represents the new standard of care frontline regimen for both esophageal adenocarcinoma and squamous cell carcinoma. Advances in targeting HER2 and other molecular targets have also expanded our therapeutic landscape. This article aims to provide an overview of recent advances in immunotherapy and targeted therapy for esophageal cancer as well as summarize ongoing clinical trials and future directions.

Akira Dobashi, Darrick K. Li, Georgios Mavrogenis, Kavel H. Visrodia, and Fateh Bazerbachi

Esophageal cancer is the eighth most common malignancy worldwide with more than 600,000 new cases diagnosed annually. Although curative approaches to early-stage esophageal cancer have historically been surgical, advances in endoscopic techniques resulted in the identification of patients who may benefit from minimally invasive endoscopic therapies. In this exposition, we discuss the identification of patients who are candidates for endoscopic resection and detail different aspects of endoscopic curative techniques for esophageal neoplasia. We also discuss therapies directed at the palliation of esophageal cancer sequelae.

Po-Kuei Hsu, Yi-Ying Lee, Lin-Chi Chuang, and Yu-Chung Wu

Lymph node metastasis is one of the most important prognostic factors in esophageal squamous cell carcinoma. However, the optimal extent of lymph node dissection is still under debate. We specifically address several controversies regarding lymph node dissection, for example, recurrent laryngeal node lymphadenectomy, cervical lymphadenectomy, and thoracic duct resection, in esophageal squamous cell carcinoma. We also describe new concepts in surgical anatomy of the upper mediastinum and technologies, for example, near-infrared image-guided lymphatic mapping and intraoperative neural monitoring that facilitate recurrent laryngeal node lymphadenectomy.

Esophagectomy and colon interposition in the adult patient, either for primary alimentary reconstruction or as a secondary replacement after initial resection/reconstruction for malignant or benign disease, remains a valuable tool in the thoracic surgeon's armamentarium. It is important for surgeons to remain versed in the complexities of the operation, including preoperative preparation and decision making, operative procedural and technical variations, and recognition and timely treatment of postoperative complications. In this article, we present technical details of the procedure, a review of selected published studies, long-term results, and indications and outcomes for revisional surgery.

Complex esophageal reconstruction represents a high risk and challenging procedure. A dedicated pathway with multispecialty teams can facilitate a systematic checklist approach to perioperative management and evaluation of long-term outcomes. Refinements in the operative technique for supercharged pedicled jejunum (SPJ) for long segment interposition in esophageal reconstruction are reviewed in this article. Medical and surgical complications among this complex niche group of patients are significant and require care in specialist centers with a focused team. Patient-reported outcomes (PROs) in long-segment SPJ interposition are recognized to provide additional monitoring of surgical outcomes and may help guide interventions for subsequent symptom control.

Reducing perioperative morbidity and mortality following esophagectomy remains central to surgeons' intraoperative decision-making. There remains wide variation in the technical approaches to esophagectomy and the employment of prophylactic strategies to reduce postoperative complications. In this article, we discuss the ongoing controversies related to feeding tube placement, pyloroplasty, and thoracic duct clipping and the evidence regarding these procedures.

The optimal management of Siewert Type II or Junction AEG II adenocarcinoma remains a point of debate. Surgical options include an extended total gastrectomy or esophagectomy. Accurately identifying the location of the esophagogastric junction (GEJ) is important as the epicenter of the lesion is defined in reference to the GEJ. Type II tumors, in the most recent iteration of the AJCC, describe these lesions as being within 1 cm cephalad and 2 cm caudal to GEJ. Accurate staging of the location and identification of nodal metastasis is vital to guide the optimal surgical approach. Endoscopy, endosonography, CT, and PET help guide decision-making as to what junctional subtype is present. The extent of resection and lymphadenectomy remains contestable. Both surgical approaches remain viable, as each has its own advantages and issues. The key to the management of these cancers is that the surgeon has the capability to operate on both sides of the diaphragm to manage these oftentimes challenging malignancies.

THORACIC SURGERY CLINICS

Foreword

Esophageal Cancer Management: Baby Steps Distally

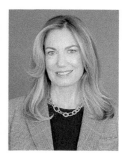

Virginia R. Litle, MD
Consulting Editor

Globally, esophageal cancer is a dismal disease accounting for more than 544,000 deaths each year[1] and with a continued increase in incidence in the United States to ~20,000 cases per year in 2021. The best chance of cure for locally advanced disease includes an esophagectomy with a concerning morbidity rate of ~50%. On the other hand, positive progress is happening on all multimodal fronts. Not only has there been the paradigm shift for curative management of superficial cancers with endoscopic resections but also we are seeing the advances with use of immunotherapy and targeted therapies beyond trastuzumab. With evolving disease management and a continued global malignancy problem, we invited Toronto esophageal experts Drs Jonathan Yeung and Elena Elimova to guest edit this issue of *Thoracic Surgery Clinics*. Dr Yeung is the Director of Thoracic Foregut Surgery at Toronto General and is the successor to Dr Gail Darling's robust esophageal program with multiple on-going prospective translational and technical studies. He is the perfect lead for that program and works closely with medical oncologist Dr Elena Elimova to move this field forward. Together they invited a panoply of experts to give us state-of-the art reviews of the ever-evolving topic of esophageal cancer care.

For food-for-thought, you will read about the continued controversies of routine biomarker testing of all tumors when diagnosed, technical considerations about routine drainage procedures and duct ligation as well as extent of recurrent nerve node dissection and duct resection for squamous cell carcinomas. Esophageal cancer is often approached by nonesophagologists and oncologists with a nihilistic approach; however, this issue of *Thoracic Surgery Clinics* reminds us that lung cancer is not the only thoracic malignancy casting a light of optimism on our field.

Thank you to all the contributors and to guest editors Drs Elimova and Yeung. Please enjoy the content as a current reference for managing a classically dismal disease with a sense of hope for our patients.

Sincerely,

Virginia R. Litle, MD
Division of Thoracic Surgery
Department of Surgery
Boston University
88 East Newton Street
Collamore Building, Suite 7380
Boston, MA 02118, USA

E-mail address:
vlitle@gmail.com

Twitter: @vlitlemd (V.R. Litle)

REFERENCE

1. Sung H, Ferlay J, Siegel RL, et al. Global Cancer Statistics 2020: GLOBOCAN estimates of incidence and mortality worldwide for 36 cancers in 185 countries. CA Cancer J Clin 2021;71(3):209–49.

Thorac Surg Clin 32 (2022) xi
https://doi.org/10.1016/j.thorsurg.2022.08.005
1547-4127/22/© 2022 Published by Elsevier Inc.

Preface
Overview of the Management of Esophageal Cancer

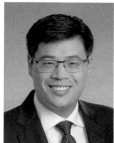

Jonathan C. Yeung, MD, PhD, FRCSC   Elena Elimova, MD, MSc, FRCPC
Editors

Esophageal cancer surgery is an exciting, but challenging, part of thoracic surgery practice. The management of esophageal cancer requires thoughtful preoperative planning, technical oncologic resection, creativity in reconstruction, and meticulous postoperative care. It is also multidisciplinary, involving expertise from therapeutic endoscopists, medical and radiation oncologists, radiologists, and pathologists. Despite this, the thoracic surgeon maintains a central role for every patient from diagnosis to palliation. We envision this issue of *Thoracic Surgery Clinics* as an update on esophageal cancer for thoracic surgeons.

Zyla and Kalimuthu start the issue by reviewing the pathologic condition of Barrett esophagus and esophageal adenocarcinoma and allow the reader to understand the pathologist's perspective on the disease. With advances in sequencing technology, we have gained a deeper understanding of the genomic landscape of esophageal cancer. The future of esophageal cancer care will be in personalizing treatment based on tumor-specific markers. Jajosky and Fels Elliott review these advances and how this may ultimately impact clinical care.

With increased survival data, esophageal cancer staging is evolving, and Marom reviews the latest staging system for esophageal cancer. The majority of resectable esophageal cancers require multimodality therapy, and the next three articles by Lewis and Lukovic, Abdelhakeem and Blum-Murphy, and Yang and Janjigian update us on adjuvant and neoadjuvant treatments, including immunotherapy.

There have been significant advances in endoscopy and endoscopic therapy for gastrointestinal malignancies, and Dobashi and colleagues review endoscopic treatment and palliation options. Though the majority of cancers seen in the Western world are adenocarcinoma, squamous cell carcinoma does still exist, and Hsu and colleagues review lymphadenectomy as performed in the East.

When the gastric conduit is not usable, colon and supercharged jejunal conduits need to be in the surgeon's toolbox, and Sanchez and colleagues and Mohan and colleagues provide comprehensive reviews on the use of these conduits, respectively. Finally, Bonner and colleagues and Carroll and Devaud review the literature on common controversies, including the need for feeding tubes, clipping the thoracic duct, and how to treat Siewert II junctional tumors.

Thorac Surg Clin 32 (2022) xiii–xiv
https://doi.org/10.1016/j.thorsurg.2022.08.001
1547-4127/22/© 2022 Published by Elsevier Inc.

We would like to thank all of the contributors and hope you enjoy this issue!

Jonathan C. Yeung, MD, PhD, FRCSC
Department of Surgery
University of Toronto
Toronto General Hospital
200 Elizabeth Street, 9N-949
Toronto, ON M5G 2C4, Canada

Elena Elimova, MD, MSc, FRCPC
Department of Medicine
University of Toronto
Princess Margaret Cancer Centre
610 University Avenue, OPG 7-715
Toronto, ON M5G 2M9, Canada

E-mail addresses:
Jonathan.yeung@uhn.ca (J.C. Yeung)
Elena.elimova@uhn.ca (E. Elimova)

Barrett's Esophagus and Esophageal Adenocarcinoma: A Histopathological Perspective

Roman E. Zyla, MD[a], Sangeetha N. Kalimuthu, MD, FRCPath, FRCPC[a,b],*

KEYWORDS

- Barrett's esophagus • Esophageal adenocarcinoma • Regression grading
- Molecular pathogenesis

KEY POINTS

- Barrett's esophagus (BE) is the putative precursor for esophageal adenocarcinoma (EAC), and both are increasing in prevalence in the Western world.
- Surgical pathologists play a key role in assessing BE and EAC specimens, with several pathologic features critically influencing therapeutic decision-making.
- There is an ongoing controversy surrounding the cell of origin of BE, but major strides have been made in elucidating the molecular pathogenesis of EAC from BE.

GLOSSARY LIST

Esophageal adenocarcinoma (EAC), Barrett's esophagus (BE), low-grade dysplasia (LGD), high-grade dysplasia (HGD), intramucosal carcinoma (IMC), gastroesophageal reflux disease (GERD)

INTRODUCTION

Esophageal adenocarcinoma (EAC) represents a growing health burden, particularly in the developed world, with the number of cases rising dramatically over the past several decades. In Canada, the annual incidence of EAC increased from approximately 1 case per 100,000 in 1992 to more than 2.5 per 100,000 in 2010, with a similar trend in the United States.[1,2] EAC carries a dismal prognosis, with a 5-year survival rate of less than 20% in patients with locally advanced or metastatic disease.[3,4] Furthermore, discouragingly, the majority of patients diagnosed with EAC present with late-stage disease.[5–7]

Barrett's esophagus (BE) is the putative precursor of EAC and is broadly defined as the metaplastic transformation of esophageal squamous epithelium to columnar epithelium. Canonically, BE has been thought to progress to EAC through a stepwise pattern, progressing from nondysplastic BE to BE with low-grade dysplasia (LGD), high-grade dysplasia (HGD), and finally invasive EAC; however, the vast majority of patients with BE never go on to develop EAC.[3,6]

Considerable efforts have been made to develop screening programs that would allow for (1) the efficient detection of patients with BE and (2) the early identification and definitive treatment of LGD, HGD, and early EAC in patients with BE, before the presentation of the "red-flag" symptoms which typically portend advanced, incurable disease. The current standard for EAC screening in those with BE involves costly and time-consuming endoscopic inspection of the distal esophagus in conjunction with histologic examination of random biopsy samples for evidence of dysplasia or malignancy. The American College of Gastroenterology

[a] Department of Laboratory Medicine and Pathobiology, University of Toronto, 27 King's College Cir, Toronto, ON M5S 1A1, Canada; [b] University Health Network, Toronto, Ontario, Canada
* Corresponding author. Department of Pathology, University Health Network, Rm 11E210, 200 Elizabeth Street, Toronto, Ontario.
E-mail address: sangeetha.kalimuthu@uhn.ca

Thorac Surg Clin 32 (2022) 413–424
https://doi.org/10.1016/j.thorsurg.2022.06.005
1547-4127/22/© 2022 Elsevier Inc. All rights reserved.

(ACG) recommends at least eight biopsies taken randomly across all four quadrants of the circumferentially abnormal esophagus, because an increased number of biopsies correlates with an increased rate of identifying intestinal metaplasia (IM).[3,8] The prevalence of BE in Western countries is high, estimated at between 0.3% and 7% of the general population, including up to 12% of those with long-standing gastroesophageal reflux disease (GERD).[3–5,9,10] Most professional gastroenterological associations, therefore, recommend restricting screening for BE and EAC to patients with long-standing GERD and multiple other risk factors for progression to EAC.[3]

It is critical for pathologists examining BE specimens to accurately identify LGD and HGD, because these findings have major treatment and surveillance implications. The risk of progression from nondysplastic BE, LGD, and HGD increases from 0.33% to 0.54% to 6%, respectively.[11–13] Whereas patients with LGD may be managed with increased surveillance frequency alone or with definitive endoscopic therapy, HGD is an indication for definitive therapy, typically through endoscopic resection of any visible lesions as well as radiofrequency ablation of all background mucosa endoscopically compatible with BE.[9]

In this review, we summarize the pathologic features and diagnostic challenges of BE and EAC and discuss controversial areas that are still evolving, such as the cell of origin of BE and risk stratification for malignant progression in BE.

BARRETT'S ESOPHAGUS
Anatomic Location

The normal esophagus is lined by squamous epithelium with scattered submucosal glands comprising mucin-containing cells. The esophago–gastric junction (EGJ) is defined as the site where the most distal portion of the esophagus meets the stomach, which can also be referred to as the Z-line (a term for a faint zig–zag impression at the EGJ that demarcates the transition between the stratified squamous epithelium in the esophagus and the intestinal epithelium of the gastric cardia). Endoscopically, the EGJ can be determined by identifying the proximal margin of the gastric folds. Previously, the distal 1 to 2 cm of the esophagus was thought to be lined by columnar epithelium. However, this belief has been refuted and it is now accepted that the presence of columnar epithelium located proximal to the anatomic EGJ is metaplastic in origin and has developed secondary to chronic injury due to GERD.[9]

BE exemplifies the final stage of metaplastic conversion of the normal squamous epithelium to columnar epithelium. However, knowledge of the endoscopic impression is imperative before making a histologic diagnosis of BE (discussed later), including the distance of the site of the biopsy from incisors and the presence or absence of hiatus hernia. BE can be further arbitrarily divided into long- and short-segment BE, based on the endoscopic length of the abnormal epithelium; >3 cm and <3 cm, respectively.[14] The endoscopic appearances of the long segment are effectively diagnostic for BE; however, in short-segment BE there may be a greater role for histologic assessment.[15] An ultrashort segment BE has also been described. This entity is fraught with interpretative challenges as some use this term to refer to BE that is not endoscopically detectable; however, the more accurate use of this term is for the presence of intestinal metaplasia in the gastric cardia. The more appropriate terminology for the latter is cardia intestinal metaplasia (CIM), because the risk of dysplasia from CIM is said to be more significant than short-segment BE.[15]

Nomenclature

The features of BE were first outlined by Norman Barrett in his seminal paper in 1950.[16] Since then, the terminology and diagnostic criteria have continued to befuddle the gastroesophageal community. In North America, we have widely accepted the terminology of BE; however, it is known by several appellations across the world, including CELLO (columnar epithelium-lined lower esophagus) in Europe, EBO (endobrachyoesophage) in France, and CLO (columnar-lined esophagus) in the United Kingdom. Perhaps, the chief contention lies in whether IM should be the defining feature in the diagnosis of BE. In North America, France, Germany, and the Netherlands, IM is required before making a histologic diagnosis of BE; however, in the United Kingdom and Japan, the need for the presence of IM has been dropped.[17] The United Kingdom makes the latter argument for the following reasons: (1) it has long been recognized that there is a spectrum of histologic phenotypes for BE beyond the presence of IM[18], (2) the absence of IM can imply a sampling bias because a study has demonstrated that there is a linear correlation with the number of biopsies sampled for the demonstration of IM[17], (3) the presence of intestinal metaplasia depends on the number of levels performed during pathologic evaluation, and (4) there is high interobserver variability among pathologists in the detection of IM.[15] In contrast, in North America, the presence of IM is still necessary for the diagnosis of BE, because it has been recognized as the phenotype to be associated with adenocarcinoma. However, recent studies have shown that adenocarcinoma can arise from cardia-type mucosa in BE, arguing against the latter assertion.[19,20] On the whole, the conflicting reporting styles of BE have resulted in inconsistent data on BE. This precludes the ability to monitor patients with BE who truly progress to adenocarcinoma and improve our understanding of the disease process. The hope would be for the experts in the field to reach a global consensus and implement standardized reporting of BE.

Histology of Barrett's esophagus

There are three main types of metaplastic epithelium that have been described in BE, including cardia-type (junctional), fundic-type, and intestinal (specialized) epithelium. The cardia and fundic types of epithelium are morphologically similar to their equivalents in the stomach. The intestinal (specialized) epithelium demonstrates surface maturation with preserved architecture. The surface shows the uniform, undulating, and villiform

architecture, and the lining cells show intestinal metaplastic type, characterized by goblet cells (**Fig. 1**A). Identifying the goblet cell is requisite to confirm the presence of intestinal metaplasia. Cytologically, goblet cells have distended, mucin-filled cytoplasm, eccentric nuclei, and a barrel-shaped configuration (see **Fig. 1**B).[1,4] Occasionally, distended columnar cells can mimic the appearance of goblet cells histologically and they are referred to as pseudogoblet cells. Given that goblet cells contain acid mucins, Alcian blue stain at pH 2.5 has been used for histologic confirmation of the same; however, this practice has been largely discontinued as Alcian blue can also stain the mucin pseudogoblet cells, albeit to a lesser extent.[9,14] Another characteristic feature in BE is the thickening and duplication of the muscularis mucosa.[17] This is particularly important when assessing potential invasion into the submucosa in endoscopic mucosal resection (EMR) for adenocarcinoma (discussed later).

Cell of Origin of Barrett's Esophagus

The cell of origin of the metaplastic columnar cell in BE remains a quandary and thus far, several

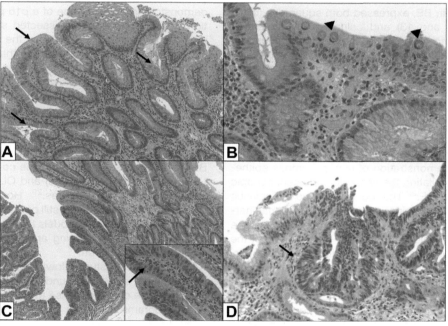

Fig. 1. (*A, B*) BE demonstrating the presence of metaplastic intestinal epithelium, characterized by intestinal epithelium (*arrow*). The surface shows a villiform architecture and the lining cells show intestinal metaplastic type, characterized by goblet cells (*arrowhead*) a characteristic feature of intestinal metaplasia. Cytologically, goblet cells have distended, mucin-filled cytoplasm, eccentric nuclei, and a barrel-shaped configuration; (*C*) BE transitioning to LGD, where there is loss of surface maturation with relative preservation of overall architecture. The stratified nuclei are mildly enlarged, hyperchromatic, and elongated with relative preservation of size and shape (*inset-arrow*); (*D*) In contrast, HGD, shows more severe cytologic atypia and architectural complexity than LGD, seen here as a cribriform growth pattern (*arrow*).

theories and different possible precursor cells have been suggested. One could argue that knowledge of the cell of origin is purely an academic curiosity; however, identifying the candidate cell of origin for BE would facilitate understanding the pathogenesis of BE, which would, in turn, lead to better diagnostic stratification, and treatment options, and targeting of therapeutic vulnerabilities.

The purported progenitor cell for BE has been thought to originate from either esophagus, gastric cardia, bone marrow, or a combination of the aforementioned.[9] One proposed mechanism for the metaplastic transformation of a squamous cell into a columnar cell in BE is "transdifferentiation." Transdifferentiation is a process whereby a mature, differentiated cell switches into another, without an intermediate pluripotent state.[9,21,22] Previously, observations in mouse models have proposed a potential role for transdifferentiation in BE. Furthermore, there has been histologic evidence of transdifferentiation observed using immunohistochemical studies.[23] Boch and colleagues observed that the multilayered epithelium (composed of multiple layers of haphazardly heaped epithelioid cells, which are stippled with mucous-containing cells), which can be occasionally seen in BE, expressed both squamous (cytokeratin 4 and 13) and columnar (cytokeratin 8 and 19) markers, suggesting dual squamous and columnar differentiation.[23] As such, this could suggest the multilayered epithelium can be a transitional state between squamous and columnar epithelium. However, the role of transdifferentiation in BE pathogenesis has been refuted by experts in the field, largely owing to the lack of evidence to support full phenotypic conversion of cultured mature squamous cells to columnar cells and the demonstration of new squamous epithelium repopulating the esophagus postendoscopic removal of BE.[22] That being said, the metaplastic conversion of acinar cells to ductal cells (acinar-ductal metaplasia) has been observed in the pancreas, which is thought to be the origin of the putative precursor of pancreatic ductal adenocarcinoma, pancreatic intraepithelial neoplasia[24] Although the latter was demonstrated in a different organ site, transdifferentiation cannot be entirely excluded in the realm of BE pathogenesis.

The more widely accepted theory suggests that the metaplastic BE epithelium arises from the shift in the commitment of pluripotent stem cells that are responsible for replenishing esophageal epithelium. This mechanism is referred to as "transcommitment," which begins with the reprogramming of progenitor cells that will differentiate into another cell type. However, the origin of these progenitor cells is contentious and there are presently at least four mechanistic theories proposed by experts in the field (see later).[9]

Given the abundance of squamous epithelium in the esophagus, one theory lends support for basal squamous epithelial stem cells as the cell of origin for BE. Barbera and colleagues concluded that the squamous esophageal cells demonstrated widespread stem cell-like properties, where the majority of the proliferative activity was observed in the interpapillary basal region of the squamous epithelium, providing validation that this could be the potential location cell for the cell of origin in BE.[25]

Bone marrow stem cells have been shown to contribute to the development of BE in rat models with GERD, where the stem cells relocate and plant themselves in the esophagus.[26] However, a later study refuted this claim by demonstrating that bone marrow progenitor cells in surgically induced GERD mouse models did not engraft the damaged regions of the mouse models.[27] As such, the true validity of the role of bone marrow stem cells in BE pathogenesis is questionable.

Esophageal submucosal gland stem cells have also been considered a contender for the cell of origin in BE. Results from a study by Leedham and colleagues supported this hypothesis by demonstrating the presence of a p16 point mutation originating in a microdissected submucosal duct that was also appreciated in the contiguous metaplastic crypt, thus concluding that the presence of an identical mutation in these two tissue types provides strong evidence to suggest that the cell of origin of BE is derived from esophageal submucosal glands.[28] In a subsequent study, Owen and colleagues used single-cell RNAseq to demonstrate the transcriptional similarities between esophageal submucosal gland cells and BE, as both these cell populations co-expressed LEFTY1 (developmental gene) and OLFM4 (stem cell-associated gene) genes.[29] However, one study has shown that it was still possible to induce BE-like epithelium in rat models that are devoid of submucosal glands, arguing against a stem cell origin from this location.[27]

In a most recent study, Nowicki-Osuch and colleagues have shown that undifferentiated gastric cells from the cardia give rise to BE via transcriptional programs driven by c-MYC and HNF4A.[30] They did this by analyzing freshly isolated tissue from the esophagus, GEJ, and gastric cardia, including normal and diseased tissue (BE, dysplasia, and tumor), and performed multi-omic profiling of different epithelial cells.[30] This led to the identification of an undifferentiated BE cell type that showed expression for intestinal and BE stem cell markers, where the BE cells most closely resemble cells from the gastric cardia.[30] Although correlation does not prove causality, these findings render stem cell origin from this location likely.

Despite the fervent efforts made to identify the cell of origin for BE (see our earlier discussion), the dizzying array of conflicting data in the literature still leaves us none the wiser; albeit, the hope is that the published work so far represents the seminal stages of unraveling the pathogenesis of BE.

Dysplasia in Barrett's Esophagus

Dysplasia is defined as the presence of neoplastic epithelium that is confined within the basement membrane of the gland from which it arises.[31] Dysplasia in BE can be recognized on low magnification due to loss of surface maturation, mucin depletion, and an increase in the number of nuclei. Caution should be exercised when interpreting BE biopsies in the presence of active inflammation as the latter can mimic the neoplastic changes. However, it is important to be aware that dysplasia and inflammation can co-exist. The presence of features, such as an abrupt transition in the architectural and nuclear features (ie, nuclear size, nuclear stratification), strongly favor dysplasia over a reactive process.[32] Dysplasia can be designated as either low grade or high grade based on the degree of abnormality present.

In LGD, there is a loss of surface maturation secondary to nuclear stratification with relative preservation of overall architecture. The stratified nuclei are mildly enlarged, hyperchromatic, and elongated; however, they are relatively equal in size and shape (see **Fig. 1**C). Furthermore, there is a retention of nuclear polarity. There is a diminished number of goblet cells; however, when present they tend to be predominantly dystrophic in nature. Dystrophic goblet cells have usually lost cellular polarity and have the appearance of a misorientated mucin bubble.[32]

In contrast, HGD shows more severe cytologic atypia and architectural complexity than LGD. The architectural complexity is characterized by glandular branching or budding and cribriform growth (see **Fig. 1**D). Cytologically, the cells show more nuclear pleomorphism and hyperchromatism and a higher nuclear to cytoplasmic (N:C) ratio than LGD. Some degree of nuclear stratification can still be appreciated but to a lesser degree than seen in LGD.

It is important to make the distinction between HGD and intramucosal carcinoma (IMC); however, this can often be extremely challenging, particularly on small biopsy samples. In IMC, neoplastic cells have penetrated through the basement membrane and infiltrated into the lamina propria, typically as single cells or groups of cells. In clinical practice, when the distinction between HGD and IMC is difficult, it is prudent to perform multiple levels on the biopsy material and seek a second opinion from a colleague, if necessary, because therapeutic strategies are based on the separation between the two diagnoses.

Finally, there is the diagnosis of "indefinite for dysplasia." The main reason for the usage of this category is when there are cytologic changes suggestive of dysplasia but the changes are associated with prominent active inflammation and it is difficult to establish whether these changes are florid reactive/regenerative changes as a result of the inflammation (**Fig. 2**A and B).[15] Another indication for the use of indefinite for dysplasia would include poorly orientated or tangentially sectioned biopsies, which preclude the assessment of surface maturation. Furthermore, a recently described form of dysplasia

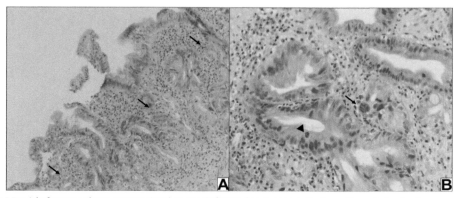

Fig. 2. (A) BE with features best categorized as "indefinite for dysplasia" given the cytologic changes suggestive of dysplasia in the presence of prominent inflammation (*arrow*); (B) most of the dysplastic changes are seen in deeper glands (*arrow*), including marked increase in nuclear to cytoplasmic ratio (N:C) and mitoses with evidence of surface maturation (*arrowhead*).

has been termed "basal crypt dysplasia-like aty-pia", where the dysplastic changes include nuclear enlargement, hyperchromasia, and prominent mitotic activity, in the absence of active inflammation, are confined to the basal crypts with evidence of surface maturation. This is thought to represent dysplasia in the early stage of development.[9] However, most pathologists would prefer to err on the side of caution and categorize this stage as "indefinite for dysplasia," because this designation will ensure appropriate management, including enhanced surveillance.

ESOPHAGEAL ADENOCARCINOMA
Histology of Esophageal Adenocarcinoma

EAC shares histologic similarities with other adenocarcinomas of the gastrointestinal tract. The morphology can be broadly divided into two histologic groups:(1) intestinal, characterized by a tubulopapillary growth pattern and (2) diffuse, characterized by diffuse sheets of pleomorphic cells or signet-ring cells with abundant extracellular mucin (**Fig. 3**A–D).[33,34] Any signet-ring cell component represents an independent, poor prognostic factor and also predicts poor response to neoadjuvant chemotherapy, and therefore this finding should be documented by the reporting pathologist.[35,36] Typically, EAC displays at least focal gland formation with variable amounts of associated intracellular mucin.[37] However, some poorly differentiated tumors may lack clear lineage-defining histologic features, requiring an immunohistochemical panel for classification (cytokeratin 7 and mucicarmine will show positivity in EAC, whereas p40 and cytokeratin 5/6

characterize SCC).[37,38] Grading of EAC follows similar parameters to those used in other tumors of the gastrointestinal tract. Briefly, well-differentiated tumors are characterized by well-formed glands making up greater than 95% of the tumor, poorly differentiated tumors have 49% or less gland formation, and moderately differentiated tumors fall between these two boundaries.[37]

Site of Origin

One area of controversy in the pathologic assessment of cancers of the EGJ is the distinction between EAC and proximal gastric adenocarcinoma. EAC arises almost exclusively in the distal esophagus, in the vicinity of the EGJ, though rare proximal cases arising in gastric inlet patches have been described.[39] The Cancer Staging Manual of the current American Joint Committee on Cancer classifies adenocarcinomas involving the EGJ as being of esophageal origin if the tumor epicenter extends no further than 2 cm into the anatomically defined gastric cardia.[37] Immunohistochemistry does not have any significant role in ascertaining esophageal versus gastric origin.[40,41] However, the emerging data on the molecular underpinnings of EAC and gastric adenocarcinomas may allow for a more precise and meaningful distinction of these tumors in the future.

Staging Considerations

There are a few different specimen types a pathologist may encounter in the assessment of EAC. The ACG recommends endoscopic therapy alone, typically through EMR, for intramucosal (pT1a) tumors.[3] More advanced, nonmetastatic disease is

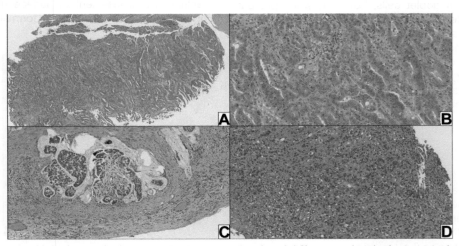

Fig. 3. The two main histotypes of EAC are intestinal type (*A, B*) and diffuse type (*C, D*). The intestinal type shows variable gland formation with frequent tubulopapillary growth architecture, whereas the diffuse type has a discohesive growth pattern (*C*) and is often associated with large, extracellular mucin pools and the presence of signet-ring cells (*D*).

typically treated with multimodal therapy, including neoadjuvant chemo(radio)therapy followed by esophagectomy and regional lymphadenectomy.[42] Regardless of the specimen type received, pathologic examination of the esophagus is aided by proper specimen handling. Many authors recommend opening the esophagus and pinning it to a corkboard before fixation, to minimize tissue distortion and preserve anatomic relationships between structures.[37,43]

Accurate pathologic staging of EAC is critical due to the role of the tumor stage in prognostication and dictating therapy.[3] In the setting of submucosal/pT1b invasion, esophagectomy is the treatment of choice for many patients, although if there is minimal submucosal invasion (<500 μm) without other high-risk features (ie, poorly differentiated component, positive resection margin, or lymphovascular invasion), endoscopic therapy alone may still be considered, particularly in those who are suboptimal surgical candidates.[3,44] Tumors with greater than 500 μm submucosal invasion have a substantially higher rate of lymph node metastases, and as such endoscopic resection is inappropriate as curative-intent therapy.[45–48] In fact, some studies have shown high rates of lymph node metastases with even superficial invasion of the submucosa, and the best treatment for pT1b tumors remains an area of controversy.[49–52] Somewhat discouragingly, there is high interobserver variability in the measurement of submucosal invasion in EAC, even when the decision is restricted to a binary cutoff of less than or greater than 500 μm[53]. Recommendations for reducing such variability include ensuring all tissue fragments are assessed, and identifying adjacent areas of muscularis mucosae (MM) in the event of MM destruction to ascertain the deepest point of MM from which invasion should be measured.[53] Furthermore, there is some evidence that depth of invasion within the mucosa itself may have prognostic significance, with invasion into the MM portending a higher risk of lymph node metastases than more superficial malignancies, but these data are limited by the very low rate of LNM in this population.[54,55]

A critical phenomenon that must be taken into account during the examination of endoscopic resections for EAC is duplication of the MM.[9] Based on the assessment of adjacent, unremarkable esophageal mucosa, it has been established that the outer layer of MM represents the original, "true" MM, whereas the inner layer is the duplicated or "neo" MM[9]. Only tumoral invasion through the outer layer is considered to represent a true submucosal invasion, and tumors that invade only through the inner MM should be classified as intramucosal, pT1a tumors.[9] This recommendation is validated by a study by Estrella and colleagues, which found that tumoral invasion through the neo-MM, but not into the submucosa, confers a similarly low risk of lymph node metastasis as more superficial intramucosal carcinoma.[56,57] Piecemeal specimen excision and incomplete MM duplication may create challenges in assessing the precise depth of invasion. Helpful clues to indicate true submucosal invasion include looking for the presence of esophageal submucosal glands and thick-walled arteries of large caliber[37] and being able to distinguish the neo-MM from the original MM by assessing the thicker caliber and greater organization of the true, outer MM[45].

Assessment of Post-neoadjuvant Tumor Regression

Neoadjuvant chemo(radio)therapy has become part of the standard of care for many patients with EAC.[5] Accurate pathologic assessment of post-neoadjuvant esophagectomy specimens is critical for prognostication. In the absence of grossly apparent residual tumor, the specimen should be carefully examined for mucosal alterations, and the entire suspected tumor bed should be submitted for histopathologic assessment (**Fig. 4**A).[37] Histologically, neoadjuvant therapy can induce characteristic changes in the residual neoplastic cells (large, irregular, hyperchromatic nuclei with minimal mitoses and frequent karyorrhectic and pyknotic debris), the background, the benign epithelium (reactive nuclear atypia), and the stroma (with changes, including variable amounts of fibrosis, stromal mucin, vascular intimal proliferation, telangiectasia, and microthrombi) (see **Fig. 4**B and C).[37,58] Neoadjuvant therapy is also associated with an increase in neuroendocrine differentiation in EAC.[58,59]

The degree of response to neoadjuvant therapy is a strong predictor of survival in EAC (see **Fig. 4**D).[60–62] Several scoring systems for categorizing the degree of post-neoadjuvant tumor regression exist. The Mandard system assesses tumor regression based on the ratio of residual tumor to treatment-related fibrosis,[63] whereas the Becker system uses a quantitative assessment of relative residual tumor as a percentage of the tumor bed.[64] The Ryan score uses a qualitative assessment of residual tumor and while initially developed for rectal adenocarcinomas, has been shown to have prognostic significance when used in EAC.[65] There is no clear consensus on which system to use, and many of the systems routinely in use have been shown to provide meaningful prognostic stratification with acceptable

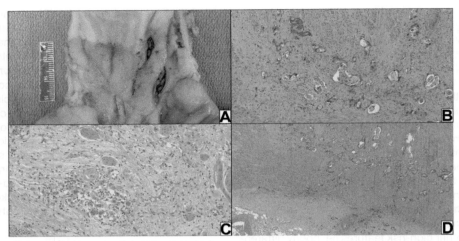

Fig. 4. Neoadjuvant therapy can result in complete macroscopic remission of the tumor; in this case, areas of mucosal alteration compatible with prior tumor must be identified macroscopically and submitted in toto where feasible, to identify any possible residual microscopic tumor (*A*); neoadjuvant chemotherapy can cause marked atypia in the neoplastic cells (*B*) and stromal changes, such as edema and vascular irregularities (*C*). Various tumor regression scores exist, which can be based on factors, such as the ratio of tumor:stroma or the percentage of previous tumor, which remains viable (*D*).

levels of interobserver variability.[66,67] Importantly, acellular mucin pools alone, in the absence of neoplastic cells, should not be treated as a residual tumor, even in cases where mucin is present at the resection margin.[68] Moreover, whereas evidence of complete tumor regression in lymph nodes, such as fibrosis or acellular mucin, does not factor into the quantification of tumor response, it should nevertheless be documented.[37] Tumors with evidence of lymph node tumor regression but no viable lymph node metastases are classified as ypN0.[37]

Other Prognostic Factors in the Pathologic Assessment of Esophageal Adenocarcinoma

Margin assessment is critical to determining the completeness of EAC excision, and a positive margin on endoscopic resection influences prognosis and may indicate the need for further therapy.[69] Pathologists assessing EAC specimens should be aware of differences in margin classification between institutions and should communicate clearly with their clinical colleagues regarding what system is employed. For example, the College of American Pathologists defines microscopic margin positivity as requiring a tumor to be present immediately at the inked resection margin, whereas the Royal College of Pathologists considers any margin to be positive if the tumor comes to within 1 mm of that margin.[37] Both of these definitions of margin positivity have been shown to be prognostically significant.[70] Microscopic margin assessment may also be required as part of an intraoperative

consultation for esophagectomy, with a positive margin potentially requiring additional tissue to be resected before reanastomosis.[37]

Tumor budding represents a new histologic parameter that may correlate with prognosis in EAC.[33,71–73] Tumor budding is defined as single cells or clusters of no more than 5 cells present at the invasive front of the tumor.[71] Tumor budding is typically classified using a three-tier score based on the highest number of "buds" identified in a 0.785 mm^2 "hotspot."[74]

The presence of lymph node metastases is an ominous prognostic factor in EAC.[37] Individuals involved in a gross examination of esophagectomy specimens must be diligent about documenting and submitting all possible regional lymph nodes, to increase the accuracy of prognostication.[37] However, peri-esophageal adipose tissue should only be removed for lymph node examination *after* submission of a full-thickness section of the tumor and assessment and submission of the adventitial resection margin, to avoid disrupting the relationship between tissues.[37] Extracapsular tumor extension in lymph node metastases is an independent predictor of poor overall survival.[75] In the absence of pathologically confirmed lymph node metastases, lymphovascular invasion is also a poor prognostic factor in EAC.[76]

Biomarker Assessment

The role of pathologists in routinely guiding targeted therapy for EAC is currently limited to an assessment of HER2 status. The anti-HER2 antibody trastuzumab has been shown to improve survival in HER2-positive locally advanced and metastatic tumors.[77,78] HER2 overexpression is seen in 15% to 19% of EACs but is typically not identified in nondysplastic BE or BE with LGD, suggesting HER2 amplification plays a late role in EAC pathogenesis.[79] Key differences between HER2 immunohistochemical staining patterns in EAC compared with breast carcinoma (in which HER2 immunohistochemistry was first extensively studied) include increased intratumoral heterogeneity, as well as more frequent basolateral staining without complete, circumferential immunoreactivity.[79] Routine assessment of HER2 status in EAC is based on immunohistochemistry, with in situ hybridization-based techniques for gene amplification reserved for cases that are borderline (2+) by IHC.[79] Several papers outline the scoring parameters and technical considerations for interpretation of HER2 status in EAC.[79–81]

Future Perspectives

Given the growing incidence of EAC and the persistent limitations associated with identifying and treating those at the highest risk of malignant transformation in BE, further insights into the molecular and pathologic characteristics of BE and EAC are essential, if this challenge is to be met successfully in the 21st century. Better systems to model the relationship between BE, dysplasia, and EAC, such as mouse models, mouse xenografts, and organoids would be necessary to achieve this goal. Finally, leveraging the histologic heterogeneity of EAC may be of value in understanding the mechanisms underpinning these different morphologic features, which can facilitate converting these features to a more therapeutically targetable subtype.

CLINICS CARE POINTS

- An abrupt transition into a region of suspicious architectural and nuclear features in Barrett's esophagus favors a diagnosis of dysplasia, even in the presence of background inflammation.
- Even when an esophageal adenocarcinoma shows predominantly tubulopapillary architecture, care must be taken to identify any small foci of signet-ring differentiation, as any signet-ring component is associated with a poorer prognosis.
- When assessing invasion in a biopsy for esophageal adenocarcinoma, submucosal

invasion can be erroneously diagnosed if the reporting pathologist does not take into account the frequent presence of duplicated muscularis mucosae in this setting.
- When assessing response to neoadjuvant chemo(radio)therapy in an esophagectomy specimen, thorough sampling and accurate identification of residual neoplastic cells are more important than the particular classification score used.

DISCLOSURE

The authors have nothing to disclose.

REFERENCES

1. Cattelan L, Ghazawi FM, Le M, et al. Epidemiologic trends and geographic distribution of esophageal cancer in Canada: A national population-based study. Cancer Med 2020;9(1):401–17.
2. Hur C, Miller M, Kong CY, et al. Trends in esophageal adenocarcinoma incidence and mortality. Cancer 2013;119(6):1149–58.
3. Shaheen NJ, Falk GW, Iyer PG, et al. ACG Clinical Guideline: Diagnosis and management of Barrett's esophagus. Am J Gastroenterol 2016;111(1):30–50.
4. Cook MB, Thrift AP. Epidemiology of Barrett's esophagus and esophageal adenocarcinoma - implications for screening and surveillance. Gastrointest Endosc Clin N Am 2021;31(1):1–26.
5. Rustgi AK, El-Serag HB. Esophageal carcinoma. N Engl J Med 2014;371(26):2499–509.
6. Groulx S, Limburg H, Doull M, et al. Guideline on screening for esophageal adenocarcinoma in patients with chronic gastroesophageal reflux disease. Can Med Assoc J 2020;192(27):E768–77.
7. Then EO, Lopez M, Saleem S, et al. Esophageal cancer: An updated Surveillance Epidemiology and End Results database analysis. World J Oncol 2020;11(2):55–64.
8. Harrison R, Perry I, Haddadin W, et al. Detection of intestinal metaplasia in Barrett's esophagus: an observational comparator study suggests the need for a minimum of eight biopsies. Am J Gastroenterol 2007;102(6):1154–61.
9. Naini BV, Souza RF, Odze RD. Barrett's esophagus: a comprehensive and contemporary review for pathologists. Am J Surg Pathol 2016;40(5):e45–66.
10. Coleman HG, Xie SH, Lagergren J. The epidemiology of esophageal adenocarcinoma. Gastroenterology 2018;154(2):390–405.
11. Desai TK, Krishnan K, Samala N, et al. The incidence of oesophageal adenocarcinoma in nondysplastic Barrett's oesophagus: a meta-analysis. Gut 2012;61(7):970–6.

12. Singh S, Manickam P, Amin AV, et al. Incidence of esophageal adenocarcinoma in Barrett's esophagus with low-grade dysplasia: a systematic review and meta-analysis. Gastrointest Endosc 2014;79(6): 897–909. e4.

13. Rastogi A, Puli S, El-Serag HB, et al. Incidence of esophageal adenocarcinoma in patients with Barrett's esophagus and high-grade dysplasia: a meta-analysis. Gastrointest Endosc 2008;67(3): 394–8.

14. Goldblum JR. Barrett's esophagus and Barrett's-related dysplasia. Mod Pathol 2003;16(4):316–24.

15. Hopcroft SA, Shepherd NA. The changing role of the pathologist in the management of Barrett's oesophagus. Histopathology 2014;65(4):441–55.

16. Barrett NR. Chronic peptic ulcers of the œsophagus and 'œsophagitis. Br J Surg 1950;38(150):175–82.

17. Lowes H, Somarathna T, Shepherd NA. Definition, derivation, and diagnosis of Barrett's esophagus: pathological perspectives. In: Jansen M, Wright NA, editors. Stem cells, Pre-neoplasia, and early cancer of the Upper gastrointestinal tract. Switzerland: Springer International Publishing; 2016. p. 111–36.

18. Paull A, Trier JS, Dalton MD, et al. The histologic spectrum of Barrett's esophagus. N Engl J Med 1976;295(9):476–80.

19. Watanabe G, Ajioka Y, Takeuchi M, et al. Intestinal metaplasia in Barrett's oesophagus may be an epiphenomenon rather than a preneoplastic condition, and CDX2-positive cardiac-type epithelium is associated with minute Barrett's tumour. Histopathology 2015;66(2):201–14.

20. Takubo K, Aida J, Naomoto Y, et al. Cardiac rather than intestinal-type background in endoscopic resection specimens of minute Barrett adenocarcinoma. Hum Pathol 2009;40(1):65–74.

21. Slack JMW. Metaplasia and transdifferentiation: from pure biology to the clinic. Nat Rev Mol Cell Biol 2007;8(5):369–78.

22. Geboes K, Hoorens A. The cell of origin for Barrett's esophagus. Science 2021;373(6556):737–8.

23. Boch J, Shields H, Antonioli D, et al. Distribution of cytokeratin markers in Barrett's specialized columnar epithelium. Gastroenterology 1997; 112(3):760–5.

24. Aichler M, Seiler C, Tost M, et al. Origin of pancreatic ductal adenocarcinoma from atypical flat lesions: a comparative study in transgenic mice and human tissues. J Pathol 2012;226(5):723–34.

25. Barbera M, Pietro M di, Walker E, et al. The human squamous oesophagus has widespread capacity for clonal expansion from cells at diverse stages of differentiation. Gut 2015;64(1):11–9.

26. Sarosi G, Brown G, Jaiswal K, et al. Bone marrow progenitor cells contribute to esophageal regeneration and metaplasia in a rat model of Barrett's esophagus. Dis Esophagus 2008;21(1):43–50.

27. Aikou S, Aida J, Takubo K, et al. Columnar metaplasia in a surgical mouse model of gastro-esophageal reflux disease is not derived from bone marrow-derived cell. Cancer Sci 2013;104(9): 1154–61.

28. Leedham SJ, Preston SL, McDonald SAC, et al. Individual crypt genetic heterogeneity and the origin of metaplastic glandular epithelium in human Barrett's oesophagus. Gut 2008;57(8):1041–8.

29. Owen RP, White MJ, Severson DT, et al. Single cell RNA-seq reveals profound transcriptional similarity between Barrett's oesophagus and oesophageal submucosal glands. Nat Commun 2018; 9(1):4261.

30. Nowicki-Osuch K, Zhuang L, Jammula S, et al. Molecular phenotyping reveals the identity of Barrett's esophagus and its malignant transition. Science 2021;373(6556):760–7.

31. Riddell RH, Goldman H, Ransohoff DF, et al. Dysplasia in inflammatory bowel disease: standardized classification with provisional clinical applications. Hum Pathol 1983;14(11):931–68.

32. van der Wel MJ, Jansen M, Vieth M, et al. What makes an expert Barrett's histopathologist?. In: Jansen M, Wright NA, editors. Stem cells, Pre-neoplasia, and early cancer of the Upper gastrointestinal tract. Switzerland: Springer International Publishing; 2016. p. 137–59.

33. Yin F, Hernandez Gonzalo D, Lai J, et al. Histopathology of Barrett's esophagus and early-stage esophageal adenocarcinoma: an updated review. Gastrointest Disord 2019;1(1):147–63.

34. Kumarasinghe MP, Armstrong M, Foo J, et al. The modern management of Barrett's oesophagus and related neoplasia: role of pathology. Histopathology 2021;78(1):18–38.

35. Corsini EM, Foo WC, Mitchell KG, et al. Esophageal adenocarcinoma with any component of signet ring cells portends poor prognosis and response to neoadjuvant therapy. J Thorac Cardiovasc Surg 2021; 162(5):1404–12.

36. Patel VR, Hofstetter WL, Correa AM, et al. Signet ring cells in esophageal adenocarcinoma predict poor response to preoperative chemoradiation. Ann Thorac Surg 2014;98(3):1064–71.

37. Rice TW, Patil DT, Blackstone EH. 8th edition AJCC/UICC staging of cancers of the esophagus and esophagogastric junction: application to clinical practice. Ann Cardiothorac Surg 2017;6(2):119–30.

38. Bejarano PA, Berho M. Examination of surgical specimens of the esophagus. Arch Pathol Lab Med 2015;139(11):1446–54.

39. Orosey M, Amin M, Cappell MS. A 14-year study of 398 esophageal adenocarcinomas diagnosed among 156,256 EGDs performed at two large

hospitals: an inlet patch is proposed as a significant risk factor for proximal esophageal adenocarcinoma. Dig Dis Sci 2018;63(2):452–65.

40. Taniere P, Borghi-Scoazec G, Saurin JC, et al. Cytokeratin expression in adenocarcinomas of the esophagogastric junction: a comparative study of adenocarcinomas of the distal esophagus and of the proximal stomach. Am J Surg Pathol 2002; 26(9):1213–21.

41. Driessen A, Nafteux P, Lerut T, et al. Identical cytokeratin expression pattern CK7+/CK20- in esophageal and cardiac cancer: etiopathological and clinical implications. Mod Pathol 2004;17(1):49–55.

42. Shah MA, Kennedy EB, Catenacci DV, et al. Treatment of locally advanced esophageal carcinoma: ASCO Guideline. J Clin Oncol 2020;38(23):2677–94.

43. Muir JA, Marcon N, Aranda-Hernandez J, et al. Endoscopic mucosal resection (EMR) in Barrett's esophagus associated neoplasia: recommendations for pathological evaluation and reporting. Can J Pathol 2015;7(4):25–36.

44. Sharma P, Shaheen NJ, Katzka D, et al. AGA clinical practice update on endoscopic treatment of Barrett's esophagus with dysplasia and/or early cancer: expert review. Gastroenterology 2020;158(3):760–9.

45. Kumarasinghe MP, Bourke MJ, Brown I, et al. Pathological assessment of endoscopic resections of the gastrointestinal tract: a comprehensive clinicopathologic review. Mod Pathol 2020;33(6):986–1006.

46. Othman MO, Lee JH, Wang K. AGA clinical practice update on the utility of endoscopic submucosal dissection in T1b esophageal cancer: expert review. Clin Gastroenterol Hepatol 2019;17(11):2161–6.

47. Manner H, Pech O, Heldmann Y, et al. The frequency of lymph node metastasis in early-stage adenocarcinoma of the esophagus with incipient submucosal invasion (pT1b sm1) depending on histological risk patterns. Surg Endosc 2015;29(7):1888–96.

48. Manner H, Pech O, Heldmann Y, et al. Efficacy, safety, and long-term results of endoscopic treatment for early stage adenocarcinoma of the esophagus with low-risk sm1 invasion. Clin Gastroenterol Hepatol 2013;11(6):630–5.

49. Nentwich MF, von Loga K, Reeh M, et al. Depth of submucosal tumor infiltration and its relevance in lymphatic metastasis formation for T1b squamous cell and adenocarcinomas of the esophagus. J Gastrointest Surg 2014;18(2):242–9.

50. Griffin SM, Burt AD, Jennings NA. Lymph node metastasis in early esophageal adenocarcinoma. Ann Surg 2011;254(5):731–7.

51. Cen P, Hofstetter WL, Correa AM, et al. Lymphovascular invasion as a tool to further subclassify T1b esophageal adenocarcinoma. Cancer 2008;112(5):1020–7.

52. Badreddine RJ, Prasad GA, Lewis JT, et al. Depth of submucosal invasion does not predict lymph node metastasis and survival of patients with esophageal carcinoma. Clin Gastroenterol Hepatol 2010;8(3):248–53.

53. Karamchandani DM, Gonzalez RS, Westerhoff M, et al. Measuring depth of invasion of submucosa – invasive adenocarcinoma in oesophageal endoscopic specimens: how good are we? Histopathology 2022;80(2):420–9.

54. Dunbar KB, Spechler SJ. The risk of lymph node metastases in patients with high grade dysplasia or intramucosal carcinoma in Barrett's esophagus: a systematic review. Am J Gastroenterol 2012;107(6):850–63.

55. Zemler B, May A, Ell C, et al. Early Barrett's carcinoma: the depth of infiltration of the tumour correlates with the degree of differentiation, the incidence of lymphatic vessel and venous invasion. Virchows Archiv 2010;456(6):609–14.

56. Estrella JS, Hofstetter WL, Correa AM, et al. Duplicated muscularis mucosae invasion has similar risk of lymph node metastasis and recurrence-free survival as intramucosal esophageal adenocarcinoma. Am J Surg Pathol 2011;35(7):1045–53.

57. Kaneshiro DK, Post JC, Rybicki L, et al. Clinical significance of the duplicated muscularis mucosae in Barrett esophagus-related superficial adenocarcinoma. Am J Surg Pathol 2011;35(5):697–700.

58. Chang F, Deere H, Mahadeva U, et al. Histopathologic examination and reporting of esophageal carcinomas following preoperative neoadjuvant therapy: practical guidelines and current issues. Am J Clin Pathol 2008;129(2):252–62.

59. Wang KL, Yang Q, Cleary KR, et al. The significance of neuroendocrine differentiation in adenocarcinoma of the esophagus and esophagogastric junction after preoperative chemoradiation. Cancer 2006;107(7):1467–74.

60. Alnaji RM, Du W, Gabriel E, et al. Pathologic complete response is an independent predictor of improved survival following neoadjuvant chemoradiation for esophageal adenocarcinoma. J Gastrointest Surg 2016;20(9):1541–6.

61. Langer R, Ott K, Feith M, et al. Prognostic significance of histopathological tumor regression after neoadjuvant chemotherapy in esophageal adenocarcinomas. Mod Pathol 2009;22(12):1555–63.

62. Groth SS, Burt BM, Farjah F, et al. Prognostic value of neoadjuvant treatment response in locally advanced esophageal adenocarcinoma. J Thorac Cardiovasc Surg 2019;157(4):1682–93.

63. Mandard AM, Dalibard F, Mandard JC, et al. Pathologic assessment of tumor regression after preoperative chemoradiotherapy of esophageal carcinoma. Clinicopathologic correlations. Cancer 1994;73(11):2680–6.

64. Langer R, Becker K. Tumor regression grading of gastrointestinal cancers after neoadjuvant therapy. Virchows Archiv 2018;472(2):175–86.

65. Takeda FR, Tustumi F, de Almeida Obregon C, et al. Prognostic value of tumor regression grade based on Ryan score in squamous cell carcinoma and adenocarcinoma of esophagus. Ann Surg Oncol 2020;27(4):1241–7.

66. Noble F, Lloyd MA, Turkington R, et al. Multicentre cohort study to define and validate pathological assessment of response to neoadjuvant therapy in oesophagogastric adenocarcinoma. Br J Surg 2017;104(13):1816–28.

67. Karamitopoulou E, Thies S, Zlobec I, et al. Assessment of tumor regression of esophageal adenocarcinomas after neoadjuvant chemotherapy: comparison of 2 commonly used scoring approaches. Am J Surg Pathol 2014;38(11):1551–6.

68. Hornick JL, Farraye FA, Odze RD. Prevalence and significance of prominent mucin pools in the esophagus post neoadjuvant chemoradiotherapy for Barrett's-associated adenocarcinoma. Am J Surg Pathol 2006;30(1):28–35.

69. Spicer J, Benay C, Lee L, et al. Diagnostic accuracy and utility of intraoperative microscopic margin analysis of gastric and esophageal adenocarcinoma. Ann Surg Oncol 2014;21(8):2580–6.

70. Chan DSY, Reid TD, Howell I, et al. Systematic review and meta-analysis of the influence of circumferential resection margin involvement on survival in patients with operable oesophageal cancer. Br J Surg 2013;100(4):456–64.

71. Thies S, Guldener L, Slotta-Huspenina J, et al. Impact of peritumoral and intratumoral budding in esophageal adenocarcinomas. Hum Pathol 2016; 52:1–8.

72. Landau MS, Hastings SM, Foxwell TJ, et al. Tumor budding is associated with an increased risk of lymph node metastasis and poor prognosis in superficial esophageal adenocarcinoma. Mod Pathol 2014;27(12):1578–89.

73. Lohneis P, Hieggelke L, Gebauer F, et al. Tumor budding assessed according to the criteria of the International Tumor Budding Consensus Conference determines prognosis in resected esophageal adenocarcinoma. Virchows Archiv 2021;478(3): 393–400.

74. Marginean EC, Dhanpat J. Pathologic assessment of endoscopic resection specimens with superficial carcinoma of the esophagus: current practice and practical issues. Ann N Y Acad Sci 2020;1482(1): 130–45.

75. Nafteux PR, Lerut AM, Moons J, et al. International multicenter study on the impact of extracapsular lymph node involvement in primary surgery adenocarcinoma of the esophagus on overall survival and staging systems. Ann Surg 2015;262(5): 809–16.

76. Wang A, Tan Y, Geng X, et al. Lymphovascular invasion as a poor prognostic indicator in thoracic esophageal carcinoma: a systematic review and meta-analysis. Dis Esophagus 2019;32(2):doy083.

77. Lordick F, Mariette C, Haustermans K, et al. Oesophageal cancer: ESMO Clinical Practice Guidelines for diagnosis, treatment and follow-up. Ann Oncol 2016;27:v50–7.

78. Bang YJ, Van Cutsem E, Feyereislova A, et al. Trastuzumab in combination with chemotherapy versus chemotherapy alone for treatment of HER2-positive advanced gastric or gastro-oesophageal junction cancer (ToGA): a phase 3, open-label, randomised controlled trial. Lancet 2010;376(9742):687–97.

79. Hu Y, Bandla S, Godfrey TE, et al. HER2 amplification, overexpression and score criteria in esophageal adenocarcinoma. Mod Pathol 2011;24(7): 899–907.

80. Yoon HH, Shi Q, Sukov WR, et al. Association of HER2/ErbB2 expression and gene amplification with pathologic features and prognosis in esophageal adenocarcinomas. Clin Cancer Res 2012; 18(2):546–54.

81. Bartley AN, Washington MK, Ventura CB, et al. HER2 testing and clinical decision making in gastroesophageal adenocarcinoma: guideline from the College of American Pathologists, American Society for Clinical Pathology, and American Society of Clinical Oncology. Am J Clin Pathol 2016;146(6):647–69.

Esophageal Cancer Genetics and Clinical Translation

Audrey Jajosky, MD, PhD[a], Daffolyn Rachael Fels Elliott, MD, PhD[b],*

KEYWORDS

• Esophageal cancer • Genetics • Molecular biomarkers • Mutations

KEY POINTS

- Genomic heterogeneity in esophageal cancer, including differences between the 2 major histologic subtypes, likely contributes to the overall poor survival and lack of effective targeted therapies to date.
- Esophageal adenocarcinoma and squamous cell carcinoma have distinct risk factors and molecular features, supporting the consideration of unique treatment approaches.
- Genomic overlap between esophageal adenocarcinoma and the chromosomal instability subtype of gastric adenocarcinoma supports the consideration of gastroesophageal adenocarcinoma as a single diagnostic entity.
- Tissue-agnostic therapies are FDA-approved for all solid tumors that harbor defined molecular alterations (microsatellite instability-high or deficient mismatch repair, tumor mutational burden-high, *NTRK* fusions) regardless of the site of origin or histologic subtype.
- Immunohistochemistry for p53 is a promising biomarker to predict the risk of neoplastic progression in Barrett esophagus.

INTRODUCTION: CLINICAL UTILITY OF MOLECULAR BIOMARKERS

Despite therapeutic advances and improved survival in many cancer types, esophageal cancer has few effective targeted therapies and poor 5-year survival (<20%).[1,2] This is attributed to the generally advanced stage at diagnosis and genomic heterogeneity among patients, including differences between tumor histologic subtypes.[3–5] A better understanding of the genomic landscape of esophageal cancer may help to molecularly stratify patients for enrollment in clinical trials to identify optimal therapies. This article reviews the molecular landscape of esophageal cancer with emphasis on clinical translation and therapeutic relevance.

The genomic characterization of individual tumors promotes personalized cancer care. Diagnostic biomarkers may facilitate screening and early diagnosis of esophageal cancer by distinguishing high-grade dysplasia from earlier precursor lesions and/or reactive atypia (eg, immunohistochemistry (IHC) for p53 in Barrett esophagus). Prognostic biomarkers provide information about expected health outcomes irrespective of treatment, such as improved overall survival in patients with esophageal cancer with microsatellite instability-high (MSI-H) tumors. Predictive biomarkers indicate the likelihood a patient will

The authors have nothing to disclose.
[a] Department of Pathology and Laboratory Medicine, University of Rochester Medical Center, 211 Bailey Road, West Henrietta, NY 14586, USA; [b] Department of Pathology and Laboratory Medicine, University of Kansas Medical Center, 3901 Rainbow Boulevard, Mailstop 3045, Kansas City, KS 66160, USA
* Corresponding author.
E-mail address: dfelselliott@kumc.eud
Twitter: @AudreyJajosky (A.J.); @FelsElliott (D.R.F.E.)

Thorac Surg Clin 32 (2022) 425–435
https://doi.org/10.1016/j.thorsurg.2022.06.002
1547-4127/22/© 2022 Published by Elsevier Inc.

benefit from treatment, such as targeted therapy (eg, HER2 overexpression and/or *ERBB2* amplification predict response to trastuzumab) or immunotherapy (eg, PD-L1 expression predicts response to pembrolizumab).

Some predictive molecular biomarkers are linked to "tissue-agnostic" FDA-approved drugs. Regardless of histology or site of origin, unresectable or metastatic solid tumors exhibiting specific genomic signatures, such as MSI-H or tumor mutational burden-high (TMB-H), may be eligible for immune checkpoint inhibitor therapy with pembrolizumab. The National Comprehensive Cancer Network (NCCN) guidelines recommend evaluating several predictive biomarkers in patients with unresectable locally advanced, locally recurrent, or metastatic esophageal cancer who are candidates for targeted therapies or immunotherapy (**Table 1**).

EPIDEMIOLOGY, RISK FACTORS, AND PATHOGENESIS

The 2 main histologic subtypes of esophageal cancer, adenocarcinoma (EAC) and squamous cell carcinoma (ESCC) have distinct epidemiologic risk factors, geographic patterns, and molecular profiles (**Table 2**). In recent decades, the incidence of EAC has increased in Western populations and parallels a rise in proximal gastric adenocarcinoma.[11,12] Risk factors include older age, male gender, Caucasian ethnicity, abdominal obesity, and gastroesophageal reflux.[13] EAC usually arises near the gastroesophageal junction where the distal esophagus is exposed to acid reflux.[14,15] Chronic gastroesophageal reflux leads to an inflammatory microenvironment with mucosal injury, increased cell turnover and DNA damage (**Fig. 1**).[16,17] Barrett esophagus is a well-characterized precursor lesion that extends proximally from the gastroesophageal junction, visible by endoscopy and defined histologically as a metaplastic change from normal squamous to columnar epithelium.[18] Interestingly, *Helicobacter pylori* infection appears to be protective, possibly related to decreased stomach acid production.[19] Familial predisposition to Barrett esophagus and EAC has been described (~7% of cases),[20–22] but the underlying genetic factors are not well understood. Genome-wide association studies (GWAS) have identified risk loci including *FOXF1, BARX1, CRTC1,* MHC locus 16.24, and *ABCC5*.[20,23]

Although its incidence is declining in many countries, ESCC accounts for ~85% of esophageal cancer cases worldwide.[24] ESCC is highly prevalent in Asia, Southeastern Africa, and South America where diet and socioeconomic conditions are predominant risk factors.[25–27] In contrast, in nonendemic regions such as Western industrialized nations, ESCC is strongly associated with smoking and alcohol exposures.[28] ESCC arises in the upper and middle esophagus in the setting of chronic mucosal injury, progressing from basal cell hyperplasia and dysplasia to carcinoma (see **Fig. 1**). Inherited cancer predisposition syndromes, including tylosis, Fanconi anemia, and Bloom syndrome, are rare causes of ESCC. Tylosis is an autosomal dominant disorder caused by germline *RHBDF2* mutations that is characterized by thickened skin on the palms and soles, esophageal lesions (hyperkeratosis), and a high (~90%) risk of developing ESCC.[29,30] Fanconi anemia, an X-linked or autosomal recessive disorder caused by *FANC* gene mutations, is characterized by chromosomal fragility, progressive bone marrow failure, and an increased risk of developing both solid tumors and hematologic malignancies.[31] Bloom syndrome is an autosomal recessive disorder caused by loss-of-function *BLM* mutations that leads to chromosomal instability, growth and immune deficiencies and a strong propensity for early-onset cancers including ESCC.[32]

MOLECULAR CLASSIFICATION

Large-scale sequencing efforts by The Cancer Genome Atlas (TCGA) and International Cancer Genome Consortium (ICGC) have advanced our understanding of the genomic landscape of esophageal cancer. Esophageal cancer is a heterogeneous disease and the 2 main histologic subtypes, EAC and ESCC, have distinct molecular profiles. Genomic differences suggest these tumor subtypes should be considered as separate entities in clinical trials for novel therapeutics.

Esophageal Adenocarcinoma: Genomic Landscape and Molecular Subtypes

EAC is a heterogenous disease with high tumor mutational burden, copy number alterations, and structural rearrangements. Although point mutations are common in EAC, the majority of cases appear to be dominated by copy number alterations and structural rearrangements.[33]

Mutational driver events

Median tumor mutational burden is ~10 mutations/Mb, which is comparable to other highly mutated solid tumors such as bladder and lung cancers.[34–36] MSIH tumors represent a minority of EAC (3–7%)[35,37] but have important clinical implications for better prognosis and response to immunotherapy. Recurrent point mutations predominantly involve loss-of-function mutations in

Table 1
Predictive biomarkers of response to targeted therapies and immunotherapies

Biomarker	Cancer Subtype(s)	Testing Methodology (Gold Standard)	Definition	Therapeutic Implications
MSI-H (0–3%)[6]	EAC, ESCC	Polymerase chain reaction (PCR)	≥ 30% of the markers exhibit instability; ≥ 2 of the 5 National Cancer Institute (NCI) or mononucleotide markers exhibit instability	Pembrolizumab (tumor agnostic), nivolumab, dostarlimab
Deficient mismatch repair (dMMR) (0–3%)[6]	EAC, ESCC	Immunohistochemistry (IHC)	Loss of nuclear expression of one or more MMR proteins	Pembrolizumab (tumor agnostic), nivolumab, dostarlimab
TMB-H (4–18%)[6]	EAC, ESCC	Next generation sequencing (NGS)	≥ 10 mutations per megabase of DNA	Pembrolizumab (tumor agnostic), nivolumab
PD-L1 expression	EAC, ESCC	IHC (FDA-approved companion diagnostic test)	Combined positive score (CPS[a]) ≥ 10 (ESCC) or ≥ 1 (EAC)	Pembrolizumab
HER2 overexpression (12–18%)[7]	EAC	IHC (Fluorescence *in situ* hybridization (FISH) for *ERBB2* amplification in equivocal cases)	IHC: Strong complete, basolateral, or lateral membranous reactivity in ≥ 10% of cancer cells (or at least 5 cohesive cells in biopsy)[8]	Trastuzumab
NTRK 1/2/3 fusion[9] (<1%)	EAC, ESCC	IHC, NGS, PCR, or FISH	IHC: may show cytoplasmic, nuclear, and/or membranous staining patterns (at least 1% of tumor cells[10])	Larotrectinib or entrectinib (tumor agnostic)

[a] CPS (combined positive score) is the number of PD-L1-positive cells (tumor cells, lymphocytes, macrophages) divided by the total number of viable tumor cells, multiplied by 100.

tumor suppressor genes, including *TP53* (∼70%), *CDKN2A*, *ARID1A*, and *SMAD4*, with fewer activating mutations in oncogenes such as *ERBB2*.[33–35,38,39] *CDKN2A* is inactivated in a majority of EAC (∼75%) by mutation, deletion or epigenetic silencing.[35,38,39] Mutations in components of the SWI/SNF chromatin remodeling complex are also frequent in EAC (eg, *ARID1A*, *SMARCA4*, *PBRM1*).

Copy number alterations and receptor tyrosine kinases

The oncogenic driver events appear to predominantly involve amplifications of oncogenes (eg,

ERBB2, *VEGFA*, *GATA4*, *GATA6*, and *CCNE1*). Receptor tyrosine kinases (RTKs) are frequently amplified in EAC, including *ERBB2* (∼30%), *EGFR*, *MET*, and *FGFR*, and have potential for targeted therapy by RTK inhibitors.[39] The anti-ERBB2 (HER2/neu) antibody Trastuzumab was initially approved by the United States Food and Drug Administration (FDA) for the treatment of gastric and gastroesophageal junction adenocarcinomas,[40] and is used to treat ERBB2-positive EAC routinely in many centers. Inhibitors of other RTKs are under evaluation in ongoing clinical trials. Coamplification of multiple RTKs and/or downstream mitogenic activation of MAPK and PI3K

Table 2
Epidemiologic and genetic risk factors

	Adenocarcinoma	Squamous Cell Carcinoma
Geographic prevalence	Western Europe, North America, Australia	Asia, Southeastern Africa, South America
Risk factors	Older age, male gender, Caucasian, gastroesophageal reflux, obesity, smoking	Older age, male gender, tobacco, alcohol, caustic injury, recurrent thermal injury, micronutrient deficiencies, achalasia
Precursor lesions	Barrett esophagus (metaplasia) → dysplasia → carcinoma	Squamous hyperplasia → dysplasia → carcinoma
Genetic predisposition syndromes	Familial Barrett esophagus (risk loci from GWAS: *FOXF1*, *BARX1*, *CRTC1*, MHC locus 16.24. *ABCC5*)	Tylosis (*RHBDF2*), Fanconi anemia (*FANC* genes, *BRCA2*), Bloom syndrome (*BLM*)

pathways is a potential mechanism of resistance in EAC.[33] This suggests a potential role for combination RTK inhibitor therapy.

Genomic catastrophes

Whole-genome sequencing demonstrates that genomic catastrophes frequently occur in EAC,

including chromothripsis in nearly a third of cases and localized hypermutation (kataegis) in 30 to 85% of cases.[33,34] Chromothripsis involves chromosome shattering that results in 10s to 100s of structural rearrangements localized to specific regions.[41] The complex rearrangements resulting from chromothripsis and breakage-fusion-bridge

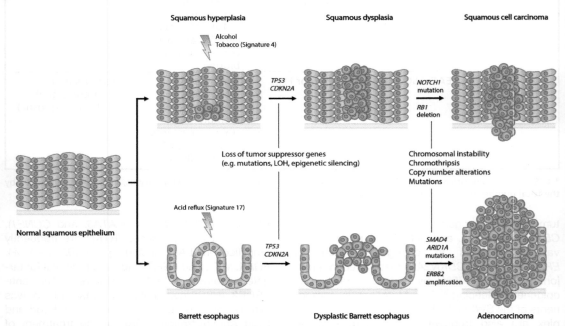

Fig. 1. Pathogenesis and molecular changes in esophageal cancer. Exposure to chronic mucosal insults triggers molecular alterations that promote the development and progression of esophageal cancer through the induction of genomic instability. Esophageal adenocarcinoma arises in the distal esophagus in the setting of chronic acid reflux via a metaplasia–dysplasia–carcinoma sequence. Squamous cell carcinoma often arises in the setting of chronic alcohol or tobacco exposure (in the West) or specific dietary factors (in the East) via a hyperplasia–dysplasia–carcinoma sequence. LOH: loss of heterozygosity. (*Adapted from* Smyth EC, Lagergren J, Fitzgerald RC, et al. Oesophageal cancer. *Nat Rev Dis Primers.* 2017;3:17048. Published 2017 Jul 27.)

events can promote tumorigenesis through the amplification of oncogenes (eg, *MYC, MDM2,* and *KRAS*).[33,34,41,42] Potential mechanisms underlying chromosomal instability include the high frequency of *TP53* mutations and telomere shortening in EAC, which may explain the higher prevalence of chromothripsis compared to other solid tumor types.[34] Additionally, mutational signature analysis suggests that chromosomal instability in EAC may be driven by *BRCA2* mutations.[34]

Mutational signatures and molecular subtypes of esophageal adenocarcinoma

Somatic mutations accumulate over a patient's lifetime and are caused by exposures to mutagens, defective DNA repair, infidelity of DNA replication, or enzymatic modification of DNA.[43] Mutational signatures offer clues to the biological processes underlying somatic mutations in cancer. More than 20 mutational signatures have been described in human cancers.[36] Some mutational signatures are observed in many cancer types (eg, age signature) while others are specific to certain cancers (eg, ultraviolet light signature in melanoma).[36] A hallmark mutational signature of EAC consists of frequent T > G nucleotide base substitutions in a CTT context (signature 17) and may be attributable to gastric acid reflux and oxidative DNA damage.[33,35,38] Signature 17 has also been detected in nondysplastic Barrett esophagus and high-grade dysplasia.[44] The APOBEC-driven hypermutated phenotype (signature 2) has also been described in EAC, likely due to over-activity of cytidine deaminases which convert cytidine to uracil.[33,36]

Using mutational signatures derived from whole-genome sequencing, Secrier and colleagues[33] defined 3 molecular subtypes of EAC with potential therapeutic relevance: (1) enriched for BRCA signature with evidence of impaired DNA damage repair; (2) mutagenic T > G mutational pattern with high tumor mutation burden possibly due to acid reflux (signature 17); and (3) C > A/T mutational pattern with an aging signature. The BRCA signature subtype had the highest degree of genomic instability. The mutagenic subtype had the highest mutational burden and neoantigen presentation,[33] which may confer better response to immunotherapy. There were no differences in *TP53* mutation status or other recurrently mutated genes between subtypes.

Esophageal Squamous Cell Carcinoma: Genomic Landscape and Molecular Subtypes

Despite the shared anatomical location, ESCC is molecularly distinct from EAC[39] and more closely resembles squamous cell carcinomas (SCC) of

other tissues, such as lung[45,46] and head and neck.[47] Unlike head and neck SCC, however, ESCC has not been definitively linked to human papillomavirus (HPV) infection.[39] HPV vaccination is, therefore, unlikely to prevent ESCC.

Mutational driver events

Genes that are recurrently mutated in ESCC cluster within several oncogenic signaling pathways, including Notch, phosphoinositide 3-kinase (PI3K), Ras, and Hippo signaling as well as pathways regulating the cell cycle, genomic integrity, and chromatin remodeling.[20] Significantly mutated genes include *TP53, KMT2D, NOTCH1, TGFBR2,* and *NFE2L2.*[39] *TP53* is mutated in a majority of ESCC and is an early driver event detectable within dysplastic precursor lesions.[48] While both ESCC and EAC demonstrate mutations in chromatin-modifying enzymes, genes encoding histone H3 modifiers (ie, *KDM6A, KMT2D,* and *KMT2C*) are mutated more frequently in ESCC while genes encoding SWI/SNF family members (ie, *ARID1A, SMARC4,* and *PBRM1*) are enriched in EAC.[39] Mutational signatures that have been described in ESCC include a C > A signature associated with tobacco use (signature 4) and APOBEC hypermutated phenotype (signatures 2 and 13).[39,49]

Copy number alterations and structural variants

Recurrent copy number alterations include amplifications of *SOX2, TERT, FGFR1, NKX2-1, MDM2, CCND1,* and *TP63* and deletion of *RB1*. Potential therapeutic targets include RTKs such as *EGFR* (activated by mutation or amplification in 19% of tumors) and downstream activators of the PI3K signaling pathway (*PIK3CA, PTEN,* and *PIK3R1* altered in a combined 24% of tumors), which can be targeted by RTK inhibitors.[39] Dysregulation of cell cycle regulators including *CDKN2A* (inactivated in 76% of tumors) and *CCND1* (amplified in 57% of tumors) suggests a potential therapeutic role for cell cycle kinase inhibitors. Genomic catastrophes generated by chromothripsis, kataegis, and breakage-fusion-bridge events have been described in up to 55% of ESCC, with complex structural rearrangements leading to the amplification of oncogenes (*FGFR1, LETM2, CCND1, EGFR, ERBB2,* and *MYC*).[50]

Molecular subtypes of esophageal squamous cell carcinoma

Using comprehensive genomic profiling, TCGA identified 3 molecular subtypes of ESCC (ESCC1, ESCC2, and ESCC3).[39] By mutational analysis and gene expression, the ESCC1 subgroup resembled the molecular subtypes of lung[46] and head and neck[47] SCC previously described by TCGA. ESCC1 was characterized by NRF2 pathway mutations (*NFE2L2*, *KEAP1*, *CUL3*, and *ATG7*), copy number alterations expected to activate the Hippo pathway (amplification of *YAP1*, deletion of *VGLL4* and/or *ATG7*), and amplifications of *SOX2* and *TP63*. ESCC2 was enriched for the APOBEC hypermutated phenotype ("signature 2") and showed prominent infiltration by white blood cells. ESCC2 showed frequent *NOTCH1* or *ZNF750* mutations, *CDK6* amplification, and inactivating *KDM6A, KDM2D, PTEN,* or *PIK3R1* alterations. ESCC3 (a minor subgroup, n = 4) showed no alterations expected to dysregulate the cell cycle and only 1 of 4 tumors had a *TP53* mutation. ESCC3 was characterized by alterations predicted to activate PI3K signaling and mutations in *KMT2D* and *SMARCA4*. Molecular subtypes appeared to be enriched within specific geographic regions: ESCC1 in Vietnamese patients (the only Asian population studied), ESCC2 in Eastern Europe/South America, and ESCC3 in North America. This data implicates geographically distinct genetic and/or environmental risk factors, such as heritable alterations in alcohol-metabolizing enzymes (ie, polymorphisms of alcohol dehydrogenases and aldehyde dehydrogenases) in East Asia.[51]

MOLECULAR DISTINCTION OF ESOPHAGEAL ADENOCARCINOMA FROM SQUAMOUS CELL CARCINOMA

Combined molecular data from TCGA and ICGC show that recurrently mutated genes differ between EAC and SCC histologic subtypes (**Table 3**), with overlap in only 4 driver genes (*TP53, CDKN2A, FBXW7,* and *PIK3CA*).[52] Clustering of genomic data across multiple platforms (copy number alterations, DNA methylation, mRNA and microRNA expression) also separates esophageal tumors by histologic subtype.[39] Gene expression data demonstrate E-cadherin signaling is increased in EAC, while Notch-p63 signaling (which promotes squamous differentiation) and Wnt/beta-catenin signaling pathways are upregulated in SCC.[39] These data suggest that distinct mutational patterns and lineage-specific signaling pathways drive tumorigenesis in EAC and SCC.

MOLECULAR DISTINCTION OF ESOPHAGEAL FROM GASTRIC CANCERS

Distinguishing the anatomic origin of esophageal and gastric adenocarcinomas arising near the gastroesophageal junction is a clinical challenge. Four molecular subtypes of gastric

adenocarcinomas have been identified by TCGA, including microsatellite unstable tumors, tumors with chromosomal instability, genomically stable tumors, and tumors positive for Epstein–Barr virus (EBV).[53] EACs are enriched for chromosomal instability (71/72 cases in TCGA dataset), with higher prevalence of chromosomal aberrations extending proximally from the gastroesophageal junction.[39] The overlap in molecular features between EACs and the chromosomal instability subtype of gastric adenocarcinomas supports the consideration of gastroesophageal adenocarcinoma as a single diagnostic entity from a genomic perspective. This has implications for therapeutic management and enrollment in clinical trials.

CLINICAL TRANSLATION: MOLECULAR BIOMARKERS TO PREDICT THE RISK OF PROGRESSION IN BARRETT ESOPHAGUS

A step-wise model of Barrett carcinogenesis suggests that early loss of tumor suppressor genes (*TP53* and *CDKN2A*) is followed by chromosomal instability and amplification of oncogenes as a later event.[4,38,54–57] Predicting the small subset of patients who will progress to EAC is a clinical challenge. The annual risk of neoplastic progression is relatively low (0.12–0.6%)[58–62] unless there is histologic evidence of dysplasia.[63–67] Currently the histologic diagnosis of dysplasia is the only validated predictive biomarker for neoplastic progression in routine clinical use. However, there is significant inter-observer variability for low-grade dysplasia and indefinite for dysplasia. Molecular biomarkers would be clinically useful to stratify patients with Barrett esophagus at high risk of progression who can benefit from increased surveillance and early endoscopic intervention.

Several molecular biomarkers and biomarker panels have been proposed in the literature to predict risk of neoplastic progression in Barrett esophagus (**Table 4**). Potential barriers to the clinical implementation of molecular biomarkers include the need for large prospective clinical trials for validation, high cost to analyze complex molecular assays, and the laboratory expertise required to analyze and score assay results. *TP53* is discussed in the subsequent section as a candidate predictive biomarker with potential for clinical application.

TP53 Predicts Neoplastic Progression of Barrett Esophagus

TP53 is commonly mutated in EAC, and mutations tend to occur early in the metaplasia–dysplasia–carcinoma sequence.[4] *TP53* mutations can be detected in endoscopic biopsies of Barrett

Table 3
Summary of recurrent molecular alterations in esophageal cancer

	Adenocarcinoma	Squamous Cell Carcinoma
Mutations	*Tumor suppressors*: TP53, CDKN2A, ARID1A, SMAD4, *Oncogenes*: ERBB2, PIK3CA	*Tumor suppressors*: TP53, KMT2D, KDM6A, KMT2C, ZNF750, TGFBR2, PTCH1 *Oncogenes*: NFE2L2, NOTCH1
Copy number alterations	*Amplifications*: receptor tyrosine kinases (ERBB2, EGFR, MET, FGFR), VEGFA, GATA4, GATA6, CCNE1 *Deletions*: SMAD4	*Amplifications*: CCND1, SOX2, TP63, TERT, FGFR1, MDM2, NKX2-1 *Deletions*: RB1, VGLL4, ATG7
Structural rearrangements and genomic catastrophes	Chromothripsis, breakage-fusion-bridge, kataegis	Chromothripsis, breakage-fusion-bridge, kataegis
Mutational signatures	S1: age signature S2: APOBEC signature S3: BRCA signature S17: hallmark signature of EAC (possible acid reflux)	S1: age signature S2 and S13: APOBEC signatures S4: smoking signature
Gene expression signatures	Upregulation of E-cadherin signaling	Upregulation of Notch-p63 and Wnt/beta-catenin signaling

esophagus before histologic evidence of dysplasia or significant changes in copy number.[72] Mutation of *TP53* may result in the complete loss or stabilization of mutant p53 protein, which can be visualized by IHC. Several studies have suggested that *TP53* mutation and/or abnormal p53 IHC is associated with increased risk of progression to high-grade dysplasia and EAC.[72,76,77,80,81]

Recently, Redston and colleagues showed that abnormal p53 IHC was associated with progression to EAC in a large retrospective cohort of patients including nondysplastic Barrett esophagus,[75] indefinite for dysplasia, and low-grade dysplasia (n = 561; p < 0.001) and predicted neoplastic progression in a prospective validation cohort (n = 1487; p < 0.001). Importantly, p53 IHC was more sensitive than histology for identifying at-risk patients, especially at earlier timepoints during surveillance endoscopy (p < 0.01). P53 IHC is readily available in most pathology laboratories and has the potential to be incorporated into routine clinical practice as a predictive biomarker.

Beyond Endoscopy: Detecting TP53 Mutations Using the Cytosponge™

Since not all *TP53* mutations result in stabilization or complete loss of mutant p53 protein, IHC may not be as sensitive as DNA sequencing to detect

Table 4
Molecular biomarkers predictive of progression in Barrett esophagus

Hierarchy of Molecular Biology	Biomarkers
Chromosomal alterations	The Reid panel: abnormal DNA ploidy, 9p LOH (p16), 17p LOH (p53)[68] FISH probes for 7p12 (EGFR), 8q24.12 (c-myc), and 20q13.2[69]
Epigenetic markers	Promoter methylation of p16, RUNX3, and HPP1[70]
DNA mutations and LOH	17p (p53) LOH[71] TP53 mutation[72]
Genetic clonal diversity	Measures of clonal diversity[73]
Gene expression and microRNAs	miRNAs (miR-193, 194, 196a and196b)[74]
Protein markers	IHC for p53[75–77] Fluorescently labeled peptide SNFYMPL[78] Fluorescently labeled lectins[79]

TP53 mutations. Weaver and colleagues[38] proposed a nonendoscopic strategy for detecting *TP53* mutations using a cell sampling device called the Cytosponge™, which can be administered in a primary care setting. The Cytosponge™ consists of a polypropylene fiber sponge compressed in a capsule attached to a string, and the device collects cells along the length of the esophagus when it is withdrawn.[82] As proof of concept, the Cytosponge™ detected *TP53* mutations in 86% (19/22) of patients with high-grade dysplasia by multiplex polymerase chain reaction (PCR) and massively parallel sequencing covering most of the *TP53* gene coding region.[38] This approach could potentially be expanded to include a larger panel of genes for risk stratification.

SUMMARY AND FUTURE DIRECTIONS

EAC and ESCC are genomically distinct with unique driver mutations and gene expression signatures, suggesting that lineage-specific signaling pathways drive tumorigenesis. A model of genomic instability is emerging in esophageal cancer where genomic catastrophes and complex rearrangements lead to the amplification of oncogenes and marked heterogeneity between patients. Personalized medicine with targeted therapy is part of current management for EAC. The anti-HER2/neu antibody Trastuzumab is the only targeted therapy that is routinely used in clinical practice, although inhibitors of other RTKs are under evaluation in clinical trials. ESCC, the predominant histologic subtype worldwide, harbors several therapeutically targetable alterations under investigation in clinical trials.

Although some tissue-agnostic drugs are FDA-approved for use in all solid tumors, the molecular alterations targeted by these therapies occur in only a subset of patients with esophageal cancer. The NCCN Guidelines for esophageal cancer recommend using a combination of IHC, FISH, and PCR to analyze multiple predictive molecular biomarkers. In the future, comprehensive next-generation sequencing (NGS) panels will likely be used more routinely to simultaneously evaluate a range of targeted molecular alterations and overarching mutational signatures that predict response to therapy. Emerging NGS applications may enable less invasive, tissue-sparing detection and monitoring of disease. Liquid biopsy of peripheral blood specimens for circulating tumor DNA may be increasingly used to screen for esophageal cancer, monitor for disease recurrence, and/or detect mechanisms of resistance to targeted therapies. IHC for p53 protein is a promising candidate biomarker to predict patients with Barrett

esophagus at high risk of neoplastic progression. Finally, evaluation of the esophageal microbiome may provide clues to the pathogenesis of esophageal cancer within an inflammatory microenvironment and possible dietary risk factors.[83,84] A more complete understanding of how to use emerging molecular data to improve the screening, diagnosis, treatment, and monitoring of esophageal cancer is needed.

CLINICS CARE POINTS

- The National Comprehensive Cancer Network guidelines recommend evaluating multiple predictive biomarkers (MSI/MMR, HER2, PD-L1, *NTRK*) in patients with unresectable locally advanced, recurrent, or metastatic esophageal cancer
- Patients with esophageal cancer whose tumors display high microsatellite instability and/or mismatch repair deficiency, high tumor mutational burden, or PD-L1 expression may be eligible for immune checkpoint inhibitor therapy
- Evaluation of HER2 overexpression by immunohistochemistry and/or *ERBB2* amplification by FISH is recommended in patients with esophageal adenocarcinoma who may benefit from targeted therapy with Trastuzumab

REFERENCES

1. De Angelis R, Sant M, Coleman MP, et al. Cancer survival in europe 1999-2007 by country and age: Results of eurocare–5-a population-based study. Lancet Oncol 2014;15:23–34.
2. Siegel RL, Miller KD, Jemal A. Cancer statistics, 2016. CA Cancer J Clin 2016;66:7–30.
3. Ross-Innes CS, Becq J, Warren A, et al. Whole-genome sequencing provides new insights into the clonal architecture of barrett's esophagus and esophageal adenocarcinoma. Nat Genet 2015;47: 1038–46.
4. Stachler MD, Taylor-Weiner A, Peng S, et al. Paired exome analysis of barrett's esophagus and adenocarcinoma. Nat Genet 2015;47:1047–55.
5. Hao JJ, Lin DC, Dinh HQ, et al. Spatial intratumoral heterogeneity and temporal clonal evolution in esophageal squamous cell carcinoma. Nat Genet 2016;48:1500–7.
6. Eso Y, Seno H. Current status of treatment with immune checkpoint inhibitors for gastrointestinal,

hepatobiliary, and pancreatic cancers. Therap Adv Gastroenterol 2020;13:1–20.

7. Hu Y, Bandla S, Godfrey TE, et al. Her2 amplification, overexpression and score criteria in esophageal adenocarcinoma. Mod Pathol 2011;24:899–907.

8. Bartley AN, Washington MK, Ventura CB, et al. Her2 testing and clinical decision making in gastroesophageal adenocarcinoma: Guideline from the college of american pathologists, american society for clinical pathology, and american society of clinical oncology. Arch Pathol Lab Med 2016;140:1345–63.

9. Westphalen CB, Krebs MG, Le Tourneau C, et al. Genomic context of ntrk1/2/3 fusion-positive tumours from a large real-world population. NPJ Precis Oncol 2021;5:69.

10. Gatalica Z, Xiu J, Swensen J, et al. Molecular characterization of cancers with ntrk gene fusions. Mod Pathol 2019;32:147–53.

11. Brown LM, Devesa SS, Chow WH. Incidence of adenocarcinoma of the esophagus among white americans by sex, stage, and age. J Natl Cancer Inst 2008;100:1184–7.

12. Devesa SS, Fraumeni JF Jr. The rising incidence of gastric cardia cancer. J Natl Cancer Inst 1999;91:747–9.

13. Prasad GA, Bansal A, Sharma P, et al. Predictors of progression in barrett's esophagus: Current knowledge and future directions. Am J Gastroenterol 2010;105:1490–502.

14. Enzinger PC, Mayer RJ. Esophageal cancer. N Engl J Med 2003;349:2241–52.

15. Lagergren J, Bergstrom R, Lindgren A, et al. Symptomatic gastroesophageal reflux as a risk factor for esophageal adenocarcinoma. N Engl J Med 1999;340:825–31.

16. Picardo SL, Maher SG, O'Sullivan JN, et al. Barrett's to oesophageal cancer sequence: a model of inflammatory-driven upper gastrointestinal cancer. Dig Surg 2012;29:251–60.

17. Poehlmann A, Kuester D, Malfertheiner P, et al. Inflammation and barrett's carcinogenesis. Pathol Res Pract 2012;208:269–80.

18. Shaheen NJ, Falk GW, Iyer PG, et al. Acg clinical guideline: diagnosis and management of barrett's esophagus. Am J Gastroenterol 2016;111:30–50 [quiz 51].

19. Weston AP, Sharma P, Mathur S, et al. Risk stratification of barrett's esophagus: updated prospective multivariate analysis. Am J Gastroenterol 2004;99:1657–66.

20. Smyth EC, Lagergren J, Fitzgerald RC, et al. Oesophageal cancer. Nat Rev Dis Primers 2017;3:17048.

21. Romero Y, Cameron AJ, Locke GR 3rd, et al. Familial aggregation of gastroesophageal reflux in patients with barrett's esophagus and esophageal adenocarcinoma. Gastroenterology 1997;113:1449–56.

22. Chak A, Lee T, Kinnard MF, et al. Familial aggregation of barrett's oesophagus, oesophageal adenocarcinoma, and oesophagogastric junctional adenocarcinoma in caucasian adults. Gut 2002;51:323–8.

23. Gharahkhani P, Fitzgerald RC, Vaughan TL, et al. Genome-wide association studies in oesophageal adenocarcinoma and barrett's oesophagus: a large-scale meta-analysis. Lancet Oncol 2016;17:1363–73.

24. Arnold M, Ferlay J, van Berge Henegouwen MI, et al. Global burden of oesophageal and gastric cancer by histology and subsite in 2018. Gut 2020;69:1564–71.

25. Domper Arnal MJ, Ferrandez Arenas A, Lanas Arbeloa A. Esophageal cancer: risk factors, screening and endoscopic treatment in western and eastern countries. World J Gastroenterol 2015;21:7933–43.

26. Torre LA, Bray F, Siegel RL, et al. Global cancer statistics, 2012. CA Cancer J Clin 2015;65:87–108.

27. Ferlay J, Soerjomataram I, Dikshit R, et al. Cancer incidence and mortality worldwide: sources, methods and major patterns in globocan 2012. Int J Cancer 2015;136:E359–86.

28. Engel LS, Chow WH, Vaughan TL, et al. Population attributable risks of esophageal and gastric cancers. J Natl Cancer Inst 2003;95:1404–13.

29. Ellis A, Risk JM, Maruthappu T, et al. Tylosis with oesophageal cancer: diagnosis, management and molecular mechanisms. Orphanet J Rare Dis 2015;10:126.

30. Marger RS, Marger D. Carcinoma of the esophagus and tylosis. A lethal genetic combination. Cancer 1993;72:17–9.

31. Velleuer E, Dietrich R. Fanconi anemia: Young patients at high risk for squamous cell carcinoma. Mol Cell Pediatr 2014;1:9.

32. Cunniff C, Bassetti JA, Ellis NA. Bloom's syndrome: clinical spectrum, molecular pathogenesis, and cancer predisposition. Mol Syndromol 2017;8:4–23.

33. Secrier M, Li X, de Silva N, et al. Mutational signatures in esophageal adenocarcinoma define etiologically distinct subgroups with therapeutic relevance. Nat Genet 2016;48:1131–41.

34. Nones K, Waddell N, Wayte N, et al. Genomic catastrophes frequently arise in esophageal adenocarcinoma and drive tumorigenesis. Nat Commun 2014;5:5224.

35. Dulak AM, Stojanov P, Peng S, et al. Exome and whole-genome sequencing of esophageal adenocarcinoma identifies recurrent driver events and mutational complexity. Nat Genet 2013;45:478–86.

36. Alexandrov LB, Nik-Zainal S, Wedge DC, et al. Signatures of mutational processes in human cancer. Nature 2013;500:415–21.

37. Farris AB 3rd, Demicco EG, Le LP, et al. Clinicopathologic and molecular profiles of microsatellite

unstable barrett esophagus-associated adenocarcinoma. Am J Surg Pathol 2011;35:647–55.

38. Weaver JMJ, Ross-Innes CS, Shannon N, et al. Ordering of mutations in preinvasive disease stages of esophageal carcinogenesis. Nat Genet 2014;46: 837–43.

39. Cancer Genome Atlas Research N, Analysis Working Group: Asan U, Agency BCC et al. Integrated genomic characterization of oesophageal carcinoma. Nature 2017;541:169–75.

40. Bang YJ, Van Cutsem E, Feyereislova A, et al. Trastuzumab in combination with chemotherapy versus chemotherapy alone for treatment of her2-positive advanced gastric or gastro-oesophageal junction cancer (toga): A phase 3, open-label, randomised controlled trial. Lancet 2010;376:687–97.

41. Stephens PJ, Greenman CD, Fu B, et al. Massive genomic rearrangement acquired in a single catastrophic event during cancer development. Cell 2011;144:27–40.

42. Zack TI, Schumacher SE, Carter SL, et al. Pan-cancer patterns of somatic copy number alteration. Nat Genet 2013;45:1134–40.

43. Stratton MR, Campbell PJ, Futreal PA. The cancer genome. Nature 2009;458:719–24.

44. Newell F, Patel K, Gartside M, et al. Complex structural rearrangements are present in high-grade dysplastic barrett's oesophagus samples. BMC Med Genomics 2019;12:31.

45. Kim Y, Hammerman PS, Kim J, et al. Integrative and comparative genomic analysis of lung squamous cell carcinomas in east asian patients. J Clin Oncol 2014;32:121–8.

46. Cancer Genome Atlas Research N. Comprehensive genomic characterization of squamous cell lung cancers. Nature 2012;489:519–25.

47. Cancer Genome Atlas N. Comprehensive genomic characterization of head and neck squamous cell carcinomas. Nature 2015;517:576–82.

48. Liu X, Zhang M, Ying S, et al. Genetic alterations in esophageal tissues from squamous dysplasia to carcinoma. Gastroenterology 2017;153:166–77.

49. Moody S, Senkin S, Islam SMA, et al. Mutational signatures in esophageal squamous cell carcinoma from eight countries with varying incidence. Nat Genet 2021;53:1553–63.

50. Cheng C, Zhou Y, Li H, et al. Whole-genome sequencing reveals diverse models of structural variations in esophageal squamous cell carcinoma. Am J Hum Genet 2016;98:256–74.

51. Matejcic M, Gunter MJ, Ferrari P. Alcohol metabolism and oesophageal cancer: A systematic review of the evidence. Carcinogenesis 2017;38: 859–72.

52. Lin DC, Dinh HQ, Xie JJ, et al. Identification of distinct mutational patterns and new driver genes in oesophageal squamous cell carcinomas and adenocarcinomas. Gut 2018;67:1769–79.

53. Cancer Genome Atlas Research N. Comprehensive molecular characterization of gastric adenocarcinoma. Nature 2014;513:202–9.

54. Galipeau PC, Prevo LJ, Sanchez CA, et al. Clonal expansion and loss of heterozygosity at chromosomes 9p and 17p in premalignant esophageal (barrett's) tissue. J Natl Cancer Inst 1999;91: 2087–95.

55. Li X, Galipeau PC, Sanchez CA, et al. Single nucleotide polymorphism-based genome-wide chromosome copy change, loss of heterozygosity, and aneuploidy in barrett's esophagus neoplastic progression. Cancer Prev Res (Phila) 2008;1:413–23.

56. Reid BJ, Barrett MT, Galipeau PC, et al. Barrett's esophagus: Ordering the events that lead to cancer. Eur J Cancer Prev 1996;5(Suppl 2):57–65.

57. Wong DJ, Paulson TG, Prevo LJ, et al. P16(ink4a) lesions are common, early abnormalities that undergo clonal expansion in barrett's metaplastic epithelium. Cancer Res 2001;61:8284–9.

58. Yousef F, Cardwell C, Cantwell MM, et al. The incidence of esophageal cancer and high-grade dysplasia in barrett's esophagus: A systematic review and meta-analysis. Am J Epidemiol 2008;168: 237–49.

59. Desai TK, Krishnan K, Samala N, et al. The incidence of oesophageal adenocarcinoma in non-dysplastic barrett's oesophagus: A meta-analysis. Gut 2012;61:970–6.

60. Hvid-Jensen F, Pedersen L, Drewes AM, et al. Incidence of adenocarcinoma among patients with barrett's esophagus. N Engl J Med 2011;365:1375–83.

61. Bhat S, Coleman HG, Yousef F, et al. Risk of malignant progression in barrett's esophagus patients: Results from a large population-based study. J Natl Cancer Inst 2011;103:1049–57.

62. Sikkema M, de Jonge PJ, Steyerberg EW, et al. Risk of esophageal adenocarcinoma and mortality in patients with barrett's esophagus: A systematic review and meta-analysis. Clin Gastroenterol Hepatol 2010; 8:235–44 [quiz e232].

63. Sharma P, Falk GW, Weston AP, et al. Dysplasia and cancer in a large multicenter cohort of patients with barrett's esophagus. Clin Gastroenterol Hepatol 2006;4:566–72.

64. Dulai GS, Shekelle PG, Jensen DM, et al. Dysplasia and risk of further neoplastic progression in a regional veterans administration barrett's cohort. Am J Gastroenterol 2005;100:775–83.

65. Weston AP, Sharma P, Topalovski M, et al. Long-term follow-up of barrett's high-grade dysplasia. Am J Gastroenterol 2000;95:1888–93.

66. Rastogi A, Puli S, El-Serag HB, et al. Incidence of esophageal adenocarcinoma in patients with

barrett's esophagus and high-grade dysplasia: A meta-analysis. Gastrointest Endosc 2008;67:394–8.

67. Schnell TG, Sontag SJ, Chejfec G, et al. Long-term nonsurgical management of barrett's esophagus with high-grade dysplasia. Gastroenterology 2001; 120:1607–19.

68. Galipeau PC, Li X, Blount PL, et al. Nsaids modulate cdkn2a, tp53, and DNA content risk for progression to esophageal adenocarcinoma. PLoS Med 2007;4: e67.

69. Rygiel AM, Milano F, Ten Kate FJ, et al. Gains and amplifications of c-myc, egfr, and 20.Q13 loci in the no dysplasia-dysplasia-adenocarcinoma sequence of barrett's esophagus. Cancer Epidemiol Biomarkers Prev 2008;17:1380–5.

70. Schulmann K, Sterian A, Berki A, et al. Inactivation of p16, runx3, and hpp1 occurs early in barrett's-associated neoplastic progression and predicts progression risk. Oncogene 2005;24:4138–48.

71. Reid BJ, Prevo LJ, Galipeau PC, et al. Predictors of progression in barrett's esophagus ii: Baseline 17p (p53) loss of heterozygosity identifies a patient subset at increased risk for neoplastic progression. Am J Gastroenterol 2001;96:2839–48.

72. Stachler MD, Camarda ND, Deitrick C, et al. Detection of mutations in barrett's esophagus before progression to high-grade dysplasia or adenocarcinoma. Gastroenterology 2018;155:156–67.

73. Maley CC, Galipeau PC, Finley JC, et al. Genetic clonal diversity predicts progression to esophageal adenocarcinoma. Nat Genet 2006;38:468–73.

74. Revilla-Nuin B, Parrilla P, Lozano JJ, et al. Predictive value of micrornas in the progression of barrett esophagus to adenocarcinoma in a long-term follow-up study. Ann Surg 2013;257:886–93.

75. Redston M, Noffsinger A, Kim A, et al. Abnormal tp53 predicts risk of progression in patients with barrett's esophagus regardless of a diagnosis of dysplasia. Gastroenterology 2021;162:468–81.

76. Kastelein F, Spaander MC, Biermann K, et al. Nonsteroidal anti-inflammatory drugs and statins have chemopreventative effects in patients with barrett's esophagus. Gastroenterology 2011;141: 2000–8 [quiz e2013-2004].

77. Murray L, Sedo A, Scott M, et al. Tp53 and progression from barrett's metaplasia to oesophageal adenocarcinoma in a uk population cohort. Gut 2006;55:1390–7.

78. Li M, Anastassiades CP, Joshi B, et al. Affinity peptide for targeted detection of dysplasia in barrett's esophagus. Gastroenterology 2010;139:1472–80.

79. Bird-Lieberman EL, Neves AA, Lao-Sirieix P, et al. Molecular imaging using fluorescent lectins permits rapid endoscopic identification of dysplasia in barrett's esophagus. Nat Med 2012;18:315–21.

80. Krishnadath KK, van Blankenstein M, Tilanus HW. Prognostic value of p53 in barrett's oesophagus. Eur J Gastroenterol Hepatol 1995;7:81–4.

81. Weston AP, Banerjee SK, Sharma P, et al. P53 protein overexpression in low grade dysplasia (lgd) in barrett's esophagus: Immunohistochemical marker predictive of progression. Am J Gastroenterol 2001;96:1355–62.

82. Kadri SR, Lao-Sirieix P, O'Donovan M, et al. Acceptability and accuracy of a non-endoscopic screening test for barrett's oesophagus in primary care: Cohort study. BMJ 2010;341:c4372.

83. Elliott DRF, Walker AW, O'Donovan M, et al. A non-endoscopic device to sample the oesophageal microbiota: A case-control study. Lancet Gastroenterol Hepatol 2017;2:32–42.

84. Munch NS, Fang HY, Ingermann J, et al. High-fat diet accelerates carcinogenesis in a mouse model of barrett's esophagus via interleukin 8 and alterations to the gut microbiome. Gastroenterology 2019;157:492–506 e492.

Esophageal Cancer Staging

Gad Marom, MD, MSc

KEYWORDS

- Esophageal cancer • Staging • Neoadjuvant • Stage groups • TNM

KEY POINTS

- Staging of esophageal cancer is imperative for determining the best treatment modality.
- Staging is determined based on diagnostic modalities, including endoscopic ultrasound, esophagogastroscopy, computed tomography (CT), and PET-CT.
- There are currently three stage groups, clinical, post-neoadjuvant, and pathologic, all based on tumor, node, and metastasis.

BACKGROUND

The management of esophageal cancer is challenging and highly complex. Different treatment modalities have evolved over the years, ranging from endoscopic resection, such as endoscopic mucosal resection (EMR) and endoscopic submucosal dissection (ESD) for superficial (T1a) lesions to up-front esophagectomy and multimodal treatment, including chemotherapy, with or without radiation, and surgery for more advanced disease.

Accurate staging is therefore essential to guide appropriate therapy and to predict prognosis. The staging of esophageal cancer is determined using the tumor, node, and metastasis (TNM) classification. The 8th Edition of the American Joint Committee on Cancer (AJCC)[1,2] is the common staging method for esophageal and esophagogastric junction (EGJ) epithelial cancers. In this edition, a few changes were made, including separate classifications for clinical (cTNM), pathologic (pTNM), and post-neoadjuvant (ypTNM) stage groups. In addition, separate stage groupings for the two major histologic subtypes, adenocarcinoma (AC) and squamous cell carcinoma (SCC), were delineated. Another change that was made was regarding the definition of the location of the epicenter of the tumor which now determines that tumors located more than 2 cm distal to the EGJ are to be considered gastric tumors—not esophageal.

In this article, we discuss the different group stagings which guide the clinician in staging esophageal cancer, and the subsequent best treatment modality for each patient.

STAGING MODALITIES

The staging of esophageal cancer is determined based on information obtained from different modalities. Histopathological evaluation is obtained via biopsy, EMR, or ESD. Staging by imaging is largely obtained from computed tomography (CT) and PET scans. Finally, endoscopic staging is performed via esophagogastroduodenoscopy (EGD) and endoscopic ultrasound (EUS). Other less frequently used image-based modalities include MRI. In select cases, minimally invasive surgical and bronchoscopic staging may be indicated. Overall, no single investigation is sufficient and these investigations complement one another to determine accurate clinical staging.

Clinical Stage Groups

The clinical-stage group refers to staging done pre-neoadjuvant and pre-operatively (**Fig. 1**). The primary esophageal tumor (T) is defined solely by the depth of invasion and further categorized between T1 and T4 (**Fig. 2**). Tis (formerly tumor in situ) is high-grade dysplasia and defined as malignant cells confined by the basement membrane. T1 cancers are tumors that invade the lamina

Department of General Surgery, Hadassah Hebrew University Medical Center and Faculty of Medicine, Hebrew University of Jerusalem, Jerusalem 91120, Israel
E-mail address: gadim@hadassah.org.il

Thorac Surg Clin 32 (2022) 437–445
https://doi.org/10.1016/j.thorsurg.2022.06.006
1547-4127/22/© 2022 Elsevier Inc. All rights reserved.

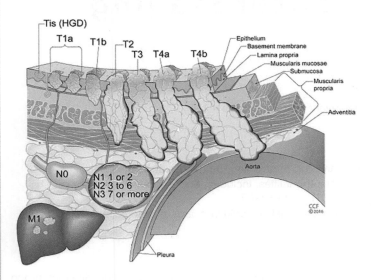

Fig. 1. Clinical TNM (cTNM) stage groups of squamous cell carcinoma (*A*) and adenocarcinoma (*B*). L—lower esophagus, U—upper esophagus, and M- mid-esophagus. (*From* Rice TW, Ishwaran H, Ferguson MK, Blackstone EH, Goldstraw P. Cancer of the Esophagus and Esophagogastric Junction: An Eighth Edition Staging Primer. J Thorac Oncol. 2017;12(1):36-42.)

propria, muscularis mucosae, or submucosa. This wide definition of T1 tumors prompted further subclassification to T1a, which are tumors invading the lamina propria or the muscularis mucosae and T1b which are tumors that invade the submucosa. One of the purposes of this subdivision is the ability to offer patients an organ-preserving treatment modality, such as EMR or ESD for T1a tumors. T2 tumors invade the muscularis propria.

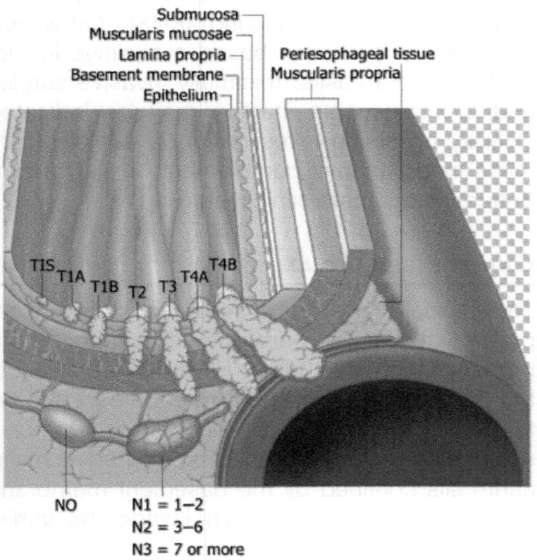

Fig. 2. Locoregional esophageal cancer staging. (*From* DaVee T, Ajani JA, Lee JH. Is endoscopic ultrasound examination necessary in the management of esophageal cancer?. World J Gastroenterol. 2017;23(5):751-762.)

T3 cancers invade beyond the esophageal muscular wall into the surrounding tissue but not into proximal organs. T4 cancers invade adjacent structures; these tumors are also subdivided into T4a which refers to an invasion of resectable structures (pleura, azygos vein, pericardium, diaphragm, and peritoneum), and T4b which refers to the invasion of the tumor to unresectable structures (trachea, aorta, and vertebral body).

Lymph node metastases (N) are a major factor in the staging of esophageal cancer. It can either show no spread to the lymph node (N0) or it can show that the tumor has spread to the regional lymph nodes (N1–3). The number of lymph nodes involved determines the overall N status (**Table 1**). This substaging to N1–3 is important with prognostics as N3 disease has survival similar to metastatic disease. One key term is "regional lymph nodes" and distinguishing it from nonregional lymph nodes is an important factor in the staging of esophageal cancer. The physician should be familiar with the regional lymph node map and be able to use it. Metastatic disease is a disease found outside of the regional lymph nodes.

STAGING MODALITIES

To assess the TNM stage, we use several investigational modalities to help us. These include EGD, EUS, CT, PET-CT, and others.

ESOPHAGOGASTRODUODENOSCOPY

EGD is a very important investigational tool used to diagnose esophageal cancer, and its value cannot be underestimated. By providing direct visualization of the mucosa, it allows for the

Table 1
Cancer staging categories for cancer of the esophagus and esophago–gastric junction

T category

TX	Tumor cannot be assessed
T0	No evidence of primary tumor
Tis	High-grade dysplasia, defined as malignant cells confined by the basement membrane
T1	Tumor invades the lamina propria, muscularis mucosa, or submucosa
T1a[a]	Tumor invades the lamina propria or muscularis mucosa
T1b[a]	Tumor invades the submucosa
T2	Tumor invades the muscularis propria
T3	Tumor invades adventitia
T4	Tumor invades adjacent structures
T4a[a]	Tumor invades the pleura, azygos vein, diaphragm, pericardium, or peritoneum
T4b[a]	Tumor invades other adjacent structures, such as trachea, vertebral body, or aorta

N category

NX	Regional lymph nodes cannot be assessed
N0	No regional lymph node metastasis
N1	Metastasis in 1–2 regional lymph nodes
N2	Metastasis in 3–6 regional lymph nodes
N3	Metastasis in 7 or more regional lymph nodes

M category

M0	No distant metastasis
M1	Distant metastasis

Adenocarcinoma G Category

GX	Differentiation cannot be assessed
G1	Well differentiated. >95% of tumor is composed of well-formed glands
G2	Moderately differentiated. 50% to 95% of tumor shows gland formation
G3[b]	Poorly differentiated. Tumors composed of nests and sheets of cells with <50% of tumor demonstrating glandular formation.

Squamous cell carcinoma G category

GX	Differentiation cannot be assessed
G1	Well-differentiated. Prominent keratinization with pearl formation and a minor component of nonkeratinizing basal-like cells. Tumor cells are arranged in sheets, and mitotic counts are low.
G2	Moderately differentiated. Variable histologic features, ranging from parakeratotic to poorly keratinizing lesions. Generally, pearl formation is absent.
G3[c]	Poorly differentiated. Consists predominantly of basal-like cells forming large and small nests with frequent central necrosis. The nests consist of sheets or pavement-like arrangements of tumor cells, and occasionally are punctuated by small numbers of parakeratotic or keratinizing cells.

Squamous cell carcinoma L category[d]

LX	Location unknown
Upper	Cervical esophagus to lower border of azygos vein
Middle	Lower border of azygos vein to lower border of inferior pulmonary vein
Lower	Lower border of inferior pulmonary vein to stomach, including esophagogastric junction

[a] Subcategories.
[b] If further testing of "undifferentiated" cancers reveals a glandular component, categorize as adenocarcinoma G3.
[c] If further testing of "undifferentiated" cancers reveals a squamous cell component, or if after further testing they remain undifferentiated, categorize as squamous cell carcinoma G3.
[d] Location is defined by epicenter of esophageal tumor.

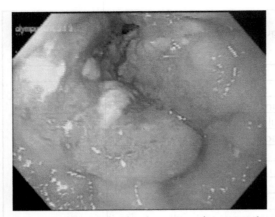

Fig. 3. Esophagogastroduodenoscopy demonstrating long circular irregular lesion. Final pathology showed moderately to poorly differentiated adenocarcinoma of gastroesophageal junction.

assessment of lesions for accurate localization (proximal, mid, or distal esophagus), evaluating the involvement of the esophago-gastric junction, and possible invasion into the stomach (**Fig. 3**). It also provides the opportunity to measure the length of the tumor and the degree of its circumference in the esophageal lumen. Additionally, EGD can evaluate for intramural metastases, especially in cases of SCC, and allows for the acquisition of biopsies which is crucial for diagnosis.

ENDOSCOPIC ULTRASOUND

EUS provides detailed information on the esophageal wall and is important for T-staging of esophageal cancer. In addition, it can also provide important information on pathologically appearing lymph nodes in the surgical field. EUS can evaluate the full thickness of the esophageal wall by visualizing its alternating hypo- and hyperechoic layers that represent the esophageal wall layers (**Fig. 4**). There is no use for trans-thoracic ultrasound in the staging of esophageal cancer.

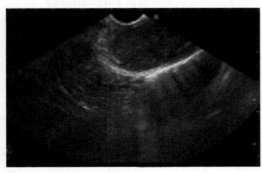

Fig. 4. Endoscopic ultrasound demonstrating esophageal cancer involving all esophageal layers. Final pathology showed T4N2M0.

For many years, EUS evaluation of esophageal cancer did not differentiate esophageal adenocarcinoma (EAC) from esophageal squamous cell carcinoma (ESCC). However, over the last few years, studies began to emerge suggesting there might be a difference when evaluating ESCC and EAC. Yang and colleagues[3] evaluated 1434 patients with ESCC using EUS pre-operatively and compared the results to the pathologic reports and found the sensitivity and accuracy of EUS for Tis, T1a, T1b, T2, T3, and T4a categories were 15.8% and 98.8%, 16.3% and 95.7%, 33.1% and 89.3%, 56.8% and 65.0%, 65.8%, and 70.0%, and 27.3% and 97.5%, respectively. In addition, they found that 58.2% were correctly classified by EUS, with 17.9% being over-staged and 23.9% being understaged when compared with pathologic staging post-op. They thereby concluded that EUS should be used with caution for discriminating between Tis, T1a, and T1b disease, as well as T4 disease. However, in their meta-analysis, Lin-na Luo and colleagues[4] found T1 stage sensitivity of 77% and when substaging to T1a and T1b it was 83% and 84%, respectively. In addition, they demonstrated 84% sensitivity for the T4 stage.

EUS staging of AC has been investigated by Klamt and colleagues,[5] who found that for T1, sensitivity was 64.7%, with an accuracy of 89.6%. For T2, sensitivity was 35.7%, with an accuracy of 87.1%. For T3, sensitivity was 82.5%, with an accuracy of 87%, and for T4, sensitivity was 38.6% and 94%, respectively with an accuracy of 66.4%.

Furthermore, via EUS, a physician can obtain tissue from peri-esophageal lymph nodes for histopathologic assessment. Endoscopic ultrasonography is used to evaluate the nodal size, shape, border, and internal echo characteristics in regional lymph node assessment. Lymph nodes that are larger than 1 cm, and have a round shape, sharp edges, or hypoechoic appearance are considered suspect and can be sampled via fine-needle aspiration (FNA). EUS-FNA further refines clinical staging by adding tissue sampling to EUS findings. This is important for N-stage assessment and is complementary to other modalities of investigations, such as CT or PET-CT that we discuss next.

Because of the large size of the scope, staging esophageal cancer in patients with a malignant stenotic esophagus by EUS is an issue. Molina and colleagues[6] enrolled 150 patients with high-grade malignant stenosis of the esophagus for esophageal dilation. They concluded that high-grade esophageal strictures preventing complete EUS are associated with advanced-stage disease

(>T3) and therefore further T-staging of such tumors is of little benefit. Therefore, the role of preoperative EUS in the setting of malignant esophageal stenosis is mainly to obtain EUS-guided FNA from proximal peri-esophageal lymph nodes which may affect treatment decisions, for example, a larger radiation field may be needed if nodes are found to be positive.

ENDOSCOPIC MUCOSAL RESECTION

Given the relatively low accuracy of EUS for early-stage cancers, the pathologic evaluation of biopsies obtained during EGD procedures, such as EMR and endoscopic submucosal dissection ESD, for patients with cT1N0M0 and cT2N0M0 is particularly important. First, the specimen allows for a pathologic diagnosis but, more importantly, will help confirm T1a from T1b pathologically. Second, a pathologic report of the grade of the tumor can help in prognostication and treatment planning. Grade 3 tumors, poorly differentiated and signet-ring cell morphology, are associated with a poorer outcome and may lead clinicians to decide on a more aggressive treatment or resection.[7]

COMPUTED TOMOGRAPHY AND PET

The role of CT scan in staging esophageal cancer is somewhat limited. First, it has a limited role in determining the T stage. This is primarily because CT cannot distinguish the esophageal wall layers. However, it can help determine if the tumor is T4. When the tumor is seen infiltrating the fat tissue on a CT scan and involving other structures, it can help classify it as T4. Second, CT can assist in determining the N stage. It can show enlarged lymph nodes in close proximity to the tumor;

however, this is not specific and can only guide an endoscopist when performing EUS in searching for suspected lymph nodes to sample via FNA. Last, CT can show metastases and help determine the M stage. When performing CT with IV contrast, it can help demonstrate metastases in areas that cannot be otherwise demonstrated by EGD or EUS.

PET scan is overall superior to CT for staging. It uses a radiolabeled substance, in this case, [18]fluorodeoxyglucose (FDG), to demonstrate tissue with high glucose metabolism with the expectation that cancer cells will demonstrate higher glucose metabolism compared with the rest of the body. Usually, PET scans are overlayed onto a noncontrast CT scan and the combination of functional data by PET and structural data by CT allows for the best identification of nodal and distant metastases.

FDG-PET has a key role in detecting lymph node involvement and determining the N stage (**Fig. 5**). Lymph nodes that are not adjacent to the tumor are better seen by FDG-PET than CT; however, when these are in close proximity to the tumor itself, they can appear to be part of the tumor itself, thereby decreasing the sensitivity in N staging. PET can also demonstrate metastases better than CT. ACOSOG z0060 is a study[8] that included 189 patients with surgically resectable esophageal cancer. Patients with preoperative evaluation based on CT, MRI, and bone scans that were staged as T1-3, N0-1, and M0-1a underwent additional PET scans. This study showed metastases in 4.8% of the patients proven by biopsy, precluding them from surgery. In addition, they found that 9.5% had suspected metastases, which were not proven by biopsy, but resulted in the cancellation of surgery based on these imaging findings. This

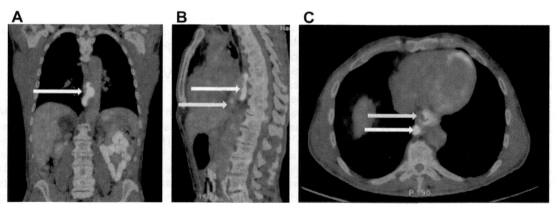

Fig. 5. PET-CT fused image of esophageal cancer with para-esophageal lymph nodes involvement. A- coronal view, B- sagittal view, and C- axial view. Yellow arrow—esophageal tumor. White arrow—para-esophageal lymph nodes. This patient had ypT3N3M0.

study set the ground for further studies looking into a better way to assess occult metastases. Indeed, occult lymph node metastases are present in 22% to 43% of patients with T1-T2 N0 in the pretreatment evaluation.[9,10]

OTHER CLINICAL STAGING MODALITIES
MRI

MRI has several advantages including a lack of ionizing radiation and contrast agents. It is currently not part of the staging imaging modalities used in esophageal cancer mainly due to wide variability in its performance in several studies. In recent years, however, many studies have been performed seeking to improve its performance. A recent systematic review and meta-analysis by Lee and colleagues,[11] demonstrated accuracy for stage T0 versus stage T1 or higher had a sensitivity of 92% and a specificity of 67%. Pooled accuracy for stage T2 or lower versus stage T3 or higher had a sensitivity of 86% and a specificity of 86%. Pooled accuracy for stage N0 versus stage N1 or higher had a sensitivity of 71% and a specificity of 72%. In Another study by Schmidlin and colleagues,[12] looked at the application of MRI in evaluating the T stage via advanced MR technology and demonstrated good staging performance post neoadjuvant treatment. This study also showed that PET-MR correlates with TNM staging in patients with esophageal carcinoma but does not show an advantage. Further technological advancements might lead MRI to become an integral part of esophageal cancer staging.

Minimally Invasive Surgical Staging

Minimally invasive surgical staging, such as laparoscopy, mediastinoscopy, and/or thoracoscopy, although not widely accepted as part of the routine staging modalities, can be performed in select cases for optimal clinical staging. This is usually done either to assess for N stage or M stage via sampling of lymph nodes and cytology. Mehta and colleagues[13] reported an added benefit for staging laparoscopy when evaluating for N1 disease and detection of distant metastases compared with EUS. The authors even suggest using intraoperative ultrasonography of the liver to assess for occult lesions. In their longitudinal study of over 7 years, De Graaf and colleagues[14] have evaluated the role of staging laparoscopy in determining the resectability of esophagogastric cancers. In 416 patients with esophageal cancers deemed to be resectable by preoperative CT and/or EUS, they found that staging laparoscopy changed the management in 84 (20.2%) patients. However, 17 patients had locally advanced

disease, 4 had extensive lymph node involvement, and 63 had distant metastases in the liver and peritoneum. Minimally invasive staging is most useful in EAC of the distal esophagus and esophagogastric junction. Staging laparoscopy was also recommended by Fountoulakis and colleagues,[15] including peritoneal washing and cytology to patients with locally advanced (T3 or T4) AC of the distal esophagus EGJ to prevent major surgery.

Bronchoscopy

Bronchoscopy is a clinical adjunct that can help establish a T4b stage. Several studies have tried to address the use of bronchoscopy in the staging of esophageal cancer. Kunal and colleagues[13] recommend that bronchoscopy should be performed in patients with proximal or mid-esophageal lesions, at or above the carina level to assess for airway involvement. They mention that bronchoscopy identified airway invasion in 6.5% of otherwise potentially operable patients. Allum and colleagues.[16] suggested that bronchoscopy should be used in patients where imaging has raised suspicion but not certainty of invasion of the airway. On bronchoscopy, tracheobronchial involvement includes a widened carina, external compression, tumor infiltration, and fistula. The last two signs contraindicate resection and radiation. In addition, the endoscopist should perform brush cytology and biopsy of suspicious areas.

Barium Contrast Study

There is limited use of barium contrast study in the staging of esophageal cancer. Although it can give some guidance to the endoscopist and may be suggest fistula to the airways, the availability of more sophisticated imaging and investigation modalities has made it nonessential.

Laboratory Studies

Blood work, including tumor markers, has shown no use in the staging of esophageal cancer.

POST-NEOADJUVANT THERAPY STAGE GROUPS

In recent years, it has become clear that cTNM staging carries less accurate prognostic information than pTNM. The Worldwide Esophageal Cancer Collaboration,[17] in an attempt to solve this, evaluated survival rates among 22,123 patients who had cTNM staging. They found that patients with early cancers had worse survival and those with advanced cancers had better survival than expected from equivalent pathologic staging based on previous staging manuals.[18,19] This led them to

	N0M0	N1M0	N2M0	N3M0	Any N M1
T0	I	IIIA	IIIB	IVA	IVB
Tis	I	IIIA	IIIB	IVA	IVB
T1	I	IIIA	IIIB	IVA	IVB
T2	I	IIIA	IIIB	IVA	IVB
T3	II	IIIB	IIIB	IVA	IVB
T4a	IIIB	IVA	IVA	IVA	IVB
t4b	IVA	IVA	IVA	IVA	IVB

Fig. 6. Post-neoadjuvant pathologic stage groups (ypTNM): adenocarcinoma and squamous cell carcinoma. (*Adapted from* Rice TW, Ishwaran H, Ferguson MK, Blackstone EH, Goldstraw P. Cancer of the Esophagus and Esophagogastric Junction: An Eighth Edition Staging Primer. J Thorac Oncol. 2017;12(1):36-42.)

the conclusion that clinical categories did not share the same prognostic implications as pathologic categories after esophagectomy alone. In an effort to understand what made the difference between the expected survival based on pTNM that was based, at that time, on esophagectomy alone and cTNM, they looked into a subgroup of patients from that cohort of 7773 who had received neoadjuvant treatment. The majority had chemoradiotherapy, 20% had chemotherapy, and 10% of the SCC esophageal cancer patients had radiotherapy alone.[20] Fifteen percent of patients received postoperative adjuvant therapy. They found that the survival of patients who were node-negative post-neoadjuvant therapy (ypN0) was *worse* than patients who were equivalently pathologically categorized post-esophagectomy alone (pN0), meaning that sterilization of metastatic regional lymph nodes by neoadjuvant therapy does not equate with cure. In addition, the prognosis of patients with node-positive disease post-neoadjuvant therapy (ypN+) was either worse or no better than equivalent patients post-esophagectomy alone (pN+).

The prefix y is used to denote the stage after neoadjuvant therapy. There is currently no yc, meaning post-therapy clinical-stage group, for esophageal cancer. As cTNM staging is based mostly on imaging, the sensitivity and specificity of restaging by FDG-PET/CT and/or EUS is not high enough to perform ycTNM staging to facilitate decision-making and may be spare patients' unnecessary surgery. Nonoperative treatment might have a role in the post-neoadjuvant setting if a staging method would be found for yc. A promising modality might be MRI.[21] There are few studies currently in progress with exciting results to come.[22,23]

Pathologic staging of the tumor in the setting of post-neoadjuvant treatment has several limitations and implications. It is noted that a wide range of morphologic changes occurs in the esophagus following neoadjuvant therapy. Grossly, the tumor beds can present as a scar, ulcer, erythema mucosal irregularity, or obvious residual tumor. Histopathologically, neoadjuvant treatment can induce tumor regression and thus fibrosis. This makes a distinction between the different layers of the esophageal wall in the area of the tumor extremely difficult, if not impossible. Obliteration of these anatomic landmarks makes assigning a reliable ypT stage very challenging. In this regard, combining T stages (eg, ypT0–2 in N0 or N1cases, ypT0–3 in N2 cases, and ypT1–4 in N3 cases) and the stage groupings in AJCC8 significantly reduces the burden for pathologists (**Fig. 6**). In addition, N staging post-neoadjuvant treatment is challenging as well, after neoadjuvant therapy,

A

			N0M0		N1M0	N2M0	N3M0	Any N M1
			L	U/M				
Tis		0						
T1a	G1		IA		IIB	IIIA	IVA	IVB
	G2/3		IB					
T1b	G1-3		IB		IIB	IIIA	IVA	IVB
T2	G1		IB		IIIA	IIIB	IVA	IVB
	G2/3		IIA					
T3	G1		IIA		IIIB	IIIB	IVA	IVB
	G2/3		IIA	IIB				
T4a			IIIB		IIIB	IVA	IVA	IVB
t4b			IVA		IVA	IVA	IVA	IVB

B

			N0M0	N1M0	N2M0	N3M0	Any N M1
Tis		0					
T1a	G1		IA	IIB	IIIA	IVA	IVB
	G2		IB				
	G3		IC				
T1b	G1		IB	IIB	IIIA	IVA	IVB
	G2						
	G3		IC				
T2	G1		IC	IIIA	IIIB	IVA	IVB
	G2						
	G3		IIA				
T3			IIB	IIIB	IIIB	IVA	IVB
T4a			IIIB	IIIB	IVA	IVA	IVB
t4b			IVA	IVA	IVA	IVA	IVB

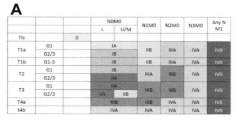

Fig. 7. Pathologic TNM (pTNM) stage groups of squamous cell carcinoma (*A*) and adenocarcinoma (*B*). L- lower esophagus, U- upper esophagus, and M- mid-esophagus. (*Adapted from* Rice TW, Ishwaran H, Ferguson MK, Blackstone EH, Goldstraw P. Cancer of the Esophagus and Esophagogastric Junction: An Eighth Edition Staging Primer. J Thorac Oncol. 2017;12(1):36-42.)

not only does the frequency of lymph node metastases decrease, but there is also a change in the distribution of lymph node metastases. In patients receiving neoadjuvant therapy, lymph nodes can atrophy and be difficult to recognize macroscopically.[24-26]

PATHOLOGIC STAGE GROUPS

As neoadjuvant therapy replaces esophagectomy alone, pathologic staging, through microscopic examination of resected specimens, remains relevant mostly in early-stage cancers and losing its relevance for advanced-stage cancer.

Pathologic stage groups are the only staging groups to include tumor grade (G). Tumor grade is separate for EAC and ESCC (**Fig. 7**). For EAC, GX means that differentiation cannot be assessed. G1 is well differentiated, with greater than 95% of the tumor composed of well-formed glands. G2 is moderately differentiated, with 50%–95% of the tumor showing gland formation. G3 is poorly differentiated, with tumors composed of nests and sheets of cells with less than 50% of the tumor demonstrating glandular formation.

For ESCC, GX means that cellular differentiation cannot be assessed, G1 is well-differentiated, with prominent keratinization with pearl formation and a minor component of nonkeratinizing basal-like cells, tumor cells arranged in sheets, and mitotic counts low. G2 is moderately differentiated, with variable histologic features ranging from parakeratotic to poorly keratinizing lesions and pearl formation generally absent. G3 is poorly differentiated, consisting predominantly of basal-like cells forming large and small nests with frequent central necrosis and with the nests consisting of sheets or pavement-like arrangements of tumor cells that are occasionally punctuated by small numbers of parakeratotic or keratinizing cells.

Pathologic staging could, in theory, provide personalized post-esophagectomy cancer care and has the potential to facilitate decision-making. However, the use of this information to direct postoperative adjuvant therapy is waning.[1,24,26]

DISCLOSURE

The author has nothing to disclose.

ACKNOWLEGEMENTS

Ronit Brodie, MPAS for assistance in manuscript preparation. Department of General Surgery Hadassah-Hebrew University Medical Center, Jerusalem, Israel.

REFERENCES

1. Amin MB, Edge S, Greene F, et al. AJCC cancer staging Manual. 8th edition. New York, (NY): Springer; 2017.
2. Amin MB, Greene F, Edge SB, et al. The Eighth Edition AJCC Cancer Staging Manual: Continuing to build a bridge from a population-based to a more "personalized" approach to cancer staging. CA Cancer J Clin 2017;67(2):93–9.
3. Yang J, Luo G, Liang RB, et al. Efficacy of Endoscopic Ultrasonography for Determining Clinical T Category for Esophageal Squamous Cell Carcinoma: Data From 1434 Surgical Cases. Ann Surg Oncol 2018;25(7):2075–82.
4. Luo LN, He L, Gao XY, et al. Endoscopic Ultrasound for Preoperative Esophageal Squamous Cell Carcinoma: a Meta-Analysis. PLoS One 2016;11(7): e0158373.
5. Klamt AL, Neyeloff J, Santos LM, et al. Echoendoscopy in Preoperative Evaluation of Esophageal Adenocarcinoma and Gastroesophageal Junction: Systematic Review and Meta-analysis. Ultrasound Med Biol 2021;47(7):1657–69.
6. Molina JC, Goudie E, Pollock C, et al. Balloon Dilation for Endosonographic Staging in Esophageal Cancer: A Phase 1 Clinical Trial. Ann Thorac Surg 2021;111(4):1150–5.
7. Peng Z, Li F, Cheng Z, et al. Comparative analysis of clinical, treatment, and survival characteristics of signet ring cell and adenocarcinoma of esophagus. J Gastrointest Oncol 2021;12(4):1643–60.
8. Meyers BF, Downey R, Decker PA, et al, American College of Surgeons Oncology Group. Z0060. The utility of positron emission tomography in staging of potentially operable carcinoma of the thoracic esophagus: results of the American College of Surgeons Oncology Group Z0060 trial. J Thorac Cardiovasc Surg 2007;133(3):738–45.
9. Shin S, Kim H, Choi YS, et al. Clinical stage T1-T2N0M0 oesophageal cancer: accuracy of clinical staging and predictive factors for lymph node metastasis. Eur J Cardiothorac Surg 2014;46(2):274–9.
10. Yun JK, Kim H, Park SI, et al. Risk prediction of occult lymph node metastasis in patients with clinical T1 through T2 N0 esophageal squamous cell carcinoma. J Thorac Cardiovasc Surg 2022;164(1): 265-275.e5.
11. Lee SL, Yadav P, Starekova J, et al. Diagnostic Performance of MRI for Esophageal Carcinoma: A Systematic Review and Meta-Analysis. Radiology 2021; 299(3):583–94.
12. Schmidlin EJ, Gill RR. New frontiers in esophageal radiology. Ann translational Med 2021;9(10):904.
13. Mehta K, Bianco V, Awais O, et al. Minimally invasive staging of esophageal cancer. Ann Cardiothorac Surg 2017;6(2):110–8.

14. de Graaf GW, Ayantunde AA, Parsons SL, et al. The role of staging laparoscopy in oesophago-gastric cancers. Eur J Surg Oncol 2007;33(8): 988–92.

15. Fountoulakis A, Souglakos J, Vini L, et al. Consensus statement of the Hellenic and Cypriot Oesophageal Cancer Study Group on the diagnosis, staging and management of oesophageal cancer. Updates Surg 2019;71(4):599–624.

16. Allum WH, Griffin SM, Watson A, et al. Guidelines for the management of oesophageal and gastric cancer. Gut 2002;50(Suppl 5):v1–23.

17. Rice TW, Apperson-Hansen C, DiPaola LM, et al. Worldwide Esophageal Cancer Collaboration: clinical staging data. Dis esophagus : official J Int Soc Dis Esophagus 2016;29(7):707–14.

18. Rice TW, Rusch VW, Apperson-Hansen C, et al. Worldwide esophageal cancer collaboration. Dis esophagus : official J Int Soc Dis Esophagus 2009; 22(1):1–8.

19. Rice TW, Rusch VW, Ishwaran H, et al. Cancer of the esophagus and esophagogastric junction: data-driven staging for the seventh edition of the American Joint Committee on Cancer/International Union Against Cancer Cancer Staging Manuals. Cancer 2010;116(16):3763–73.

20. Rice TW, Lerut TE, Orringer MB, et al. Worldwide Esophageal Cancer Collaboration: neoadjuvant pathologic staging data. Dis esophagus : official J Int Soc Dis Esophagus 2016;29(7):715–23.

21. Byrd DR, Brierley JD, Baker TP, et al. Current and future cancer staging after neoadjuvant treatment for solid tumors. CA Cancer J Clin 2021;71(2):140–8.

22. Borggreve AS, Mook S, Verheij M, et al. Preoperative image-guided identification of response to neoadjuvant chemoradiotherapy in esophageal cancer (PRIDE): a multicenter observational study. BMC cancer 2018;18(1):1006.

23. Noordman BJ, Wijnhoven BPL, Lagarde SM, et al. Neoadjuvant chemoradiotherapy plus surgery versus active surveillance for oesophageal cancer: a stepped-wedge cluster randomised trial. BMC cancer 2018;18(1):142.

24. Rice TW, Patil DT, Blackstone EH. 8th edition AJCC/UICC staging of cancers of the esophagus and esophagogastric junction: application to clinical practice. Ann Cardiothorac Surg 2017;6(2):119–30.

25. Klevebro F, Tsekrekos A, Low D, et al. Relevant issues in tumor regression grading of histopathological response to neoadjuvant treatment in adenocarcinomas of the esophagus and gastroesophageal junction. Dis esophagus : official J Int Soc Dis Esophagus 2020;33(6).

26. Zhang X, Jain D. Updates in staging and pathologic evaluation of esophageal carcinoma following neoadjuvant therapy. Ann N Y Acad Sci 2020;1482(1): 163–76.

Neoadjuvant Therapy in Esophageal Cancer

Shirley Lewis, MD, DNB[a,b,c], Jelena Lukovic, MD, MPH[b,*]

KEYWORDS

• Esophageal cancer • Surgery • Neoadjuvant • Radiation • Chemotherapy • Chemoradiation

KEY POINTS

• Surgery alone is associated with high local and distant recurrence in localized esophageal cancer ($\geq$T2 or N positive, M0).
• Neoadjuvant therapies have the potential to improve outcomes by downsizing the primary tumor and reducing the incidence of distant metastases.
• Neoadjuvant concurrent chemotherapy and radiotherapy is associated with a 10-year survival advantage of approximately 13% compared with surgery alone.
• Neoadjuvant chemotherapy improves survival compared to surgery alone but lacks superiority over neoadjuvant chemoradiation.

INTRODUCTION

Esophageal cancer is the 6th leading cause of cancer-related mortality worldwide with a five-year overall survival of less than 25%.[1,2] Patients rarely present at an early stage as symptoms do not usually arise until the tumor becomes large enough to cause obstruction or invasion of adjacent structures.[3]

Early-stage tumors may be treated with surgery alone, achieving a five-year survival of 60–85%.[4,5] Surgery alone for locally advanced disease, however, is associated with a median survival of 12 to 18 months and five-year survival of 15–39%.[6–8] Both local and systemic recurrence is common when surgical resection is performed as the sole treatment, reported in 35–50% of patients.[9] Because of the low cure rates associated with the treatment of esophageal cancer by surgery alone, multi-modality therapy has been proposed to improve survival outcome.

DISCUSSION
Neoadjuvant Strategy: Multimodality Approach

Neoadjuvant strategies including chemotherapy, radiation therapy, and concurrent chemotherapy and radiotherapy (chemoradiation–CRT) have been explored as potential ways to improve outcomes in esophageal cancer. The potential advantages of multi-modality therapy include[10]

• Early treatment of micrometastases,
• Downsizing of the primary tumor and improved locoregional control,
• Sterilizing resection margins resulting in enhanced complete (R0) resection.

Numerous randomized trials have demonstrated a survival benefit with multi-modality therapy compared with surgery alone although the optimal strategy is yet to be determined.[11,12] Patients with $\geq$cT2 and/or node-positive and M0 should be

a Radiation Medicine Program, Princess Margaret Cancer Centre, University Health Network, Toronto, Canada;
b Department of Radiation Oncology, University of Toronto, Toronto, Canada; c Department of Radiotherapy and Oncology, Manipal Comprehensive Cancer Care Centre, Kasturba Medical College, Manipal Academy of Higher Education, Manipal, India
* Corresponding author. 6-206, 700 University Avenue, Toronto, ON, M5G 1Z5, Canada
E-mail address: Jelena.lukovic@rmp.uhn.ca

Thorac Surg Clin 32 (2022) 447–456
https://doi.org/10.1016/j.thorsurg.2022.06.003
1547-4127/22/© 2022 Elsevier Inc. All rights reserved.

considered for multimodality therapy after discussion with a multidisciplinary team.[10]

Neoadjuvant radiotherapy

Preoperative radiation therapy can reduce tumor bulk by facilitating surgery and does not appear to increase perioperative morbidity nor mortality.[13] A trial conducted by the European Organization for Research and Treatment of Cancer (EORTC) compared patients receiving preoperative radiotherapy (33 Gy) with immediate surgery.[14] There were no significant differences in resectability or operative mortality. Locoregional failure was significantly decreased in the radiotherapy arm (67% vs 46%) although there was no survival benefit (10% vs 9% at 5 years).[14] A subsequent randomized trial of 206 patients compared preoperative radiotherapy (40 Gy) versus surgery alone. There was no significant difference in resectability, but local failure was reduced in the radiotherapy arm (41% vs 34%). Finally, a Norwegian trial of 186 patients with squamous cell carcinoma of the esophagus randomized patients into 4 groups: preoperative chemotherapy, preoperative radiotherapy, preoperative chemoradiation, and surgery alone.[15] This trial found significantly improved three-year overall survival in the treatment groups receiving radiotherapy. A metanalysis by Kumar and colleagues,[16] demonstrated a survival benefit for neoadjuvant radiotherapy followed by surgery versus surgery alone at three years. The available data suggest that preoperative radiotherapy for esophageal cancer results in improved local control but does not necessarily improve survival.

Neoadjuvant chemotherapy

The potential benefits of preoperative chemotherapy include downsizing to facilitate surgical resection, improvement of local control, and eradication of micrometastases. RTOG 8911 randomized 440 patients to surgery alone versus neoadjuvant chemotherapy (5-fluorouracil continuous infusion 1000 mg/m^2 and cisplatin 100 mg/m^2 x 3 cycles) followed by surgery.[17] Patients received 2 additional cycles of chemotherapy postoperatively. There was no significant difference in perioperative morbidity and mortality between the 2 groups. At a median follow-up of 55 months, there was no difference in one-year survival (59% vs 60%), two-year survival (35% vs 37%), or local or distant recurrence rates. There was no difference in the R0 resection rate (62 vs 59%) but the rate of positive resection margins was lower with neoadjuvant chemotherapy (4% vs 15%). On long-term follow-up, survival was improved in the subgroup of patients for whom an R0 resection was achieved (32% vs 5%).[18]

An Italian trial randomized patients to surgery alone versus preoperative chemotherapy (2 or 3 cycles of cisplatin (100 mg/m2 on Day 1) and 5-fluorouracil (1000 mg/m2 per day continuous infusion on Days 1–5) followed by surgery.[19] There was no difference in complete resection rates (74% vs 79%) or treatment-related mortality (4% in each arm). Responders to chemotherapy had significantly better 3/5-year and 5-year survival compared with nonresponders (74%/60% vs 24%/12%) and patients undergoing surgery alone (46%/26%).

A trial conducted by England Medical Research Council (MRC) similarly studied the use of preoperative chemotherapy versus surgery alone.[20] The rate of microscopically complete resection was significantly higher for patients undergoing preoperative chemotherapy (60% vs 54%). Postoperative complication rates were similar in both groups (41% vs 42%). Patients undergoing preoperative chemotherapy achieved significantly improved median survival (17 vs 13 months) and two-year survival (43% vs 34%) compared to surgery alone. The results of this trial are potentially confounded by the fact that preoperative radiotherapy was allowed at the discretion of the treating physician, irrespective of randomization. Long-term results demonstrated improved 5-year survival for patients receiving neoadjuvant chemotherapy (23% vs 17%); the survival benefit was seen in both histologies (adenocarcinoma: 23% vs 18%; squamous cell carcinoma: 26% vs 17%).[21] There was no difference in distant metastases rates and progression was similar between the arms.

Several metanalyses have compared neoadjuvant chemotherapy followed by surgery with surgery alone and demonstrate mixed results with some authors reporting a survival advantage and other finding no benefit.[22–25]

Neoadjuvant chemoradiation

Chemotherapy has been combined with radiotherapy to improve resectability, local control, and survival. Most reports of "trimodality therapy" describe concurrent neoadjuvant chemoradiotherapy using combinations of cisplatin and 5-fluorouracil while administering 30 Gy to 45 Gy of radiation. Some studies have used additional postoperative chemotherapy. This approach results in a pathologic complete response (pCR) rate of 15% to 30% of patients with adenocarcinoma histology and up to 50% of patients with squamous cell carcinoma histology.[12,26] The results appear comparable at most experienced centers (**Table 1**). Three major randomized trials have shown a survival benefit with neoadjuvant chemoradiation with surgery over surgery alone.

Table 1
Clinical trials of neoadjuvant chemoradiotherapy followed by surgery vs surgery alone in resectable esophageal cancer

Author and year	Patient Number	Histology	Radiation (Gy) and Chemotherapy Regimen	R0 Rates (%)	pCR (%)	Survival (%)	Postoperative Mortality (%)
Walsh et al,[27] 1996	nCRT-S: 58 S: 55	Adenocarcinoma	RT: 40/15 CT: 2 cycles CF	NA	25 NA	3y: 32 3y: 6	3 2
Tepper et al,[28] 2008	nCRT-S: 30 S: 26	Adenocarcinoma and squamous	RT: 50.4/28 CT: 2 cycles CF	NA	40 NA	5y: 39 5y: 16	0 4.2
Mariette et al,[29] FFCD 9901, 2014	nCRT-S: 98 S: 97	Adenocarcinoma and squamous	RT: 45/25 CT: 2 cycles CF	93.8 92.1	NA	5y: 41.1 5y: 33.8	11.1 3.4
CROSS, VanHagen et al,[12,30] 2012	nCRT-S: 178 S: 188	Adenocarcinoma and squamous	RT: 41.4/23 CT: 5 weekly TC	92 69	29 NA	5y: 47 5y: 34	4 4
NEOCRTEC[26]	nCRT-S: 224 S: 227	Squamous	RT: 40/20 CT: 2 cycles Cisplatin Vinorelbine	98.4 91.2	43.2 NA	5y: 59.9 5y: 49.1	2.2 0.4

CALGB 9781 randomized patients to neoadjuvant chemoradiation followed by surgery versus surgery alone but was closed due to poor accrual (56 patients accrued out of a planned 475).[28] At a follow-up of six years, the intention to treat analysis showed a median survival of 4.5 years vs 1.8 years and 5-year overall survival of 39% vs 16% favoring trimodality therapy. A larger multi-institutional randomized controlled Dutch trial (CROSS) randomized 368 patients to surgery alone or trimodality therapy with preoperative chemoradiotherapy (41.4 Gy with weekly carboplatin and paclitaxel).[12,30] An R0 resection was achieved in 92% of patients receiving neoadjuvant chemoradiotherapy versus 69% of patients undergoing surgery alone. An overall pCR rate of 29% was observed: 23% among patients with adenocarcinoma and 49% among patients with squamous cell carcinoma. There were no significant differences in postoperative complications or 30-day mortality. The long-term results demonstrated median overall survival for patients who received neoadjuvant chemoradiotherapy was 49 months compared with 24 months for patients undergoing surgery alone (P = 0.003).[12] The benefit was noted in both adenocarcinoma and squamous cell carcinoma with median overall survival, respectively, of 43 months and 82 months.[12] Eyck and colleagues,[31] confirmed a survival benefit with neoadjuvant chemoradiotherapy over surgery alone with absolute 10-year overall survival benefit of 13% (38% vs 25%). A phase III clinical trial (NEO-CRTEC5010) compared neoadjuvant chemoradiotherapy (40 Gy with concurrent cisplatin and vinorelbine) followed by surgery versus surgery alone for patients with resectable squamous cell carcinoma of the thoracic esophagus.[26] The pCR rate was 43% in chemoradiotherapy arm. Neoadjuvant chemoradiotherapy was additionally associated with a higher R0 resection rate (98% vs 91%) and median overall survival (100 vs 66 months). There was no difference in postoperative complications or mortality between the 2 arms. Several meta-analyses have found an improvement in survival with the use of neoadjuvant chemoradiotherapy–Gebski and colleagues,[22] found a 13% absolute increase in survival with neoadjuvant chemoradiotherapy over surgery alone while Sloquist and colleagues, estimated this to be 8.7% at 2 years with the number needed to treat being 11.

Sequential therapy-induction chemotherapy followed by chemoradiation and surgery

Several Phase II/III trials have investigated sequential therapy with induction chemotherapy followed chemoradiation prior to surgery and have shown promising results. A German trial (POET) compared sequential preoperative therapy followed by surgery with neoadjuvant chemotherapy and surgery in 126 patients with locally advanced adenocarcinoma of lower esophagus or gastric cardia.[32] The complete resection rates were similar between the arms with a nonsignificant increase in postoperative mortality in the sequential arm. The pCR rates were higher with sequential treatment (16% vs 2%) and there was a trend toward improved 3-year (47% vs 26%) and 5-year survival (40% vs 24%) (40). The Phase II randomized trial by Ajani and colleagues,[33] showed a nonsignificant improvement in pCR with no improvement in survival when comparing sequential therapy with neoadjuvant chemotherapy followed by surgery. The Phase II NEOSCOPE study compared preoperative regimens of radiation (45 Gy) concurrent with either oxaliplatin/capecitabine or paclitaxel/carboplatin following induction chemotherapy (oxaliplatin/capecitabine).[34] The pCR rates were higher with paclitaxel/carboplatin (29%) compared to oxaliplatin/capecitabine (11%). The recent phase II trial by Goodman and colleagues,[35] explored PET-based response to induction chemotherapy (modified oxaliplatin, leucovorin, and fluorouracil (FOLFOX) or carboplatin-paclitaxel) to tailor the chemotherapy regimen during chemoradiation (50.4 Gy) followed by the surgery. The best outcome was seen in PET responders to FOLFOX with a pCR rate of 40%, median survival of 49 months, and 5-year overall survival of 53%.

Perioperative chemotherapy for gastroesophageal junctional tumors

The treatment of gastroesophageal junction (GEJ) tumors often mirrors that of gastric cancer and is further discussed in a later article. The MRC Adjuvant Gastric Infusional Chemotherapy (MAGIC) trial is the seminal trial that established the routine use of perioperative chemotherapy–503 patients with resectable adenocarcinoma of stomach or GEJ were randomized to perioperative chemotherapy (cisplatin, epirubicin, 5-fluorouracil–ECF) and surgery or surgery alone.[11] Perioperative chemotherapy improved 5-year survival from 23% to 36% without increasing morbidity and mortality compared with surgery alone. Similar survival outcomes were shown in a French trial as well, supporting perioperative chemotherapy.[36]

More recently, Al-Batran and colleagues[37] compared 2 perioperative chemotherapy regimens (5-fluorouracil plus leucovorin, oxaliplatin, and docetaxel [FLOT] vs ECF/ECX). The FLOT arm showed significant improvement in median survival (50 vs 34 months). While majority of patients were able to complete the 3 cycles of preoperative chemotherapy, only 40–45% were able to complete postoperative chemotherapy indicating the importance of appropriate patient selection.

Neoadjuvant chemotherapy versus chemoradiation

Neoadjuvant chemoradiotherapy has been compared with neoadjuvant chemotherapy in a few randomized trials with mixed results. An Australian trial compared preoperative chemotherapy (cisplatin and 5-fluorouracil) with preoperative chemoradiation (cisplatin and 5-fluorouracil with 35 Gy) in 75 patients with resectable adenocarcinoma of the esophagus or gastroesophageal junction.[38] Median progression-free and overall survival were similar in both arms but R0 resection rate was improved in patients receiving chemoradiation (0 vs 11%).

The NeoRes trial compared neoadjuvant chemotherapy versus neoadjuvant chemoradiotherapy in 181 patients with resectable carcinoma of the esophagus or esophagogastric junction.[39] Chemotherapy in both study arms included 3 cycles of cisplatin and 5-fluorouracil. Patients in the chemoradiotherapy arm received concurrent radiotherapy (40 Gy) over 4 weeks with cycles 2 and 3. Esophagectomy was performed 4 to 6 weeks following the completion of neoadjuvant treatment. Chemoradiotherapy was associated with an improved R0 resection rate, fewer persistent lymph node metastases, and a higher rate of pCR. The progression-free and overall survival, however, were similar in both treatment arms.[40]

Several ongoing trials are comparing these 2 approaches and are discussed later in discussion.

The NEOAEGIS trial (NCT01726452) is comparing CROSS with perioperative chemotherapy MAGIC/FLOT in esophageal adenocarcinoma.[41] The preliminary results were presented at the American Society of Clinical Oncology (ASCO) Annual Meeting in 2021. In total, 377 patients were accrued (362 evaluable) – 178 received cross, 157 MAGIC, and 27 FLOT.[42] At a median follow-up of 24.5 months, the event rates were similar in both arms with estimated three-year survival probability was 56% and 57% in CROSS and perioperative chemotherapy arms, respectively. The authors concluded that these data support equipoise in clinical decision-making.

The TOPGEAR (NCT01924819) randomized controlled trial randomized patients with adenocarcinoma of stomach or gastroesophageal junction to perioperative MAGIC/FLOT regimen with or without neoadjuvant chemoradiotherapy.[43] The interim results demonstrated the safety of delivery of chemoradiotherapy; though this trial focusses primarily on

gastric cancer (>70%) and may not be applicable for all esophageal cancers.[44]

ESOPEC (NCT92509286) is a European multicenter randomized trial comparing CROSS with FLOT neoadjuvant regimens in localized adenocarcinoma of the esophagus and gastroesophageal junction.[45]

Finally, in Japan, cisplatin/5-fluorouracil is considered the standard chemotherapy regimen and the NEXT trial is a three-arm phase III trial comparing neoadjuvant chemotherapy: 2 cycles cisplatin/5-fluorouracil versus 3 cycles docetaxel/cisplatin/5-fluorouracil versus chemoradiotherapy in squamous cell carcinoma of the esophagus.[46] The results were presented at ASCO Gastrointestinal Meeting in 2022. In total, 601 patients were enrolled from 2012 to 2018 and at a median follow-up of 4.2 years, the median overall survival in cisplatin/5-fluorouracil, docetaxel/cisplatin/5-fluorouracil, and chemoradiotherapy arms were 4.6 years, not reached, and 6.0 years, respectively. The three-year overall survival was 62.6%, 72.1%, and 68.3%, respectively.[47] R0 resection was achieved in over 85% of patients in all 3 arms. The pCR rate was higher with chemoradiotherapy (38.5%) compared to chemotherapy alone (19.8% and 2.1%). The authors concluded docetaxel/cisplatin/5-fluorouracil improved overall survival over cisplatin/5-fluorouracil with manageable toxicity. The published full results are eagerly awaited.

Radiation dose

The radiation dose in the neoadjuvant trials has ranged from 30 Gy to 50.4 Gy in 15 to 28 fractions, delivered 5 days per week. A survey showed that higher dose was preferred by North American oncologists with the goal of increased pCR and R0 resection rates and additionally citing a risk of possible inadequate treatment of those patients who ultimately do not receive surgery.[48,49] In terms of outcome, a meta-analysis by Engel and colleagues,[50] found no difference in survival between lower dose (≤48.85 Gy biological effective dose) or high dose neoadjuvant regimens. A systematic review of 110 studies by Li and colleagues,[51] showed that despite higher pCR rates with high dose radiotherapy (>48.85 Gy), the progression-free survival and overall survival rates were higher with lower dose regimens and the rate of grade 3 toxicity and postoperative complications was lower. Finally, an observational propensity-matched multi-cohort study compared patients treated with neoadjuvant chemoradiation and planned surgery versus definitive chemoradiation and salvage esophagectomy due to incomplete response or local recurrence.[6] An important finding was that increased in-hospital mortality with salvage surgery was associated with radiation dose greater than 55 Gy (28% vs 4%).[52] Resultantly, doses exceeding 55 Gy in the neoadjuvant setting are not recommended.

Optimal concurrent chemotherapy regimen for chemoradiation There is variation in the use of concurrent chemotherapy regimens. Multiple retrospective studies from large institutions compared various chemotherapy regimens and found them to have similar results in terms of overall survival.[53–55] The PROTECT trial is an ongoing trial comparing 2 concurrent chemotherapy regimens–carboplatin/paclitaxel versus FOLFOX for chemoradiation (NCT 02359968) and the results are eagerly anticipated.[56]

New Developments

Response assessment with positron emission tomography

Various modalities such as endoscopy with biopsy, endoscopic ultrasound, and positron emission tomography-computed tomography (PET-CT) have been explored to assess response following neoadjuvant therapy. The role of PET-CT to assess response following neoadjuvant chemoradiotherapy is not convincing with high false positivity due to treatment-induced inflammation or high false negative due to small occult residual disease.[57] The preSANO trial was a prospective, multicenter, diagnostic cohort study that studied different diagnostic approaches after neoadjuvant chemoradiotherapy to correlate the complete clinical response with pCR.[58] About 10% of tumor regression grade 3 or 4 were missed by endoscopy bite on bite biopsies and fine-needle aspiration and 15% were missed by PET. PET-CT, however, detected 9% interval metastases. The use of PET in treatment decision making is now being evaluated in the (SANO) trial.[59]

Response to PET-CT may play a role in personalizing therapy. In the neoadjuvant chemotherapy trials, PET-CT has been used to assess response to induction chemotherapy, discriminating responders from nonresponders. In MUNICON I, patients treated with neoadjuvant chemotherapy received a PET-CT on day 14 to identify nonresponders [<35% decrease in standardized uptake value (SUV)].[60] The response on PET-CT with ≥ 35% decrease in SUV on day 14 was shown to have prognostic value and was predictive of higher pCR and OS.[61] A recent trial by Goodman and colleagues showed that early assessment of response by PET-CT may be used to identify nonresponders to chemotherapy and help tailor therapy.

Omission of surgery in responders to chemoradiation: wait and watch/surveillance The pCR rates in patients treated with neoadjuvant chemoradiotherapy followed by surgery are high and the added utility of surgery in the subset of patient who achieves complete clinical response is debatable. A retrospective study in 98 patients with complete clinical response to neoadjuvant chemoradiotherapy showed no difference in the 3-year progression-free and overall survival with active surveillance versus planned surgery.[62] A wait and watch approach with active surveillance of the complete responders with diagnostic evaluations and salvage surgery in those with locoregional residual or regrowth is being evaluated prospectively.

Few trials compared neoadjuvant chemoradiation followed by surgery vs active surveillance after chemoradiation.[63–66] All used induction chemotherapy and radiation therapy (50.4 to 66 Gy). Overall survival was similar in all 3 studies while the ESOPRESSO study showed a nonsignificant lower disease-free survival in the surveillance arm. Clinical nonresponders who underwent surgery had better overall survival than those who did not (17 vs 6 months) in FFCD 9102 trial.[67] A meta-analysis by Chow and colleagues,[68,69] showed better survival with neoadjuvant chemoradiation and surgery vs chemoradiation alone while a Cochrane meta-analysis showed surgery added no additional benefit to chemoradiation. Based on these trials, definitive chemoradiation may be a potential option and the European Society of Medical Oncology (ESMO) considers definitive CTRT as a standard alternative to neoadjuvant trimodality therapy in locally advanced esophageal squamous cancers.

Targeted therapy and immunotherapy

Epidermal growth factor (EGFR) is overexpressed in some esophageal cancers making it a potential target for neoadjuvat therapy. A phase III trial by Ruhstaller (SAKK 75/08) of induction chemotherapy followed by neoadjuvant chemoradiotherapy with or without cetuximab failed to improved progression-free or overall survival.[70] Similarly the vascular endothelial growth factor (VEGF) inhibitor bevacizumab too failed to improve outcomes when added to perioperative chemotherapy.[71]

Immunotherapy with immune checkpoint inhibitors, such as nivolumab and pembrolizumab, has improved outcomes in various solid tumors. The checkmate 577 trial explored adjuvant nivolumab after neoadjuvant chemoradiotherapy and surgery versus placebo and demonstrated an improvement in disease-free survival.[72]

The roles of targeted therapy and immunotherapy are discussed in greater detail in a later article.

RECOMMENDATIONS

Neoadjuvant therapy prior to surgery should be offered to all patients with resectable locally advanced esophageal cancer ($\geq$T2 or N positive, M0).

Neoadjuvant chemoradiation followed by surgery is a commonly used treatment paradigm. Perioperative chemotherapy is also a reasonable treatment approach, especially for tumors of the gastroesophageal junction.

Multidisciplinary care with patient selection is crucial and key to success with neoadjuvant treatment.

CONCLUSION/SUMMARY

Neoadjuvant treatment prior to surgery is the standard of care in resectable localized esophageal cancer. Neoadjuvant chemoradiation offers the best outcomes in terms of survival over surgery alone and the benefit is sustained over 10 years.

CLINICS CARE POINTS

- Neoadjuvant chemoradiation followed by surgery is recommended for resectable esophageal cancer. Perioperative chemotherapy may be considered for patients with gastroesophageal junction cancers.
- Appropriate selection of patients along with multidisciplinary coordination of care is crucial to the outcome.
- Radiation dose of 41.4 Gy in 23 fractions or equivalent with paclitaxel carboplatin or cisplatin 5 Fluorouracil is reasonable treatment regimens. Radiation dose should not exceed 55 Gy in the neoadjuvant setting as there is evidence of worse surgical outcomes in the case of salvage surgery.

DISCLOSURE

The authors have nothing to disclose.

REFERENCES

1. Sung H, Ferlay J, Siegel RL, et al. Global cancer statistics 2020: GLOBOCAN estimates of incidence and mortality worldwide for 36 cancers in 185 countries. CA: A Cancer J Clinicians 2021;71(3):209–49.
2. Then EO, Lopez M, Saleem S, et al. Esophageal cancer: an updated surveillance epidemiology and end results database analysis. World J Oncol 2020;11(2):55–64.
3. Napier KJ, Scheerer M, Misra S. Esophageal cancer: a review of epidemiology, pathogenesis, staging workup and treatment modalities. World J Gastrointest Oncol 2014;6(5):112–20.
4. Plum PS, Hölscher AH, Pacheco Godoy K, et al. Prognosis of patients with superficial T1 esophageal cancer who underwent endoscopic resection before esophagectomy-A propensity score-matched comparison. Surg Endosc 2018;32(9):3972–80.
5. Pennathur A, Farkas A, Krasinskas AM, et al. Esophagectomy for T1 esophageal cancer: outcomes in 100 patients and implications for endoscopic therapy. Ann Thorac Surg 2009;87(4):1048–54 [discussion: 54-5].
6. Hulscher JB, van Sandick JW, de Boer AG, et al. Extended transthoracic resection compared with limited transhiatal resection for adenocarcinoma of the esophagus. N Engl J Med 2002;347(21):1662–9.
7. Omloo JM, Lagarde SM, Hulscher JB, et al. Extended transthoracic resection compared with limited transhiatal resection for adenocarcinoma of the mid/distal esophagus: five-year survival of a randomized clinical trial. Ann Surg 2007;246(6):992–1000 [discussion -1].
8. Oppedijk V, van der Gaast A, van Lanschot JJ, et al. Patterns of recurrence after surgery alone versus preoperative chemoradiotherapy and surgery in the CROSS trials. J Clin Oncol 2014;32(5):385–91.
9. Chen G, Wang Z, Liu XY, et al. Recurrence pattern of squamous cell carcinoma in the middle thoracic esophagus after modified Ivor-Lewis esophagectomy. World J Surg 2007;31(5):1107–14.
10. Shah MA, Kennedy EB, Catenacci DV, et al. Treatment of locally advanced esophageal carcinoma: ASCO guideline. J Clin Oncol 2020;38(23):2677–94.
11. Cunningham D, Allum WH, Stenning SP, et al. Perioperative chemotherapy versus surgery alone for resectable gastroesophageal cancer. N Engl J Med 2006;355(1):11–20.
12. Shapiro J, van Lanschot JJB, Hulshof M, et al. Neoadjuvant chemoradiotherapy plus surgery versus surgery alone for oesophageal or junctional cancer (CROSS): long-term results of a randomised controlled trial. Lancet Oncol 2015;16(9):1090–8.
13. Mei W, Xian-Zhi G, Weibo Y, et al. Randomized clinical trial on the combination of preoperative irradiation and surgery in the treatment of esophageal carcinoma: report on 206 patients. Int J Radiat Oncol Biol Phys 1989;16(2):325–7.
14. Gignoux M, Roussel A, Paillot B, et al. The value of preoperative radiotherapy in esophageal cancer: results of a study of the E.O.R.T.C. World. J Surg 1987; 11(4):426–32.
15. Nygaard K, Hagen S, Hansen HS, et al. Pre-operative radiotherapy prolongs survival in operable esophageal carcinoma: a randomized, multicenter study of pre-operative radiotherapy and

chemotherapy. The second Scandinavian trial in esophageal cancer. World J Surg 1992;16(6):1104–9 [discussion: 10].

16. Kumar T, Pai E, Singh R, et al. Neoadjuvant strategies in resectable carcinoma esophagus: a meta-analysis of randomized trials. World J Surg Oncol 2020;18(1):59.

17. Kelsen DP, Ginsberg R, Pajak TF, et al. Chemotherapy followed by surgery compared with surgery alone for localized esophageal cancer. N Engl J Med 1998;339(27):1979–84.

18. Kelsen DP, Winter KA, Gunderson LL, et al. Long-term results of RTOG trial 8911 (USA Intergroup 113): a random assignment trial comparison of chemotherapy followed by surgery compared with surgery alone for esophageal cancer. J Clin Oncol 2007;25(24):3719–25.

19. Ancona E, Ruol A, Santi S, et al. Only pathologic complete response to neoadjuvant chemotherapy improves significantly the long term survival of patients with resectable esophageal squamous cell carcinoma: final report of a randomized, controlled trial of preoperative chemotherapy versus surgery alone. Cancer 2001;91(11):2165–74.

20. MRCOCW. Surgical. resection with or without preoperative chemotherapy in oesophageal cancer: a randomised controlled trial. The Lancet 2002;359(9319):1727–33.

21. Allum WH, Stenning SP, Bancewicz J, et al. Long-term results of a randomized trial of surgery with or without preoperative chemotherapy in esophageal cancer. J Clin Oncol 2009;27(30):5062–7.

22. Gebski V, Burmeister B, Smithers BM, et al. Survival benefits from neoadjuvant chemoradiotherapy or chemotherapy in oesophageal carcinoma: a meta-analysis. Lancet Oncol 2007;8(3):226–34.

23. Sjoquist KM, Burmeister BH, Smithers BM, et al. Survival after neoadjuvant chemotherapy or chemoradiotherapy for resectable oesophageal carcinoma: an updated meta-analysis. Lancet Oncol 2011;12(7):681–92.

24. Fan N, Wang Z, Zhou C, et al. Comparison of outcomes between neoadjuvant chemoradiotherapy and neoadjuvant chemotherapy in patients with locally advanced esophageal cancer: a network meta-analysis. eClinicalMedicine 2021;42:101183.

25. Zhou HY, Zheng SP, Li AL, et al. Clinical evidence for association of neoadjuvant chemotherapy or chemoradiotherapy with efficacy and safety in patients with resectable esophageal carcinoma (NewEC study). EClinicalMedicine 2020;24:100422.

26. Yang H, Liu H, Chen Y, et al. Neoadjuvant chemoradiotherapy followed by surgery versus surgery alone for locally advanced squamous cell carcinoma of the esophagus (NEOCRTEC5010): a phase III multicenter, randomized, open-label clinical trial. J Clin Oncol 2018;36(27):2796–803.

27. Walsh TN, Noonan N, Hollywood D, et al. A comparison of multimodal therapy and surgery for esophageal adenocarcinoma. N Engl J Med 1996;335(7):462–7.

28. Tepper J, Krasna MJ, Niedzwiecki D, et al. Phase III trial of trimodality therapy with cisplatin, fluorouracil, radiotherapy, and surgery compared with surgery alone for esophageal cancer: CALGB 9781. J Clin Oncol 2008;26(7):1086–92.

29. Mariette C, Dahan L, Mornex F, et al. Surgery alone versus chemoradiotherapy followed by surgery for stage I and II esophageal cancer: final analysis of randomized controlled phase III trial FFCD 9901. J Clin Oncol 2014;32(23):2416–22.

30. van Hagen P, Hulshof MCCM, van Lanschot JJB, et al. Preoperative chemoradiotherapy for esophageal or junctional cancer. N Engl J Med 2012;366(22):2074–84.

31. Eyck BM, Lanschot JJBv, Hulshof MCCM, et al. Ten-year outcome of neoadjuvant chemoradiotherapy plus surgery for esophageal cancer: the randomized controlled CROSS trial. J Clin Oncol 2021;39(18):1995–2004.

32. Stahl M, Walz MK, Riera-Knorrenschild J, et al. Preoperative chemotherapy versus chemoradiotherapy in locally advanced adenocarcinomas of the oesophagogastric junction (POET): Long-term results of a controlled randomised trial. Eur J Cancer 2017;81:183–90.

33. Ajani JA, Xiao L, Roth JA, et al. A phase II randomized trial of induction chemotherapy versus no induction chemotherapy followed by preoperative chemoradiation in patients with esophageal cancer. Ann Oncol 2013;24(11):2844–9.

34. Mukherjee S, Hurt CN, Gwynne S, et al. NEO-SCOPE: a randomised phase II study of induction chemotherapy followed by oxaliplatin/capecitabine or carboplatin/paclitaxel based pre-operative chemoradiation for resectable oesophageal adenocarcinoma. Eur J Cancer 2017;74:38–46.

35. Goodman KA, Ou FS, Hall NC, et al. Randomized phase II study of PET response-adapted combined modality therapy for esophageal cancer: mature results of the CALGB 80803 (Alliance) trial. J Clin Oncol 2021;39(25):2803–15.

36. Ychou M, Boige V, Pignon JP, et al. Perioperative chemotherapy compared with surgery alone for resectable gastroesophageal adenocarcinoma: an FNCLCC and FFCD multicenter phase III trial. J Clin Oncol 2011;29(13):1715–21.

37. Al-Batran SE, Homann N, Pauligk C, et al. Perioperative chemotherapy with fluorouracil plus leucovorin, oxaliplatin, and docetaxel versus fluorouracil or capecitabine plus cisplatin and epirubicin for locally advanced, resectable gastric or gastro-oesophageal junction adenocarcinoma (FLOT4): a randomised, phase 2/3 trial. Lancet 2019;393(10184):1948–57.

38. Burmeister BH, Thomas JM, Burmeister EA, et al. Is concurrent radiation therapy required in patients receiving preoperative chemotherapy for adenocarcinoma of the oesophagus? A randomised phase II trial. Eur J Cancer 2011;47(3):354–60.

39. Klevebro F, Alexandersson von Döbeln G, Wang N, et al. A randomized clinical trial of neoadjuvant chemotherapy versus neoadjuvant chemoradiotherapy for cancer of the oesophagus or gastro-oesophageal junction. Ann Oncol 2016;27(4):660–7.

40. von Döbeln GA, Klevebro F, Jacobsen AB, et al. Neoadjuvant chemotherapy versus neoadjuvant chemoradiotherapy for cancer of the esophagus or gastroesophageal junction: long-term results of a randomized clinical trial. Dis Esophagus 2019;32(2).

41. Keegan N, Keane F, Cuffe S, et al. ICORG 10-14: Neo-AEGIS: A randomized clinical trial of neoadjuvant and adjuvant chemotherapy (modified MAGIC regimen) versus neoadjuvant chemoradiation (CROSS protocol) in adenocarcinoma of the esophagus and esophagogastric junction. J Clin Oncol 2014;32(15_suppl). TPS4145-TPS.

42. Reynolds JV, Preston SR, O'Neill B, et al. Neo-AEGIS (Neoadjuvant trial in Adenocarcinoma of the Esophagus and Esophago-Gastric Junction International Study): preliminary results of phase III RCT of CROSS versus perioperative chemotherapy (Modified MAGIC or FLOT protocol). (NCT01726452). J Clin Oncol 2021;39(15_suppl):4004.

43. Leong T, Smithers BM, Michael M, et al. TOPGEAR: a randomised phase III trial of perioperative ECF chemotherapy versus preoperative chemoradiation plus perioperative ECF chemotherapy for resectable gastric cancer (an international, intergroup trial of the AGITG/TROG/EORTC/NCIC CTG). BMC Cancer 2015;15:532.

44. Leong T, Smithers BM, Haustermans K, et al. TOPGEAR: a randomized, phase III Trial of perioperative ECF chemotherapy with or without preoperative chemoradiation for resectable gastric cancer: interim results from an international, intergroup trial of the AGITG, TROG, EORTC and CCTG. Ann Surg Oncol 2017;24(8):2252–8.

45. Hoeppner J, Lordick F, Brunner T, et al. ESOPEC: prospective randomized controlled multicenter phase III trial comparing perioperative chemotherapy (FLOT protocol) to neoadjuvant chemoradiation (CROSS protocol) in patients with adenocarcinoma of the esophagus (NCT02509286). BMC Cancer 2016;16:503.

46. Nakamura K, Kato K, Igaki H, et al. Three-arm phase III trial comparing cisplatin plus 5-FU (CF) versus docetaxel, cisplatin plus 5-FU (DCF) versus radiotherapy with CF (CF-RT) as preoperative therapy for locally advanced esophageal cancer (JCOG1109, NExT study). Jpn J Clin Oncol 2013;43(7):752–5.

47. Kato K, Ito Y, Daiko H, et al. A randomized controlled phase III trial comparing two chemotherapy regimen and chemoradiotherapy regimen as neoadjuvant treatment for locally advanced esophageal cancer, JCOG1109 NExT study. J Clin Oncol 2022;40(4_suppl):238.

48. Elliott DA, Nabavizadeh N, Kusano AS, et al. Locally Advanced Esophageal Chemoradiation Therapy Practice Patterns: Results From a National Survey of ASTRO Members. Int J Radiat Oncol Biol Phys 2015;93(3):S219.

49. Ising MS, Marino K, Trivedi JR, et al. Influence of neoadjuvant radiation dose on patients undergoing esophagectomy and survival in locally advanced esophageal cancer. J Gastrointest Surg 2019;23(4):670–8.

50. Engel S, Awerbuch A, Kwon D, et al. Optimal radiation dosing in concurrent neoadjuvant chemoradiation for resectable esophageal cancer: a meta-analysis. J Gastrointest Oncol 2019;10(3):391–9.

51. Li Y, Liu H, Sun C, et al. Comparison of clinical efficacy of neoadjuvant chemoradiation therapy between lower and higher radiation doses for carcinoma of the esophagus and gastroesophageal junction: a systematic review. Int J Radiat Oncol Biol Phys 2021;111(2):405–16.

52. Markar S, Gronnier C, Duhamel A, et al. Salvage surgery after chemoradiotherapy in the management of esophageal cancer: is it a viable therapeutic option? J Clin Oncol 2015;33(33):3866–73.

53. Jiang DM, Sim HW, Espin-Garcia O, et al. Chemoradiotherapy using carboplatin plus paclitaxel versus cisplatin plus fluorouracil for esophageal or gastroesophageal junction cancer. Oncology 2021;99(1):49–56.

54. Lopez A, Harada K, Chen HC, et al. Taxane-based or platinum-based combination chemotherapy given concurrently with radiation followed by surgery resulting in high cure rates in esophageal cancer patients. Medicine (Baltimore) 2020;99(9):e19295.

55. Wang T, Yu J, Liu M, et al. The benefit of taxane-based therapies over fluoropyrimidine plus platinum (FP) in the treatment of esophageal cancer: a meta-analysis of clinical studies. Drug Des Devel Ther 2019;13:539–53.

56. Messager M, Mirabel X, Tresch E, et al. Preoperative chemoradiation with paclitaxel-carboplatin or with fluorouracil-oxaliplatin—folinic acid (FOLFOX) for resectable esophageal and junctional cancer: the PROTECT-1402, randomized phase 2 trial. BMC Cancer 2016;16(1):318.

57. Wu AJ, Goodman KA. Positron emission tomography imaging for gastroesophageal junction tumors. Semin Radiat Oncol 2013;23(1):10–5.

58. Noordman BJ, Spaander MCW, Valkema R, et al. Detection of residual disease after neoadjuvant chemoradiotherapy for oesophageal cancer (preSANO):

a prospective multicentre, diagnostic cohort study. Lancet Oncol 2018;19(7):965–74.

59. Eyck BM, van der Wilk BJ, Noordman BJ, et al. Updated protocol of the SANO trial: a stepped-wedge cluster randomised trial comparing surgery with active surveillance after neoadjuvant chemoradiotherapy for oesophageal cancer. Trials 2021;22(1):345.

60. Lordick F, Ott K, Krause BJ, et al. PET to assess early metabolic response and to guide treatment of adenocarcinoma of the oesophagogastric junction: the MUNICON phase II trial. Lancet Oncol 2007; 8(9):797–805.

61. Ott K, Weber WA, Lordick F, et al. Metabolic imaging predicts response, survival, and recurrence in adenocarcinomas of the esophagogastric junction. J Clin Oncol 2006;24(29):4692–8.

62. van der Wilk BJ, Noordman BJ, Neijenhuis LKA, et al. Active surveillance versus immediate surgery in clinically complete responders after neoadjuvant chemoradiotherapy for esophageal cancer: a multicenter propensity matched study. Ann Surg 2021; 274(6):1009–16.

63. Noordman BJ, Wijnhoven BPL, Lagarde SM, et al. Neoadjuvant chemoradiotherapy plus surgery versus active surveillance for oesophageal cancer: a stepped-wedge cluster randomised trial. BMC Cancer 2018;18(1):142.

64. Stahl M, Stuschke M, Lehmann N, et al. Chemoradiation with and without surgery in patients with locally advanced squamous cell carcinoma of the esophagus. J Clin Oncol 2005;23(10):2310–7.

65. Bedenne L, Michel P, Bouché O, et al. Chemoradiation followed by surgery compared with chemoradiation alone in squamous cancer of the esophagus: FFCD 9102. J Clin Oncol 2007;25(10):1160–8.

66. Park SR, Yoon DH, Kim JH, et al. A randomized phase III trial on the role of esophagectomy in complete responders to preoperative chemoradiotherapy for esophageal squamous cell carcinoma (ESOPRESSO). Anticancer Res 2019;39(9): 5123–33.

67. Vincent J, Mariette C, Pezet D, et al. Early surgery for failure after chemoradiation in operable thoracic oesophageal cancer. Analysis of the non-randomised patients in FFCD 9102 phase III trial: chemoradiation followed by surgery versus chemoradiation alone. Eur J Cancer 2015;51(13):1683–93.

68. Chow R, Murdy K, Vaska M, et al. Definitive chemoradiotherapy versus neoadjuvant chemoradiotherapy and esophagectomy for the treatment of esophageal and gastroesophageal carcinoma - A systematic review and meta-analysis. Radiother Oncol 2021;165:37–43.

69. Vellayappan BA, Soon YY, Ku GY, et al. Chemoradiotherapy versus chemoradiotherapy plus surgery for esophageal cancer. Cochrane Database Syst Rev 2017;8(8):Cd010511.

70. Ruhstaller T, Thuss-Patience P, Hayoz S, et al. Neoadjuvant chemotherapy followed by chemoradiation and surgery with and without cetuximab in patients with resectable esophageal cancer: a randomized, open-label, phase III trial (SAKK 75/08). Ann Oncol 2018;29(6):1386–93.

71. Cunningham D, Stenning SP, Smyth EC, et al. Peri-operative chemotherapy with or without bevacizumab in operable oesophagogastric adenocarcinoma (UK Medical Research Council ST03): primary analysis results of a multicentre, open-label, randomised phase 2–3 trial. Lancet Oncol 2017;18(3):357–70.

72. Kelly RJ, Ajani JA, Kuzdzal J, et al. Adjuvant nivolumab in resected esophageal or gastroesophageal junction cancer. N Engl J Med 2021;384(13): 1191–203.

Adjuvant Therapies for Esophageal Cancer

Ahmed Abdelhakeem, MD[a], Mariela Blum Murphy, MD[b],*

KEYWORDS

- Esophageal cancer • Gastroesophageal junction cancer • Adjuvant • Chemoradiation
- Chemotherapy

KEY POINTS

- In North America and Europe, the results of the Intergroup-0116 (INT-0116) trial established postoperative chemoradiation as a standard of care for resected gastric and GEJ adenocarcinomas.
- The degree of lymph node dissection during surgical resection may influence the efficacy of postoperative chemoradiation. Adjuvant chemoradiation should be considered for patients who received a limited lymphadenectomy. However, postoperative chemotherapy should be considered for patients who received a D2 lymphadenectomy.
- Level 1 evidence established perioperative chemotherapy (FLOT/NEOAGIS) or preoperative chemoradiation (CROSS) followed by surgery for the treatment of localized EC.
- The CheckMate 577 trial is the first study to show the benefit of adding adjuvant immunotherapy in patients with localized esophageal or GEJ cancer who had concurrent chemoradiation followed by surgery.

INTRODUCTION

Globally, esophageal cancer (EC) remains the sixth most common cause of cancer mortality, with estimated 544,000 deaths.[1] In the United States (US), the estimated number of new cases and the number of deaths in 2021 were approximately 19,260 and 15,530, respectively.[2] Nearly 70% of the cases occur in men[1] and the risk for developing E.C. increases with age, with a mean age at diagnosis of 67 years.[3] The cumulative risk of esophageal cancer, from birth to age 74, is 1.01% for men and 0.38% for women.[1] E.C. has a poor survival rate in the US with a 5-year survival rate for all stages of approximately 19.9%,[2] while survival rates are even lower in the European countries with a 5-year survival rate of 9.8%.[4] The most common histologic subtypes of EC include squamous cell carcinoma followed by adenocarcinoma. Esophageal squamous cell carcinoma (ESCC) is the most prevalent histologic type in

Asian countries, while esophageal adenocarcinoma (EAC) is more common in the US and other Western countries.[5,6]

ESCC usually arises in the proximal to middle esophagus, whereas adenocarcinomas are usually found in the distal esophagus close to the gastroesophageal junction (GEJ). ESCC arises from denuded epithelial cells and plaques. EAC arises from columnar glandular cells replacing the squamous epithelial lining of the esophagus.[7] Other less common subtypes of esophageal cancers include sarcomas, leiomyosarcomas, small cell carcinomas, carcinoids, and lymphomas.[8]

Treatment of esophageal cancer depends on patients' characteristics, including performance status and coexisting morbidities and tumor characteristics. High-grade dysplasia and very early stages tumors are suitable for local therapy that includes endoscopic resection and ablation or surgery, while advanced stages are treated with single or multimodality approaches, including

[a] Baptist Hospitals of Southeast Texas, 3282 College Street, Beaumont, TX 77701, USA; [b] The University of Texas, MD Anderson Cancer Center, 1515 Holcombe Blvd, Houston, TX 77030, USA
* Corresponding author.
E-mail addresses: abdelhakeem@shsu.edu (A.A.); mblum1@mdanderson.org (M.B.M.)

Thorac Surg Clin 32 (2022) 457–465
https://doi.org/10.1016/j.thorsurg.2022.06.004
1547-4127/22/© 2022 Elsevier Inc. All rights reserved.

chemotherapy, chemoradiotherapy followed by surgical resection, or immunotherapy.

Level 1 evidence established perioperative chemotherapy (FLOT/NEOAGIS) [9,10] or preoperative chemoradiation (CROSS) [11] followed by surgery for the treatment of localized EC. However, in some cases, when surgery has been conducted upfront, additional therapy should be considered depending on the pathologic staging.

This article will focus on adjuvant (postoperative) therapies for locally advanced esophageal and GEJ adenocarcinomas and SCCs, namely postoperative chemoradiation or chemotherapy when treatment has not been given upfront. We will also discuss the newly established level 1 approach for adjuvant treatment after concurrent chemoradiation followed by surgery.

ADJUVANT THERAPY FOR ESOPHAGEAL ADENOCARCINOMA
Adjuvant Chemoradiation for Esophageal Adenocarcinoma

In North America and Europe, the results of the Intergroup-0116 (INT-0116) trial established postoperative chemoradiation as a standard of care for resected gastric and GEJ adenocarcinomas.[12] In this trial, A total of 556 patients, including 111 (20%) patients with GEJ adenocarcinoma, were randomized to adjuvant chemotherapy and chemoradiation with 5-fluorouracil (5-FU) and leucovorin (LV) versus observation following surgical resection. The median overall survival (O.S.) for patients who received chemoradiation was 36 months compared with 27 months in the surgery-only group (P = .005). The relapse-free survival (RFS) in the chemoradiation group was 27 months compared with only 19 months in the surgery-only group (p=<0.001).[12] The study design proposed D1 resection as a primary surgical intervention. However, more than 50% of patients underwent a D0 resection, and only 10% of patients underwent a D2 nodal dissection. In that case, the chemoradiotherapy in addition to the suboptimal surgery is the reason for the difference in survival.

The Cancer and Leukemia Group B (CALGB) 80,101, a US intergroup trial, was designed to evaluate the efficacy of postoperative 5-FU and LV with 5-FU plus concurrent radiation versus postoperative epirubicin, cisplatin, and 5-FU (ECF) before and after 5-FU plus concurrent radiation in patients with gastric or GEJ adenocarcinomas after surgical resection.[13] Five hundred forty-six patients, including 120 cases (22%) of GEJ adenocarcinoma, were enrolled. Study results show similar outcomes in both arms. Five-

year overall survival rates were 44% in F.U. plus LV arm versus 44% in ECF arm, and 5-year disease-free survival rates were 39% in F.U. plus LV arm versus 37% in ECF arm. These results indicate that ECF before and after radiation does not improve survival compared with standard F.U. and LV before and after radiation.[13] The degree of lymph node dissection during surgical resection may influence the efficacy of postoperative chemoradiation. In a retrospective analysis evaluating the outcome of postoperative chemoradiation in patients with gastric adenocarcinoma who had either D1 or D2 lymphadenectomy, the study concluded that postoperative chemoradiation was associated with significantly lower recurrence after D1 lymphadenectomy. However, there was no significant difference in recurrence rate between the 2 groups following D2 lymphadenectomy.[14] The results from the ARTIST (Adjuvant Chemoradiation Therapy in Stomach Cancer) phase III trial also concluded that postoperative chemoradiation did not significantly reduce the recurrence rate after D2 lymphadenectomy when compared with postoperative chemotherapy only. The study also concluded that postoperative chemoradiation was associated with prolonged 3-year DFS compared with postoperative chemotherapy alone in patients with positive lymph nodes (78% vs 72%; P = .0365).[14] However, the subsequent ARTIST-II trial demonstrated no superior benefit of postoperative chemoradiation when compared with chemotherapy alone in patients with lymph node-positive, D2 lymphadenectomy, 3-year DFS was 74.3% versus 72.8% for postoperative chemotherapy and postoperative chemoradiation, respectively; HR, 0.971;.P = .879 [15]

Results from these studies are extrapolated for the treatment of EC. The authors do recommend considering adjuvant chemoradiation when patients receive limited lymph node dissection. However, postoperative chemotherapy should be considered for patients who received a D2 lymphadenectomy or extended lymphadenectomy.

Adjuvant Chemotherapy for Esophageal Adenocarcinoma

Few studies have been conducted to evaluate the efficacy of postoperative chemotherapy versus surgery alone. Most of these trials have been conducted in gastric and GEJ cancers. The Adjuvant Chemotherapy Trial of TS-1 for Gastric Cancer (ACTS-GC) study enrolled 1059 patients with completely resected stage II and III gastric cancer. Patients were randomized to receive adjuvant S-1, a mixture of tegafur, gimeracil, and oteracil for 1 year versus observation.[16] Five-year outcomes confirmed that the administration of S-1 for 1 year was associated with 71.7% 5-year overall survival rate compared with 61.1% with observation group (hazard ratio (HR), 0.669; 95% confidence interval (CI): 0.540–0.828). The relapse-free survival rate at 5 years was 65.4% in the S-1 group and 53.1% in the surgery-only group (HR: 0.653; 95% CI: 0.537–0.793).[17]

The capecitabine and oxaliplatin adjuvant study in stomach cancer (CLASSIC) trial was conducted in South Korea, China, and Taiwan, enrolling 1035 patients with stage II–IIIB gastric cancer who had curative D2 resection.[18] Patients were randomized for 6 months of adjuvant capecitabine/oxaliplatin versus observation. The study concluded that the adjuvant chemotherapy group has a better 3-year disease-free survival (DFS) of 74% compared with 59% in the observation group HR: 0.56, 95% CI: 0.44 to 0.72; $P < .0001$. The ARTIST II trial was designed to evaluate the benefits of postoperative chemoradiation therapy compared with postoperative chemotherapy in curatively D2 resected stage II/III, patients with node-positive gastric cancer. Study results showed that the addition of radiation therapy to postoperative S-1 and oxaliplatin didn't significantly reduce the recurrence rate after D2 gastrectomy.[15]

Phase II trial of the Eastern Cooperative Oncology Group (E8296) evaluated the effects of postoperative paclitaxel and cisplatin in 55 patients with completely resected EAC, GEJ, and gastric adenocarcinoma.[19] Forty-nine patients (89%) had node-positive disease. Study results show 2-year survival was 60% despite N1 disease.

Recently, The RESOLVE trial evaluated perioperative and postoperative S-1 and oxaliplatin (SOX) compared with postoperative capecitabine and oxaliplatin (CAPOX) in 1094 Chinese patients with locally patients with advanced gastric or GEJ adenocarcinoma undergoing D2 gastrectomy.[20] The study results show that perioperative SOX has a better outcome when compared with adjuvant CAPOX, while adjuvant SOX was noninferior to adjuvant CAPOX. 3-year DFS was 51·1% (95% CI: 45·5–56·3) in the adjuvant CAPOX group, 56·5% (51·0–61·7) in the adjuvant SOX group, and 59·4% (53·8–64·6) in the perioperative SOX group. HR was 0·77 (95% CI: 0·61–0·97; Wald $P = 0·028$) for the perioperative SOX group compared with the adjuvant-CAPOX group and 0·86 (0·68–1·07; Wald $P = 0·17$) for the adjuvant SOX group compared with the adjuvant CAPOX group.

The National Comprehensive Cancer Network (NCCN) recent guidelines recommend postoperative chemotherapy with 5-FU, Oxaliplatin, and Leucovorin (FOLFOX) in patients with resectable esophageal or GEJ cancer who had not received preoperative chemotherapy or underwent D2 lymphadenectomy.[21]

Perioperative chemotherapy for esophageal adenocarcinoma

Perioperative chemotherapy became a common approach in the US and Europe in the early 2000s, based primarily on the phase III Medical Research Council Adjuvant Gastric Infusional Chemotherapy (MAGIC) trial. The study enrolled 503 patients with gastric and GEJ (26%) adenocarcinoma.[22] Patients were randomized to receive 3 cycles of perioperative chemotherapy ECF followed by surgery, followed by 3 more cycles of ECF, or undergo surgery followed by observation. Study results confirmed improvement on 5-year OS (36% vs 23%, $P = .009$).

A French study supports the findings of the MAGIC trial. The Fédération Nationale des Centers de Lutte Contre le Cancer (FNCLCC) and the Fédération Francophone de Cancérologie Digestive (FFCD) multicenter phase III trial.[23] A total of 224 patients with resectable adenocarcinoma of the lower esophagus (11%), GEJ (64%), or stomach were randomly assigned to either perioperative chemotherapy (with cisplatin and 5-FU) and surgery followed by 3 to 4 cycles of cisplatin and 5-FU or surgery alone. the chemotherapy and surgery group had a significantly higher OS (HR for death: 0.69; 95% CI: 0.50–0.95; $P = .02$) and disease-free survival (DFS; HR for recurrence or death: 0.65; 95% CI: 0.48–0.89; $P = .003$). Five-year survival rates were 38% (95% CI: 29%–47%) in the chemotherapy and surgery group compared with 24% (95% CI: 17%–33%) in the surgery group. These results are quite similar to those of the MAGIC trial and support the use of epirubicin to cisplatin and 5-FU.

The Arbeitsgemeinschaft Internistische Onkologie (AIO) German group conducted a randomized phase II/III trial (FLOT4) comparing 4 pre- and four postoperative cycles of conventional ECF versus FLOT (5-FU, Leucovorin, Oxaliplatin, and docetaxel) in 716 patients with resectable gastric (44%) or GEJ (56%) adenocarcinoma.[9] The O.S. was significantly improved with FLOT versus ECF (50 vs 35 months; HR: 0.77; $P = .012$), with a projected improvement in 5-year O.S. (45% vs 36%). DFS was also improved with FLOT (30 vs 18 months; HR, 0.75; $P = .0036$), as were rates of R0 resection (85% vs 78%), tumor stage $\leq$ T1 (25% vs 15%), and nodal status N0 (49% vs 41%). Rates of adverse events were comparable for the 2 regimens. The FLOT4 study has established FLOT as the new standard of care for perioperative chemotherapy in patients with resectable gastric cancer who can tolerate a triplet chemotherapy regimen.[9]The Neoadjuvant trial in Adenocarcinoma of the Esophagus and Esophago-Gastric Junction International Study (NEO-AEGIS) phase III trial was designed to assess the efficacy and safety of preoperative CROSS trial chemoradiation compared with the MAGIC trial or FLOT4 trial perioperative chemotherapy regimens in patients with resectable esophageal or GEJ adenocarcinoma.[10] The study revealed that perioperative chemotherapy alone is noninferior to chemoradiation; 3-year OS was 57% for chemotherapy versus 56% for chemoradiation; HR 1.02 (95% CI: 0.74–1.42). However, it is important to highlight that few patients in the MAGIC/FLOT arm received the FLOT regimen; 27 out of 184 patients when the MAGIC regimen no longer represents the standard of care, making it hard to have a direct comparison between the CROSS regimen and FLOT regimen. Fortunately, The ESOPEC trial's design will help answer that question and hopefully will present more relevant data.

Adjuvant Therapy for Esophageal Squamous Cell Carcinoma

Multiple studies have been conducted to evaluate the role of postoperative chemotherapy and chemoradiotherapy after surgical resection for localized ESCC. These studies show limited survival benefits of postoperative treatment. The limited contribution of postoperative therapy is probably due to the moderate toxicity, which leads to treatment-related complications or an inability to complete therapy.

Adjuvant chemoradiation for esophageal squamous cell carcinoma

Little is known about the efficacy of postoperative chemoradiation therapy for patients with localized ESCC. One retrospective study of 290 localized patients with ESCC evaluated the benefit of postoperative cisplatin, 5-FU, and leucovorin with concurrent external beam radiation compared with surgery alone.[24] Survival benefit was observed for node-positive patients receiving postoperative chemoradiation. 3-year OS was 45.8% versus 14.1% (p=<0.001) and 3-year DFS was 24.1% versus 11.5% (P = .002). A recent phase III trial has been conducted in China to compare the benefits of postoperative radiation therapy versus postoperative chemoradiation versus surgery alone in 172 patients with localized (stage IIB–III) ESCC.[25] The 3-year OS for postoperative chemoradiation, postoperative radiation therapy, and

surgery alone were 66.5%, 60.8%, and 48.0%, respectively (P = .048) while 3-year DFS were 57.3%, 50.0%, and 36.7%, respectively (P = .048).

Adjuvant chemotherapy for esophageal squamous cell carcinoma

Few studies have been conducted to evaluate the role of chemotherapy after surgical resection of localized ESCC. In 1996, Pouliquen and colleagues conducted a multicenter randomized trial on 124 patients with ESCC that didn't show improvement in patients who received postoperative cisplatin plus 5-FU (C.F.).[26]

Another study designed by the Japanese Clinical Oncology Group evaluated adjuvant chemotherapy with cisplatin plus vindesine for resected patients with ESCC and found no effect on survival in patients with ESCC compared with surgery alone.[27]

In contrast, The Japanese Clinical Oncology Group (JCOG) 9204 randomized trial compared the outcomes of patients who underwent surgery followed by adjuvant C.F. versus surgery only.[28] The 5-year DFS with surgery plus C.F. was 55% compared with 45% in the surgery-only group (P = .037). The 5-year O.S. was 61% versus 52%, but it was statistically insignificant (P = .13).

Heroor and colleagues conducted a retrospective case-control study to evaluate the effect of postoperative chemotherapy in patients with ESCC who underwent R0 esophagectomy with radical lymphadenectomy. The study enrolled 211 patients; 94 received postoperative chemotherapy, whereas 117 had surgery alone.[29] On the stratification of study results, in a subgroup of patients with 8 or more positive lymph nodes, the postoperative chemotherapy group had a better O.S. than the surgery-only group (P = .013). No significant difference was found in survival between the 2 groups in any other stratified subgroup.

Adjuvant Radiation Therapy for Esophageal Squamous Cell Carcinoma

Multiple studies have been conducted to evaluate the efficacy of postoperative radiation therapy versus surgery-only. In 1991, Ténière and colleagues studied the effect of postoperative radiation therapy in 221 patients with ESCC. The study showed that postoperative radiation did not improve survival.[30]

Fok and colleagues study resulted in shorter survival of patients who underwent postoperative radiotherapy due to irradiation-related death and the early appearance of metastatic diseases.[31]

Table 1
Key studies for postoperative, perioperative, and preoperative therapy for esophageal cancer

Study	No. of Patients	Treatment Arms	Histology	HR for OS (*P* value)	Primary End Point Comparison
Postoperative Chemoradiation					
INT-0116[12]	556	Surgery → FL/CTRT (45 Gy + FL)/FL vs Surgery	Adenocarcinoma	1.32 (.004)	OS: 36 vs 27
CALGB 80101[13]	546	Surgery → ECF/CTRT + FL/ECF vs Surgery → FL/CTRT + FL/FL	Adenocarcinoma	1.03 (.80)	OS: 38 vs 37
ARTIST[14]	458	Surgery → XP/XRT/XP vs Surgery → XP	Adenocarcinoma	1.130 (.5272); N+ patients; HR for DFS, 0.70 (.04)	5-y OS: 75% vs 73%; N+ patients: 3-y DFS: 76% vs 72%
Postoperative Chemotherapy					
ACTS-GC[16]	1059	Surgery → S-1 vs Surgery	Adenocarcinoma	0.68 (.003); HR at 5 y: 0.669	3-y OS: 80.1% vs 70.1%; 3-y RFS: 72.2% vs 59.6%
CLASSIC[18]	1035	Surgery → CAPOX vs Surgery	Adenocarcinoma	0.56 (<.0001)	3-y DFS: 74% vs 59%
RESOLVE[20]	1094	Surgery → CAPOX vs Surgery → SOX vs SOX → Surgery → SOX, S-1	Adenocarcinoma	0.77 (<0.028)	3-y DFS: 51.1% vs 56.5% vs 59.4%
JCOG 9204[28]	242	Surgery → CF vs Surgery	SCC	0.13 (NR)	5-y OS: 52% vs 61%
Postoperative Immunotherapy					
CheckMate 577[38]	794	CTRT → Surgery → Nivolumab CTRT → Surgery → Placebo	Adenocarcinoma (71%) SCC (29%)	0.69 (<0.001)	OS: 22.4 mo vs 11.0 mo
Perioperative Chemotherapy					
MAGIC[22]	503	ECF → surgery → ECF vs Surgery	Adenocarcinoma	0.75 (.009)	5-y OS: 36.3% vs 23%
FNLCC/FFCP[23]	224	CF → surgery → CF vs Surgery	Adenocarcinoma	0.69 (0.02)	5-y OS: 38% vs 24%
FLOT4[9]	716	ECF → surgery → ECF vs FLOT → surgery → FLOT	Adenocarcinoma	0.77 (.012)	OS: 25 mo vs 50 mo 5-y OS: 36% vs 45%
NEO-AEGIS[10]	362	FLOT/ECF → Surgery →FLOT/ECF vs Carboplatin/paclitaxel;	Adenocarcinoma	1.02 (NR)	3-yea OS: 57% vs 56%

(continued on next page)

Table 1
(continued)

Study	No. of Patients	Treatment Arms	Histology	HR for OS (*P* value)	Primary End Point Comparison
		41.4 Gy → Surgery			
Preoperative Chemoradiation					
CALGB 9871[35]	56	CF; 50.4 Gy → Surgery vs Surgery	Adenocarcinoma (77%) SCC (23%)	1.46–5.69 (NR)	5-y OS: 39% vs 16%
CROSS[11]	366	Carboplatin/ paclitaxel; 41.4 Gy → Surgery vs Surgery	Adenocarcinoma (75) SCC (23%)	0.657 (0.003)	5-y OS: 47% vs 34%

Abbreviations: 5-fluorouracil, CTRT; CAPOX, capecitabine and oxaliplatin; CF, cisplatin; chemoradiation, DFS; cisplatin, and 5-fluorouracil; disease, free survival; docetaxel, HR; ECF, epirubicin; FL, 5-fluorouracil and leucovorin; FLOT, 5-fluoro- uracil; hazard, ratio; leucovorin, oxaliplatin; N+, lymph node positive; OS, overall survival; SCC, squamous cell carcinoma; SOX, S-1 and oxaliplatin; XP, capecitabine and cisplatin; XRT, capecitabine and radiation.

Xiao and colleagues evaluated the benefit of ra- diation therapy after radical resection in 495 pa- tients diagnosed with stage III ESCC. Study results showed improved 5-year OS in patients with ESCC with positive lymph node metastases when they received radiation therapy after surgery compared with surgery alone.[32]

Malthaner and colleagues[33] performed a meta- analysis of 34 randomized controlled trials and 6 meta-analyses in which patients with locally advanced esophageal cancer underwent pre or postoperative chemotherapy, radiotherapy, or chemoradiotherapy. No significant difference in survival was observed in the postoperative radio- therapy group. In contrast, a recent meta- analysis by Lin and colleagues concluded that postoperative radiation improves O.S. and DFS in patients with ESCC compared with surgery alone.[34]

PREOPERATIVE CHEMORADIOTHERAPY

Multiple studies have discussed the role of preop- erative chemoradiation in locally advanced esoph- ageal and GEJ cancer as an approach to improve pathologic response rates besides offering better locoregional control and improving patients' sur- vival rates. The CALGB 9871 trial included only 56 patients who were randomized to either CF chemotherapy with concurrent radiotherapy fol- lowed by surgery or surgery alone.[35] The study re- sults showed a median OS of 4.5 years in the chemoradiation followed by surgery group versus 1.8 years in the surgery alone group (*P* = .002). The 5-year OS was 39% (95% CI: 21%–57%) in the chemoradiation followed by the surgery group

versus 16% (95% CI: 5%–33%) in the surgery-only group. In a metanalysis conducted by Gebski and colleagues evaluating the benefits of preoperative chemotherapy or chemoradiation versus surgery alone,[36] the HR for all-cause mortality with preop- erative chemoradiation versus surgery alone was 0.81 (95% CI: 0.70–0.93; *P* = .002), corre- sponding to a 13% absolute difference in survival at 2 years, with similar results for different histolog- ic tumor types (squamous cell cancer: HR, 0.84, *P* = .04; adenocarcinomas: HR, 0.75, *P* = .02). The HR for preoperative chemotherapy was 0.90 (95% CI: 0.81–1.00; *P* = .05), which indicates a 2-year absolute survival benefit of 7%. There was no significant effect on all-cause mortality of chemotherapy for patients with SCC (HR 0.88; *P* = .12), although there was a significant benefit for those with adenocarcinoma (HR 0.78; *P* = .014).

The results of the Chemoradiotherapy for Esoph- ageal Cancer Followed by Surgery Study (CROSS) trial established preoperative chemoradiation as a standard of care in localized patients with esoph- ageal/GEJ cancer. Three hundred sixty-eight patients with localized esophageal cancer (adeno- carcinoma or squamous) were randomized to receive either preoperative paclitaxel or carboplatin with concurrent radiation or surgery alone. The me- dian OS for preoperative chemoradiotherapy group was 49.4 months versus 24.0 months for the surgery-alone group (HR, 0.657; 95% CI: 0.495– 0.871; *P* = .003). Five-year OS was better in the chemoradiotherapy group (47%) versus the surgery-alone group (34%).[11] The complete resec- tion rate was higher in the chemoradiotherapy group (92%) versus the surgery-alone group

(69%). In a subgroup analysis, the patients with squamous cancer demonstrated the best outcomes (HR was 0.453 for squamous cancer vs 0.732 for adenocarcinoma)[11,37]

Adjuvant Immunotherapy

Immunotherapy and targeted therapy have gained valuable roles in the management of metastatic gastric and esophageal cancers. The CheckMate 577 trial is the first study to show the benefit of adding adjuvant immunotherapy in patients with localized esophageal or GEJ cancer.[38] Seven hundred ninety-four patients with resected stage II or III esophageal or GEJ cancer who had preoperative chemoradiation and didn't achieve pathologic complete response were randomized to receive nivolumab 240 mg every 2 weeks for 16 weeks, followed by nivolumab 480 mg every 4 weeks or placebo. Nivolumab showed a better DFS, 22.4 months compared with 11 months in the placebo group.[38] Serious adverse events related to Nivolumab were 8% compared with 3% in the placebo group. The most common nivolumab adverse events reported were fatigue and diarrhea. The study results are promising and pave the way to establish nivolumab as a new standard of care for adjuvant therapy in localized patients with esophageal/GEJ cancer who had concurrent chemoradiation followed by surgery. Another advantage of adding nivolumab is the difficulty of administering postoperative chemotherapy in these patients due to considerable side effects and toxicity afterward. Several ongoing trials are investigating the role of immunotherapy in localized GEJ cancer, including EORTC 1707 VESTIGE, KEYNOTE-585, and AIO-STO-0317 DANTE.

SUMMARY

In North America and Europe, the results of the Intergroup-0116 (INT-0116) trial established postoperative chemoradiation as a standard of care for resected gastric and GEJ adenocarcinomas.

The degree of lymph node dissection during surgical resection may influence the efficacy of postoperative chemoradiation. Adjuvant chemoradiation should be considered for patients who received a limited lymphadenectomy. However, postoperative chemotherapy should be considered for patients who received a D2 lymphadenectomy.

The results of the Chemoradiotherapy for Esophageal Cancer Followed by Surgery Study (CROSS) trial established preoperative chemoradiation as a standard of care in localized patients with esophageal/GEJ cancer. However, the NEO-

AEGIS study revealed that perioperative chemotherapy alone is noninferior to chemoradiation.

The CheckMate 577 trial is the first study to show the benefit of adding adjuvant immunotherapy in patients with localized esophageal or GEJ cancer who had concurrent chemoradiation followed by surgery.

Table 1 summarizes the key studies for postoperative, perioperative, and preoperative therapy for esophageal cancer.

CLINICS CARE POINTS

- Perioperative chemotherapy or preoperative chemoradiation followed by surgery are established standard treatments for localized esophageal cancer.

- For localized patients with esophageal and gastroesophageal cancer who hadn't received preoperative therapy and had limited lymph node dissection postoperative chemoradiation should be considered. Otherwise, adjuvant chemotherapy is the preferred approach.

- For patients who have residual disease following preoperative chemoradiotherapy and surgical resection, nivolumab (PD-1 inhibitor) is preferred as adjuvant therapy.

DISCLOSURE

The authors have no conflicts of interest to disclose.

REFERENCES

1. Sung H, Ferlay J, Siegel RL, et al. Global Cancer Statistics 2020: GLOBOCAN Estimates of Incidence and Mortality Worldwide for 36 Cancers in 185 Countries. CA Cancer J Clin 2021;71(3):209–49.
2. National Cancer Institute Surveillance. Epidemiology, and End Results Program. Cancer stat facts: Esophageal cancer. Available at: https://seer.cancer.gov/statfacts/html/esoph.html. Accessed December 31, 2021.
3. Cummings LC, Cooper GS. Descriptive epidemiology of esophageal carcinoma in the Ohio Cancer Registry. Cancer Detect Prev 2008;32(1):87–92.
4. Gavin AT, Francisci S, Foschi R, et al. Oesophageal cancer survival in Europe: a EUROCARE-4 study. Cancer Epidemiol 2012;36(6):505–12.
5. Uhlenhopp DJ, Then EO, Sunkara T, et al. Epidemiology of esophageal cancer: update in global

trends, etiology and risk factors. Clin J Gastroenterol 2020;13(6):1010–21.

6. Umar SB, Fleischer DE. Esophageal cancer: epidemiology, pathogenesis and prevention. Nat Clin Pract Gastroenterol Hepatol 2008;5(9):517–26.

7. Blot WJ, Devesa SS, Fraumeni JF Jr. Continuing climb in rates of esophageal adenocarcinoma: an update. Jama 1993;270(11):1320.

8. Enzinger PC, Mayer RJ. Esophageal cancer. N Engl J Med 2003;349(23):2241–52.

9. Al-Batran SE, Homann N, Pauligk C, et al. Perioperative chemotherapy with fluorouracil plus leucovorin, oxaliplatin, and docetaxel versus fluorouracil or capecitabine plus cisplatin and epirubicin for locally advanced, resectable gastric or gastro-oesophageal junction adenocarcinoma (FLOT4): a randomised, phase 2/3 trial. Lancet (London, England) 2019;393(10184):1948–57.

10. Reynolds JV, Preston SR, O'Neill B, et al. Neo-AEGIS (Neoadjuvant trial in Adenocarcinoma of the Esophagus and Esophago-Gastric Junction International Study): Preliminary results of phase III RCT of CROSS versus perioperative chemotherapy (Modified MAGIC or FLOT protocol). (NCT01726452). J Clin Oncol 2021;39(15_suppl):4004.

11. van Hagen P, Hulshof MC, van Lanschot JJ, et al. Preoperative chemoradiotherapy for esophageal or junctional cancer. N Engl J Med 2012;366(22):2074–84.

12. Macdonald JS, Smalley SR, Benedetti J, et al. Chemoradiotherapy after surgery compared with surgery alone for adenocarcinoma of the stomach or gastroesophageal junction. N Engl J Med 2001;345(10):725–30.

13. Fuchs CS, Niedzwiecki D, Mamon HJ, et al. Adjuvant chemoradiotherapy with epirubicin, cisplatin, and fluorouracil compared with adjuvant chemoradiotherapy with fluorouracil and leucovorin after curative resection of gastric cancer: results from CALGB 80101 (Alliance). J Clin Oncol 2017;35(32):3671–7.

14. Dikken JL, Jansen EP, Cats A, et al. Impact of the extent of surgery and postoperative chemoradiotherapy on recurrence patterns in gastric cancer. J Clin Oncol 2010;28(14):2430–6.

15. Park SH, Lim DH, Sohn TS, et al. A randomized phase III trial comparing adjuvant single-agent S1, S-1 with oxaliplatin, and postoperative chemoradiation with S-1 and oxaliplatin in patients with node-positive gastric cancer after D2 resection: the ARTIST 2 trial(☆). Ann Oncol 2021;32(3):368–74.

16. Sakuramoto S, Sasako M, Yamaguchi T, et al. Adjuvant chemotherapy for gastric cancer with S-1, an oral fluoropyrimidine. N Engl J Med 2007;357(18):1810–20.

17. Sasako M, Sakuramoto S, Katai H, et al. Five-year outcomes of a randomized phase III trial comparing adjuvant chemotherapy with S-1 versus surgery alone in stage II or III gastric cancer. J Clin Oncol 2011;29(33):4387–93.

18. Bang YJ, Kim YW, Yang HK, et al. Adjuvant capecitabine and oxaliplatin for gastric cancer after D2 gastrectomy (CLASSIC): a phase 3 open-label, randomised controlled trial. Lancet 2012;379(9813):315–21.

19. Armanios M, Xu R, Forastiere AA, et al. Adjuvant chemotherapy for resected adenocarcinoma of the esophagus, gastro-esophageal junction, and cardia: phase II trial (E8296) of the Eastern Cooperative Oncology Group. J Clin Oncol 2004;22(22):4495–9.

20. Zhang X, Liang H, Li Z, et al. Perioperative or postoperative adjuvant oxaliplatin with S-1 versus adjuvant oxaliplatin with capecitabine in patients with locally advanced gastric or gastro-oesophageal junction adenocarcinoma undergoing D2 gastrectomy (RESOLVE): an open-label, superiority and non-inferiority, phase 3 randomised controlled trial. Lancet Oncol 2021;22(8):1081–92.

21. NCCN. Clinical Practice Guidelines in Oncology - Esophageal and Esophagogastric Junction Cancer. 2022. Available at: https://www.nccn.org/professionals/physician_gls/pdf/esophageal.pdf. Accessed January 26, 2022.

22. Cunningham D, Allum WH, Stenning SP, et al. Perioperative Chemotherapy versus Surgery Alone for Resectable Gastroesophageal Cancer. New Engl J Med 2006;355(1):11–20.

23. Ychou M, Boige V, Pignon JP, et al. Perioperative chemotherapy compared with surgery alone for resectable gastroesophageal adenocarcinoma: an FNCLCC and FFCD multicenter phase III trial. J Clin Oncol : official J Am Soc Clin Oncol 2011;29(13):1715–21.

24. Hsu PK, Huang CS, Wang BY, et al. Survival benefits of postoperative chemoradiation for lymph node-positive esophageal squamous cell carcinoma. Ann Thorac Surg 2014;97(5):1734–41.

25. Ni W, Yu S, Xiao Z, et al. Postoperative adjuvant therapy versus surgery alone for stage IIB–III Esophageal squamous cell carcinoma: a phase III randomized controlled trial. Oncologist 2021;26(12):e2151–60.

26. Pouliquen X, Levard H, Hay JM, et al. 5-Fluorouracil and cisplatin therapy after palliative surgical resection of squamous cell carcinoma of the esophagus. A multicenter randomized trial. French Associations for Surgical Research. Ann Surg 1996;223(2):127–33.

27. Ando N, Iizuka T, Kakegawa T, et al. A randomized trial of surgery with and without chemotherapy for localized squamous carcinoma of the thoracic esophagus: the Japan Clinical Oncology Group Study. J Thorac Cardiovasc Surg 1997;114(2):205–9.

28. Ando N, Iizuka T, Ide H, et al. Surgery plus chemotherapy compared with surgery alone for localized squamous cell carcinoma of the thoracic

esophagus: a Japan Clinical Oncology Group Study–JCOG9204. J Clin Oncol 2003;21(24): 4592–6.

29. Heroor A, Fujita H, Sueyoshi S, et al. Adjuvant chemotherapy after radical resection of squamous cell carcinoma in the thoracic esophagus: who benefits? A retrospective study. Dig Surg 2003;20(3): 229–35 [discussion: 236-227].

30. Ténière P, Hay JM, Fingerhut A, et al. Postoperative radiation therapy does not increase survival after curative resection for squamous cell carcinoma of the middle and lower esophagus as shown by a multicenter controlled trial. French University Association for Surgical Research. Surg Gynecol Obstet 1991;173(2):123–30.

31. Fok M, Sham JST, Choy D, et al. Postoperative radiotherapy for carcinoma of the esophagus: a prospective, randomized controlled study. Surgery 1993; 113(2):138–47.

32. Xiao ZF, Yang ZY, Liang J, et al. Value of radiotherapy after radical surgery for esophageal carcinoma: a report of 495 patients. Ann Thorac Surg 2003;75(2):331–6.

33. Malthaner RA, Wong RK, Rumble RB, et al. Neoadjuvant or adjuvant therapy for resectable esophageal cancer: a clinical practice guideline. BMC cancer 2004;4:67.

34. Lin HN, Chen LQ, Shang QX, et al. A meta-analysis on surgery with or without postoperative radiotherapy to treat squamous cell esophageal carcinoma. Int J Surg 2020;80:184–91.

35. Tepper J, Krasna MJ, Niedzwiecki D, et al. Phase III trial of trimodality therapy with cisplatin, fluorouracil, radiotherapy, and surgery compared with surgery alone for esophageal cancer: CALGB 9781. J Clin Oncol 2008;26(7):1086–92.

36. Gebski V, Burmeister B, Smithers BM, et al. Survival benefits from neoadjuvant chemoradiotherapy or chemotherapy in oesophageal carcinoma: a meta-analysis. Lancet Oncol 2007;8(3):226–34.

37. Oppedijk V, van der Gaast A, van Lanschot JJ, et al. Patterns of recurrence after surgery alone versus preoperative chemoradiotherapy and surgery in the CROSS trials. J Clin Oncol : official J Am Soc Clin Oncol 2014;32(5):385–91.

38. Kelly RJ, Ajani JA, Kuzdzal J, et al. Adjuvant nivolumab in resected esophageal or gastroesophageal junction cancer. New Engl J Med 2021;384(13): 1191–203.

Immune Checkpoint Blockade and Targeted Therapies in Esophageal Cancer

Jessica Yang, MD[a,b],*, Yelena Y. Janjigian, MD[a,b,1]

KEYWORDS

- Esophageal cancer • Esophageal adenocarcinoma • Esophageal squamous cell carcinoma
- Immunotherapy • Targeted therapy

KEY POINTS

- Chemotherapy plus anti-PD-1 therapy represents the new standard of care frontline regimen for advanced esophageal adenocarcinoma and squamous cell carcinoma.
- Anti-PD-1 therapy in combination with chemotherapy and trastuzumab is the emerging new standard for HER2-positive esophageal adenocarcinoma.
- Biomarker testing including MMR, PD-L1, and HER2 expression should be obtained in all patients with newly diagnosed esophageal cancer.

INTRODUCTION

Esophageal cancer is the seventh most common cancer globally and accounts for more than 544,000 deaths each year.[1] Histologically, esophageal cancer is classified as adenocarcinoma (AC) or squamous cell carcinoma (SCC). Although the incidence of esophageal SCC is declining due to reductions in cigarette smoking in Western countries, the incidence of AC continues to increase, driven by obesity, gastroesophageal reflux disease, and its associated precancerous state Barrett's esophagus.[1] Up until the early-mid 2000s, most clinical trials evaluating cytotoxic chemotherapy enrolled all patients with esophageal and gastroesophageal junction (GEJ) cancer, regardless of histologic subtype. However, emerging data points to significant differences in tumor biology and genomics between SCC and AC, paving the way for histology-specific therapeutic approaches.[2] In this article, we aim to provide an overview of recent advances in immunotherapy and targeted therapy for esophageal cancer, with an emphasis on the treatment of advanced, metastatic disease.

ESOPHAGEAL ADENOCARCINOMA
Frontline Therapy

Several practice-changing trials have established chemotherapy plus immunotherapy as the new standard of care for advanced esophageal cancer, irrespective of histology. Rationale for combining chemotherapy with immunotherapy stems from data suggesting that chemotherapy may increase tumor immunogenicity via release of tumor antigens, subsequent T cell priming, and depletion of immunosuppressive cells.[3]

The pivotal CheckMate 649 trial showed that the addition of the antiprogrammed death-1 (PD-1) antibody nivolumab to chemotherapy improved survival outcomes compared with chemotherapy alone, leading to Food and Drug Administration (FDA) approval of nivolumab for this indication. In

---

[a] Department of Medicine, Memorial Sloan Kettering Cancer Center, 300 E66th Street, Room 1001, New York, NY 10065, USA; [b] Department of Medicine, Weill Cornell Medical College, 300 E66th Street, Room 1001, New York, NY 10065, USA

[1] Present address: 300 East 66th Street, Room 1001, New York, NY 10065.

* Corresponding author. 136 Mountainview Boulevard, Basking Ridge, NJ 07920.

E-mail address: yangj10@mskcc.org

Thorac Surg Clin 32 (2022) 467–478
https://doi.org/10.1016/j.thorsurg.2022.07.002
1547-4127/22/© 2022 Published by Elsevier Inc.

the study, 1581 patients with previously untreated, advanced esophagogastric (EG) AC, irrespective of PD-L1 status, were randomized to receive nivolumab plus folinic acid, 5-fluorouracil (5-FU) and oxaliplatin (FOLFOX), or chemotherapy alone.[4] The study originally included a third arm evaluating dual immune checkpoint blockade with nivolumab plus the cytotoxic T-lymphocyte antigen-4 inhibitor ipilimumab but this arm was terminated early due to a high rate of adverse events (AEs) and death relative to the other 2 arms. The addition of nivolumab improved the overall survival (OS) in all patients (hazard ratio [HR] 0.80, 99% confidence interval [CI] 0.68–0.94, P = .0002), with a higher degree of benefit in the PD-L1 combined positive score (CPS) of 5 or greater population (HR 0.71, 98% CI 0.59–0.86, P < .0001). Updated analysis demonstrates an even more pronounced benefit in the PD-L1 CPS of 10 or greater population (median OS 15.0 vs 10.9 months, HR 0.66).[5] Patients with PD-L1-low tumors may derive less benefit, with OS HR 0.92 (95% CI 0.70–1.23) and 0.94 (95% CI 0.78–1.13) for patients with CPS less than 1 and CPS less than 5 disease, respectively. Nivolumab improved progression-free survival (PFS; HR 0.68, 98% CI 0.56–0.81, P < .0001) and objective response rate (ORR) across all patients, regardless of PD-L1 score (CPS ≥5: 60% vs 45%; CPS <5: 55% vs 46%; CPS <1: 51% vs 41%). Although nivolumab plus ipilimumab showed meaningful antitumor activity in heavily pretreated patients in a prior study, the combination did not improve OS compared with chemotherapy in the PD-L1 CPS of 5 or greater population (HR 0.89, 96.5% CI 0.71–1.10, P = .23).[6] The toxicity profile of FOLFOX plus nivolumab reflects both chemotherapy side effects and immune-mediated AEs, with grade 3 or greater treatment-related AEs occurring in 59% of patients in the combination arm versus 44% in the chemotherapy alone arm. Nivolumab is now approved in the United States, Japan, and many countries worldwide in combination with first-line fluorouracil/platinum chemotherapy irrespective of PD-L1 status. The European Medicines Agency's (EMA) approval for nivolumab is restricted to patients with PD-L1 CPS of 5 or greater.

The phase III KEYNOTE-590 trial included predominantly SCC patients and led to recent approval of pembrolizumab in combination with chemotherapy, independent of histology or PD-L1 status.[7] In this study, treatment-naïve patients with advanced esophageal/GEJ AC or SCC were randomized to pembrolizumab plus 5-FU/cisplatin versus 5-FU/cisplatin alone. A significant improvement in OS was observed in all patients but the

magnitude of benefit was highest among SCC patients with PD-L1 CPS of 10 or greater (HR 0.59, 95% CI 0.45–0.76). A similar degree of benefit was seen in all patients with PD-L1 CPS of 10 or greater (HR 0.64, 95% CI 0.51–0.80) but more than 70% of patients in the trial had SCC. Post hoc analysis demonstrated no survival benefit with the addition of pembrolizumab in the PD-L1 CPS of less than 10 population (HR 0.86, 95% CI 0.68–1.10). The EMA only approved pembrolizumab for patients with PD-L1 CPS of 10 or greater.

Similar results supporting combined chemotherapy plus immunotherapy have been reported in phase III trials (ORIENT-16, ATTRACTION-4) conducted in Asia.[8,9] **Table 1** summarizes the key frontline trials in esophageal AC.

Subgroup analyses from CheckMate 649, KEYNOTE-062, and KEYNOTE-590 would support selective use of frontline immunotherapy based on PD-L1 status to avoid unnecessary treatment toxicity and economic burden given the high costs associated with pembrolizumab and nivolumab.[10] However, arguments for broader use of immunotherapy include the improvement in response rate, observed across all PD-L1 subgroups, minimal benefit with anti-PD-1 therapy in subsequent lines of therapy for esophageal AC, interobserver variability and inconsistencies in CPS scoring, and differences in PD-L1 stromal staining among the 4 clinical laboratory improvement amendments (CLIA)-approved PD-L1 assays: Dako 22C3, Dako 28 to 8, Ventana SP263, and Ventana SP142.

Mismatch Repair Deficient/Microsatellite Instability-High Tumors

Up to 13% of localized EG ACs are mismatch repair deficient or microsatellite instability-high (MSI-H).[2] Patients with MSI-H tumors have favorable outcomes with surgery alone and may not benefit from perioperative therapy due to intrinsic chemotherapy resistance. A meta-analysis of patients with MSI-H EG cancer enrolled in perioperative and adjuvant trials showed no survival benefit with chemotherapy plus surgery compared with surgery alone.[11] Therefore, MMR/MSI testing is critical, and upfront surgery should be considered in patients with resectable disease. Future strategies include selection of patients for adjuvant pembrolizumab based on postoperative circulating tumor DNA status (NCT03832569) and neoadjuvant nivolumab/ipilimumab, which showed a 60% pathologic complete response (pCR) rate.[12]

Roughly 3% of metastatic EG ACs are MSI-H, which is predictive of poor survival outcomes with chemotherapy alone and a remarkable OS

Table 1
Frontline immunotherapy trials in esophageal adenocarcinoma

Study Name	KEYNOTE-062	CheckMate 649	ORIENT-16	ATTRACTION-4
Study design	Pembrolizumab vs chemo pembrolizumab/ chemo vs chemo	Nivolumab/chemo vs chemo	Sintilimab/chemo vs chemo	Nivolumab/ chemo vs chemo
Study population	United States/Europe/ Australia	United States/ Asia/Other	China	Japan/ South Korea/ Taiwan
PD-L1 CPS	37% CPS $\geq$10	60% CPS $\geq$5	62% CPS $\geq$5	NA
OS HR	CPS $\geq$1 0.91 (0.69–1.18) CPS $\geq$1 0.85 (0.70–1.03)	ITT 0.79 (0.71–0.88) CPS $\geq$5 0.71 (0.59–0.86) CPS <5 0.94 (0.78–1.13)	ITT 0.77 (0.63–0.94) CPS $\geq$5 0.66 (0.51–0.86)	ITT 0.90 (0.75–1.08)
PFS HR ITT	CPS $\geq$1 1.66 (1.37–2.01) CPS $\geq$1 0.84 (0.70–1.02)	0.79 (0.70–0.89)	0.64 (0.53–0.77)	0.68 (0.51–0.90)
ORR ITT	15% vs 37% 49% vs 37%	58% vs 46%	58% vs 48%	57% vs 48%
Grade 3–5 AEs	17% vs 69% 73% vs 69%	60% vs 44%	60% vs 52%	58% vs 49%

benefit with frontline immunotherapy.[13–15] In CheckMate 649, both nivolumab plus chemotherapy and nivolumab plus ipilimumab led to a dramatic improvement in OS compared with chemotherapy (HR 0.38 and 0.28, respectively). Data from KEYNOTE-062 suggests a chemotherapy-free strategy may be considered in select patients with low volume MSI-H disease (pembrolizumab vs chemotherapy: OS HR 0.29 [95% CI 0.11–0.81]; pembrolizumab plus chemotherapy vs chemotherapy: OS HR 0.37 [95% CI 0.14–0.97]). 24-month OS rates approximated 70% in the pembrolizumab arms versus 26% in the chemotherapy arm.[16]

Immunotherapy in Later Lines of Therapy

Pembrolizumab was initially approved in patients with PD-L1-positive chemotherapy refractory AC based on nonrandomized data.[17] Subsequent confirmatory studies failed to demonstrate superiority over chemotherapy (HR 0.82, 95% CI 0.66–1.03), and therefore the approval for third line pembrolizumab in AC was withdrawn.[18] Of note, nivolumab is approved in Asia in heavily pretreated patients with gastric/GEJ AC, irrespective of PD-L1 status, based on an improvement in OS with nivolumab versus placebo (HR 0.63, 95% CI 0.51–0.78).[19]

Targeting Human Epidermal Growth Factor Receptor 2 in the Frontline Setting

Human epidermal growth factor receptor 2 (HER2) overexpression and amplification occur in ~20%

of EG AC.[20–23] Per guidelines jointly devised by the American Society of Clinical Oncology and College of American Pathologists, HER2 positivity is defined as immunohistochemistry (IHC) 3+ or IHC 2+ with fluorescence in situ hybridization (FISH) positivity (ratio of HER2 to centromere (CEP17) signal $\geq$2).[24]

The benefit of HER2-targeted therapy in EG AC was first established by the seminal ToGA study, which showed improved outcomes with the addition of trastuzumab, a monoclonal anti-HER2 antibody, to standard chemotherapy.[25] Preclinical and clinical data provide convincing rationale for combined immunotherapy and HER2-targeted therapy. HER2 receptor internalization and cross-presentation by dendritic cells drive HER2-specific T-cell responses.[26–28] Trastuzumab also increases tumor expression of PD-1 and PD-L1, which may diminish T-cell response and mediate trastuzumab resistance.[29]

The combination of pembrolizumab, trastuzumab, and chemotherapy demonstrated promising activity with response rates nearing or exceeding 80% in 2 separate phase II studies conducted in the United States and Korea.[30,31] These results were confirmed in the practice-changing phase III KEYNOTE-811 trial.[32] Preplanned interim analysis of the first 264 participants demonstrated a significant improvement in ORR (74% vs 52%). More patients in the pembrolizumab group achieved a CR (11% vs 3%) and had durable response lasting 6 months or greater (70% vs

61%). A greater improvement in ORR was seen in the PD-L1 CPS of 1 or greater cohort compared with the CPS of less than 1 cohort (25% vs 5%) but there was overlap in 95% CI between the 2 subgroups, and only 35 (16%) patients had a PD-L1 CPS of less than 1. There was a similar incidence of AEs in the 2 arms, with diarrhea, nausea, and anemia being the most common events. Based on these findings, the FDA granted accelerated approval to pembrolizumab in combination with trastuzumab and chemotherapy for the treatment of unresectable or metastatic HER2-positive gastric and GEJ AC in May 2021. Patients with preexisting heart failure were excluded from these studies, and we would generally avoid HER2-targeted therapy in patients with symptomatic heart failure, valvular disease, and severe conduction abnormalities.

Other novel anti-HER2 agents are under investigation. For example, zanidatamab (ZW25), a humanized bispecific antibody directed against both the juxtamembrane extracellular domain and dimerization domain of HER2, showed promising activity in a phase I study and is being evaluated in combination with chemotherapy in an ongoing phase II study (NCT03929666).[33]

Targeting HER2 in Subsequent Lines of Therapy

Until recently, there was no strong evidence to support continued anti-HER2 therapy after progression on a first-line trastuzumab-containing regimen. Studies failed to show any benefit for continuation of trastuzumab, lapatinib, or ado-trastuzumab emtansine over taxane chemotherapy, possibly due to loss of tumoral HER2 expression, which has been observed in up to 70% of patients.[34–38] Fam-trastuzumab deruxtecan (T-DXd) is a novel antibody–drug conjugate (ADC) composed of an anti-HER2 antibody attached by a cleavable peptide-based linker to a topoisomerase I inhibitor that is 10 times more potent than irinotecan. With a high drug-to-antibody ratio approaching 8 and membrane permeable payload, T-DXd may lead to increased antitumor activity via a significant cytotoxic bystander effect regardless of HER2 expression.[39]

The open label, randomized, phase II DESTINY-Gastric01 trial showed a significant improvement in ORR (51% vs 14%), PFS (HR 0.47, 95% CI 0.31–0.71), and OS (HR 0.59, 95% CI 0.39–0.88) with T-DXd versus either irinotecan or paclitaxel in patients with HER2-positive gastric/GEJ AC who have received a prior trastuzumab-based regimen, leading to FDA approval of T-DXd for this indication.[40] The most common Grade 3 to 4

treatment-related AEs include neutropenia, anemia, thrombocytopenia, and interstitial lung disease (ILD). Fatal cases of ILD have been reported in patients with colorectal cancer treated with T-DXd, and treatment should be permanently discontinued for Grade 2 or higher pneumonitis/ILD. The follow-up DESTINY-Gastric02 study conducted in Europe and the United States confirmed the activity of T-DXd in a Western population.[41] **Table 2** lists other novel anti-HER2 strategies under investigation.

ESOPHAGEAL SQUAMOUS CELL CARCINOMA
Frontline Therapy

On a genomic level, esophageal SCC more closely resembles SCC arising from other organs than esophageal AC. Data from the previously discussed KEYNOTE-590 trial lends support to first-line chemotherapy plus immunotherapy in advanced esophageal SCC. CheckMate 648 further explored a frontline chemotherapy-free strategy. In this study, 970 patients with advanced esophageal SCC were randomized 1:1:1 to receive nivolumab plus chemotherapy, nivolumab plus ipilimumab, or chemotherapy alone.[42] There was a significant OS benefit observed with nivolumab plus chemotherapy (HR 0.54, 95% CI 0.37–0.80, $P < .0001$) and nivolumab plus ipilimumab (HR 0.64, 95% CI 0.46–0.90, $P = .0010$) compared with chemotherapy alone in the 49% of patients with PD-L1-positive disease (defined as tumor proportion score [TPS] $\geq 1\%$). Notably, the CR rate was 3-fold higher in the nivolumab-containing arms (nivolumab plus chemotherapy 16%, nivolumab plus ipilimumab 18%, chemotherapy 5%). However, there was crossover of the survival curves in the nivolumab plus ipilimumab arm, reflecting an increased incidence of early death among patients who had rapid disease progression on a chemotherapy-free regimen. In our opinion, we would only consider the use of nivolumab plus ipilimumab in the presence of minimal disease burden or in a patient who refuses or is unable to tolerate chemotherapy.

Among patients with PD-L1-negative disease, there was no survival benefit with immunotherapy compared with chemotherapy. The survival outcomes were similar when the subgroups were stratified according to PD-L1 CPS; the highest degree of benefit was seen in the PD-L1 CPS of 10 or greater population, as observed in KEYNOTE-590. A recent systematic review and meta-analysis of studies conducted in esophageal SCC came to a similar conclusion and found minimal to no benefit with the addition of immunotherapy in the PD-L1 CPS of less than 10 population.[43]

Table 2
Ongoing trials evaluating anti-HER2 therapy in second-line setting and beyond

Trial Number	Phase	Study Population	Study Treatment	Mechanism of Action	Status
NCT03821233	I	HER2+ solid tumor	ZW49	Bispecific anti-HER2 ADC (Ab sequence identical to ZW25)	Active, recruiting
NCT04147819	I	HER2+ gastric/GEJ, breast cancer	BAY 2701439	Thorium-227 labeled Ab-chelator conjugate	Active, recruiting
NCT03740256	I	HER2+ solid tumor	CaDVEC + CAR T cell therapy	Oncolytic adenovirus + HER2-specific CAR T cell therapy	Active, recruiting
NCT04704661	I	HER2+ solid tumor	Ceralasertib (AZD6738) + T-DXd	ATR inhibitor	Active, recruiting
NCT05190445	II	HER2+ gastric/GEJ cancer	Cinrebafusp Alfa (PRS-343) + ramucirumab, paclitaxel	Bispecific molecule against HER2 and CD137	Active, recruiting
NCT05002127	II/III	HER2+ gastric/GEJ cancer	Evorpacept (ALX148) + ramucirumab, paclitaxel, trastuzumab vs ramucirumab, paclitaxel ± trastuzumab	CD47 blocker	Active, recruiting
NCT04499924	II/III	HER2+ gastric/GEJ cancer	Tucatinib, trastuzumab, ramucirumab, and paclitaxel vs ramucirumab and paclitaxel	HER2 tyrosine kinase inhibitor	Active, recruiting

Three separate phase III trials conducted in Asia lend further support to combined immunotherapy plus chemotherapy in advanced esophageal SCC. ESCORT-1st, ORIENT 15, and JUPITER-06 all evaluated the addition of a novel anti-PD-1 antibody to cisplatin plus paclitaxel chemotherapy.[44–46] High response rates of 70% to 75% were consistently reported in the combination arms. Considering the limitations of cross-trial comparisons, these figures are numerically higher than the reported ORR in KEYNOTE-590 and CheckMate 648, raising the question of whether a platinum-containing and taxane-containing backbone is more appropriate for esophageal SCC. **Table 3** summarizes the frontline immunotherapy trials in esophageal SCC.

Immunotherapy in Later Lines of Therapy

Nivolumab is approved for second-line treatment of esophageal SCC, regardless of PD-L1 expression, based on data from the ATTRACTION-3 study, which demonstrated a significant improvement in OS with nivolumab versus paclitaxel or docetaxel (HR 0.77, 95% CI 0.62–0.96).[47] Two separate Asian studies, ESCORT and RATIONALE 302, showed similar superiority of the monoclonal anti-PD-1 antibodies camrelizumab and tislelizumab, respectively, over second-line chemotherapy.[48,49]

IMMUNOTHERAPY IN THE PERIOPERATIVE AND ADJUVANT SETTING

The demonstrated activity of immunotherapy in the metastatic setting has garnered interest in earlier use for localized disease. Standard chemoradiation with the concurrent carboplatin and paclitaxel regimen yields a pCR in 49% of patients with esophageal SCC, but only 23% in AC patients.[50] Response in AC may be augmented by using a PET-response adapted strategy.[51] Patients with an incomplete response to neoadjuvant chemoradiation have a high risk of relapse.

In patients with high-risk disease, the median disease-free survival (DFS) doubled from 11.0 to 22.4 months with 1 year of adjuvant nivolumab (HR 0.69, 95% CI 0.56–0.86, $P < .001$) in the CheckMate 577 study. In May 2021, the FDA approved adjuvant nivolumab for patients with residual disease following trimodality therapy, independent of histology or PD-L1 status. Although a survival benefit was observed in both SCC and AC, the degree of benefit was higher among patients with esophageal SCC (HR 0.61, 95% CI 0.42–0.88) compared with those with AC (HR 0.78, 95% CI 0.59–0.96). Post hoc analysis also indicates the survival benefit is driven by the PD-L1

CPS of 5 or greater population (median DFS 29.4 vs 10.2 months, HR 0.62 [95% CI 0.46–0.83]). Only a marginal trend toward improved DFS was seen in patients with CPS of less than 5 (HR 0.89 [95% CI 0.65–1.22]). The approval of adjuvant nivolumab raises the important question of who may still benefit from reintroduction of immunotherapy at the time of disease recurrence.

The use of immune checkpoint inhibition in the neoadjuvant rather than adjuvant setting may further enhance antitumor immunity via increased T cell expansion and diversity, leading to increased interest in perioperative immunotherapy strategies.[52,53] **Table 4** summarizes several of the ongoing trials evaluating immunotherapy for localized EG cancer.

FUTURE TARGETS

Given the molecular similarity between esophageal AC and gastric cancer with chromosomal instability, there is likely overlap in expression of novel biomarkers.[2] Targeted therapies under investigation in gastric and GEJ cancer would have clinical application in esophageal AC.

Claudin 18.2 (CLDN18.2) is a tight junction protein expressed in EG and pancreatic cancers. Zolbetuximab, a chimeric antibody directed against CLDN18.2, has shown promising activity in combination with chemotherapy (ORR 63%; median PFS 13.7 months).[54] The ongoing ILUSTRO study is evaluating zolbetuximab as monotherapy and in combination with immunotherapy or chemotherapy (NCT03505320). Other agents targeting CLDN18.2 are under active investigation, for example, TJ033721, a bispecific antibody targeting CLDN18.2 and the costimulatory molecule 4-1BB (NCT04900818).

Activating fibroblast growth factor receptor 2 (FGFR2) alterations have been documented in 4% to 9% of EG AC.[55,56] The phase II FIGHT trial demonstrated that the addition of bemarituzumab, a monoclonal antibody against FGFR2b, to chemotherapy in patients with untreated FGFR2b-overexpressing or FGFR2b-amplified tumors led to improvements in ORR (53% vs 40%), PFS (HR 0.68, $P = .07$), and OS (HR 0.58, $P = .03$).[57] Clinical benefit seemed to correlate with FGFR2b expression. Findings will be validated in 2 phase III trials. Other FGFR inhibitors are under investigation, such as the fibroblast growth factor receptor 1-3 (FGFR1-3) inhibitor derazantinib (NCT04604132).

Epidermal growth factor receptor (EGFR) is overexpressed in approximately 30% of EG cancers, and *EGFR* amplification is detected in 4% to 7% of cases.[2,58–60] EGFR inhibitors for

Table 3
Frontline immunotherapy trials in advanced esophageal SCC

Study Name	KEYNOTE-590	CheckMate 648	ESCORT-1st	ORIENT-15	JUPITER-06
Study design	Pembrolizumab/chemo vs chemo	Nivolumab/chemo vs chemo Nivolumab/ipilimumab vs chemo	Camrelizumab/chemo vs chemo	Sintilimab/chemo vs chemo	Toripalimab/chemo vs chemo
Study population	53% Asia	70% Asia	China	China	China
PD-L1 CPS	51% CPS ≥10	30% TPS ≥10	34% TPS ≥10	58% CPS ≥10; 36% TPS ≥10	NA
OS HR	ITT 0.73 (0.63–0.86) CPS ≥10 0.64 (051–0.80)	0.74 (0.58–0.96) 0.78 (0.62–0.98)	ITT 0.70 (0.56–0.88) TPS ≥10% 0.52 (0.35–0.79) TPS <10% 0.78 (0.59–1.02)	ITT 0.63 (0.51–0.78) CPS ≥10 0.64 (0.48–0.85)	0.58 (0.43–0.78)
PFS HR ITT	ITT 0.64 (0.55–0.75) CPS ≥10 0.51 (0.41–0.65)	0.81 (0.64–1.04) 1.02 (0.73–1.43)	0.56 (0.46–0.68)	0.56 (0.46–0.67)	0.58 (0.46–0.74)
ORR ITT	45% vs 29%	47% vs 27% 28% vs 27%	72% vs 62%	76% vs 57%	NA
Grade 3–5 AEs	86% vs 83%	49% vs 37% 34% vs 37%	63% vs 68%	60% vs 54%	73% vs 70%

Table 4
Ongoing immunotherapy trials for localized esophagogastric cancer

Name	Trial Number	Phase	Study Population	Study Treatment	Status
KEYNOTE-585	NCT03221426	III	Gastric/GEJ adenocarcinoma	Perioperative cisplatin and 5-FU or capecitabine ± pembrolizumab	Active, not recruiting
MATTERHORN	NCT04592913	III	Gastric/GEJ adenocarcinoma	Perioperative FLOT ± durvalumab	Active, recruiting
VESTIGE	NCT03443856	II	Gastric/GEJ adenocarcinoma	Preoperative chemotherapy → adjuvant chemotherapy vs ipilimumab/nivolumab	Active, recruiting
KEYNOTE-975	NCT04210115	III	Esophageal/GEJ SCC, adenocarcinoma	Definitive CRT (FOLFOX or cisplatin/5-FU) +/− pembrolizumab	Active, recruiting
SKYSCRAPER-07	NCT04543617	III	Esophageal SCC	Atezolizumab ± tiragolumab (anti-TIGIT Ab) after definitive CRT	Active, recruiting
—	NCT02962063	Ib/II	Esophageal/GEJ adenocarcinoma	Induction chemotherapy + durvalumab + tremelimumab with CRT	Active, recruiting
—	NCT04391049	I	Esophageal/GEJ SCC, adenocarcinoma (medically inoperable)	Definitive CRT (carboplatin, paclitaxel) + intratumoral telomelysin (oncolytic virus)	Active, recruiting

example, cetuximab and panitumumab, have produced disappointing results in unselected patients but may have meaningful activity in those with *EGFR*-amplified tumors (ORR 43% in one retrospective cohort study).[61,62] Moreover, the pan-HER kinase inhibitor afatinib yielded significant tumor regression in patients with coamplification of *ERBB2* and *EGFR*, suggesting added benefit with EGFR inhibition.[63] Based on the available data, we would consider off-protocol EGFR inhibition in patients with *EGFR*-amplified EG cancer if there is no appropriate clinical trial.

FUTURE DIRECTIONS

Combination immunotherapy plus chemotherapy has led to sustained improvements in survival for patients with PD-L1 expressing esophageal cancers. However, roughly 50% of patients will have PD-L1-low or PD-L1-negative disease, and most patients will experience disease progression within 1 year, highlighting the need for newer strategies.

Vascular endothelial growth factor (VEGF) signaling promotes an immunosuppressive tumor microenvironment.[64] Preclinical and clinical data support synergistic antitumor activity with combined VEGFR-2 and PD-1 blockade.[65–67] Several ongoing studies are exploring regorafenib or lenvatinib plus checkpoint inhibition and chemotherapy in the first-line setting (NCT04757363, NCT04662710). Other promising strategies include personalized neoantigen vaccines (NCT03639714) and chimeric antigen receptor (CAR) or modified T cell receptor T cells directed against various biomarkers for example, MUC1, HER2, EpCAM, Claudin18.2, NY-ESO-1, and MAGE-A4 (NCT04044859).

SUMMARY

Progress and innovation in the treatment of esophageal cancer has been made in 2021. Chemotherapy plus nivolumab or pembrolizumab represents the new standard of care frontline regimen for patients with advanced esophageal AC and SCC. PD-L1 status is a continuous variable, with the greatest survival benefit from immunotherapy seen in the PD-L1-high population (specifically CPS of 5 or greater in AC). Targeted therapy and immune checkpoint inhibition seem to have synergistic activity in HER2-positive disease, producing dramatic responses and leading to FDA approval of pembrolizumab plus trastuzumab and chemotherapy. Ignited by the success in HER2-positive disease, targeted therapies against Claudin18.2 and FGFR2 are also moving into the frontline arena in combination with chemotherapy and immunotherapy. With a growing armamentarium of treatment options, biomarker selection remains critical and should be routinely performed.

CLINICS CARE POINTS

- Biomarker testing including MMR, PD-L1, and HER2 expression should be obtained in all patients with newly diagnosed esophageal cancer.
- Chemotherapy plus anti-PD-1 therapy represents the new standard of care frontline regimen for advanced esophageal adenocarcinoma and squamous cell carcinoma.
- PD-L1 status is a continuous variable, with the greatest survival benefit from immunotherapy seen in the PD-L1-high population (specifically CPS of 5 or greater in esophageal adenocarcinoma).
- Anti-PD-1 therapy in combination with chemotherapy and trastuzumab is the emerging new standard for HER2-positive esophageal adenocarcinoma.
- Fam-trastuzumab deruxtecan is approved for second-line treatment of patients with HER2-positive disease who have received a prior trastuzumab-based regimen.

DISCLOSURE

J. Yang: No relevant disclosures. J.Y. Yelena: Reports receiving research funding from Bayer, Bristol Myers Squibb, Cycle for Survival, Department of Defense, Fred's Team, Genentech/Roche Lilly, Merck & Co, National Cancer Institute, and Rgenix; serving as a consultant or in an advisory role for Basilea Pharmaceutical, Bayer, Bristol Myers Squibb, Daiichi Sankyo, Imugene, Lilly, Merck, Merck Serono, Michael J Hennessy Associates, Paradigm Medical Communications, Pfizer, Rgenix, Seagen, and Zymeworks; receiving stock options from Rgenix; and nonfinancial relationships with Clinical Care Options, Axis Medical Education, and Research to Practice.

REFERENCES

1. Sung H, Ferlay J, Siegel RL, et al. Global cancer statistics 2020: GLOBOCAN estimates of incidence and mortality worldwide for 36 cancers in 185 countries. CA Cancer J Clin 2021;71(3):209–49.

2. Cancer Genome Atlas Research N, Analysis Working Group, Asan U, Agency BCC, et al. Integrated genomic characterization of oesophageal carcinoma. Nature 2017;541(7636):169–75.
3. Hato SV, Khong A, de Vries IJ, et al. Molecular pathways: the immunogenic effects of platinum-based chemotherapeutics. Clin Cancer Res 2014;20(11):2831–7.
4. Janjigian YY, Shitara K, Moehler M, et al. First-line nivolumab plus chemotherapy versus chemotherapy alone for advanced gastric, gastro-oesophageal junction, and oesophageal adenocarcinoma (CheckMate 649): a randomised, open-label, phase 3 trial. Lancet 2021;398(10294):27–40.
5. Shitara K, Ajani JA, Moehler M, et al. Nivolumab plus chemotherapy or ipilimumab in gastro-oesophageal cancer. Nature 2022;603(7903):942–8.
6. Janjigian YY, Bendell J, Calvo E, et al. CheckMate-032 study: efficacy and safety of nivolumab and nivolumab plus ipilimumab in patients with metastatic esophagogastric cancer. J Clin Oncol 2018;36(28):2836–44.
7. Sun JM, Shen L, Shah MA, et al. Pembrolizumab plus chemotherapy versus chemotherapy alone for first-line treatment of advanced oesophageal cancer (KEYNOTE-590): a randomised, placebo-controlled, phase 3 study. Lancet 2021;398(10302):759–71.
8. Xu J, Jiang H, Pan Y, et al. Sintilimab plus chemotherapy (chemo) versus chemo as first-line treatment for advanced gastric or gastroesophageal junction (G/GEJ) adenocarcinoma (ORIENT-16): First results of a randomized, double-blind, phase III study. Ann Oncol 2021;32(supplement 5):S1331.
9. Boku N, Ryu MH, Oh D-Y, et al. Nivolumab plus chemotherapy versus chemotherapy alone in patients with previously untreated advanced or recurrence gastric/gastroesophageal junction (G/GEJ) cancer: ATTRACTION-4 (ONO-4538-37) study. Ann Oncol 2020;31(suppl_4):S1142–215.
10. Zhao JJ, Yap DWT, Chan YH, et al. Low Programmed Death-Ligand 1-Expressing Subgroup Outcomes of First-Line Immune Checkpoint Inhibitors in Gastric or Esophageal Adenocarcinoma. J Clin Oncol 2022;40(4):392–402.
11. Pietrantonio F, Miceli R, Raimondi A, et al. Individual patient data meta-analysis of the value of microsatellite instability as a biomarker in gastric cancer. J Clin Oncol 2019;37(35):3392–400.
12. Andre T, Tougeron D, Piessen G, et al. Neoadjuvant nivolumab plus ipilimumab and adjuvant nivolumab in patients (pts) with localized microsatellite instability-high (MSI)/mismatch repair deficient (dMMR) oeso-gastric adenocarcinoma (OGA): The GERCOR NEONIPIGA phase II study. J Clin Oncol 2022;40(4):244.
13. Bonneville R, Krook MA, Kautto EA, et al. Landscape of Microsatellite Instability Across 39 Cancer Types. JCO Precis Oncol 2017;2017.
14. Chao J, Fuchs CS, Shitara K, et al. Assessment of pembrolizumab therapy for the treatment of microsatellite instability-high gastric or gastroesophageal junction cancer among patients in the KEYNOTE-059, KEYNOTE-061, and KEYNOTE-062 clinical trials. JAMA Oncol 2021;7(6):895–902.
15. Janjigian YY, Sanchez-Vega F, Jonsson P, et al. Genetic predictors of response to systemic therapy in esophagogastric cancer. Cancer Discov 2018;8(1):49–58.
16. Shitara K, Van Cutsem E, Bang YJ, et al. Efficacy and safety of pembrolizumab or pembrolizumab plus chemotherapy vs chemotherapy alone for patients with first-line, advanced gastric cancer: the KEYNOTE-062 phase 3 randomized clinical trial. JAMA Oncol 2020;6(10):1571–80.
17. Fuchs CS, Doi T, Jang RW, et al. Safety and efficacy of pembrolizumab monotherapy in patients with previously treated advanced gastric and gastroesophageal junction cancer: phase 2 clinical KEYNOTE-059 Trial. JAMA Oncol 2018;4(5):e180013.
18. Fuchs CS, Ozguroglu M, Bang YJ, et al. Pembrolizumab versus paclitaxel for previously treated PD-L1-positive advanced gastric or gastroesophageal junction cancer: 2-year update of the randomized phase 3 KEYNOTE-061 trial. Gastric Cancer 2022;25(1):197–206.
19. Kang YK, Boku N, Satoh T, et al. Nivolumab in patients with advanced gastric or gastro-oesophageal junction cancer refractory to, or intolerant of, at least two previous chemotherapy regimens (ONO-4538-12, ATTRACTION-2): a randomised, double-blind, placebo-controlled, phase 3 trial. Lancet 2017;390(10111):2461–71.
20. Yoon HH, Shi Q, Sukov WR, et al. Adverse prognostic impact of intratumor heterogeneous HER2 gene amplification in patients with esophageal adenocarcinoma. J Clin Oncol 2012;30(32):3932–8.
21. Gowryshankar A, Nagaraja V, Eslick GD. HER2 status in Barrett's esophagus & esophageal cancer: a meta analysis. J Gastrointest Oncol 2014;5(1):25–35.
22. Koopman T, Smits MM, Louwen M, et al. HER2 positivity in gastric and esophageal adenocarcinoma: clinicopathological analysis and comparison. J Cancer Res Clin Oncol 2015;141(8):1343–51.
23. Plum PS, Gebauer F, Kramer M, et al. HER2/neu (ERBB2) expression and gene amplification correlates with better survival in esophageal adenocarcinoma. BMC Cancer 2019;19(1):38.
24. Bartley AN, Washington MK, Colasacco C, et al. HER2 testing and clinical decision making in gastroesophageal adenocarcinoma: guideline from the college of american pathologists, american society for clinical pathology, and the american society of clinical oncology. J Clin Oncol 2017;35(4):446–64.
25. Bang YJ, Van Cutsem E, Feyereislova A, et al. Trastuzumab in combination with chemotherapy versus chemotherapy alone for treatment of HER2-positive

advanced gastric or gastro-oesophageal junction cancer (ToGA): a phase 3, open-label, randomised controlled trial. Lancet 2010;376(9742):687–97.

26. Park S, Jiang Z, Mortenson ED, et al. The therapeutic effect of anti-HER2/neu antibody depends on both innate and adaptive immunity. Cancer Cell 2010;18(2):160–70.

27. Gall VA, Philips AV, Qiao N, et al. Trastuzumab increases HER2 uptake and cross-presentation by dendritic cells. Cancer Res 2017;77(19):5374–83.

28. Taylor C, Hershman D, Shah N, et al. Augmented HER-2 specific immunity during treatment with trastuzumab and chemotherapy. Clin Cancer Res 2007; 13(17):5133–43.

29. Chaganty BKR, Qiu S, Gest A, et al. Trastuzumab upregulates PD-L1 as a potential mechanism of trastuzumab resistance through engagement of immune effector cells and stimulation of IFNgamma secretion. Cancer Lett 2018;430:47–56.

30. Janjigian YY, Maron SB, Chatila WK, et al. First-line pembrolizumab and trastuzumab in HER2-positive oesophageal, gastric, or gastro-oesophageal junction cancer: an open-label, single-arm, phase 2 trial. Lancet Oncol 2020;21(6):821–31.

31. Rha SY, Lee C-K, Kim HS, et al. A multi-institutional phase Ib/II trial of first-line triplet regimen (Pembrolizumab, Trastuzumab, Chemotherapy) for HER2-positive advanced gastric and gastroesophageal junction cancer (PANTHERA Trial): Molecular profiling and clinical update. J Clin Oncol 2021;39: 218.

32. Janjigian YY, Kawazoe A, Yanez P, et al. The KEYNOTE-811 trial of dual PD-1 and HER2 blockade in HER2-positive gastric cancer. Nature 2021;600(7890):727–30.

33. Meric-Bernstam F, Hamilton EP, Beeram M, et al. Zanidatamab (ZW25) in HER2-expressing gastroesophageal adenocarcinoma (GEA): Results from a phase I study. J Clin Oncol 2021;39(3):164.

34. Makiyama A, Sukawa Y, Kashiwada T, et al. Randomized, phase II study of trastuzumab beyond progression in patients with HER2-positive advanced gastric or gastroesophageal junction cancer: WJOG7112G (T-ACT Study). J Clin Oncol 2020; 38(17):1919–27.

35. Satoh T, Xu RH, Chung HC, et al. Lapatinib plus paclitaxel versus paclitaxel alone in the second-line treatment of HER2-amplified advanced gastric cancer in Asian populations: TyTAN–a randomized, phase III study. J Clin Oncol 2014;32(19):2039–49.

36. Thuss-Patience PC, Shah MA, Ohtsu A, et al. Trastuzumab emtansine versus taxane use for previously treated HER2-positive locally advanced or metastatic gastric or gastro-oesophageal junction adenocarcinoma (GATSBY): an international randomised, open-label, adaptive, phase 2/3 study. Lancet Oncol 2017;18(5):640–53.

37. Seo S, Ryu MH, Park YS, et al. Loss of HER2 positivity after anti-HER2 chemotherapy in HER2-positive gastric cancer patients: results of the GASTric cancer HER2 reassessment study 3 (GASTHER3). Gastric Cancer 2019;22(3):527–35.

38. Pietrantonio F, Caporale M, Morano F, et al. HER2 loss in HER2-positive gastric or gastroesophageal cancer after trastuzumab therapy: Implication for further clinical research. Int J Cancer 2016; 139(12):2859–64.

39. Ogitani Y, Hagihara K, Oitate M, et al. Bystander killing effect of DS-8201a, a novel anti-human epidermal growth factor receptor 2 antibody-drug conjugate, in tumors with human epidermal growth factor receptor 2 heterogeneity. Cancer Sci 2016; 107(7):1039–46.

40. Shitara K, Bang YJ, Iwasa S, et al. Trastuzumab deruxtecan in previously treated HER2-positive gastric cancer. N Engl J Med 2020;382(25): 2419–30.

41. Cutsem EV, Di Bartolomeo M, Smyth E, et al. Primary analysis of a phase II single-arm trial of trastuzumab deruxtecan (T-DXd) in western patients (Pts) with HER2-positive (HER2+) unresectable or metastatic gastric or gastroesophageal junction (GEJ) cancer who progressed on or after a trastuzumab-containing regimen. Ann Oncol 2021;21(suppl_5): S1283–346.

42. Doki Y, Ajani JA, Kato K, et al. Nivolumab combination therapy in advanced esophageal squamous-cell carcinoma. N Engl J Med 2022;386(5):449–62.

43. Leone AG, Petrelli F, Ghidini A, et al. Efficacy and activity of PD-1 blockade in patients with advanced esophageal squamous cell carcinoma: a systematic review and meta-analysis with focus on the value of PD-L1 combined positive score. ESMO Open 2022; 7(1):100380.

44. Luo H, Lu J, Bai Y, et al. Effect of Camrelizumab vs Placebo Added to Chemotherapy on Survival and Progression-Free Survival in Patients With Advanced or Metastatic Esophageal Squamous Cell Carcinoma: The ESCORT-1st Randomized Clinical Trial. JAMA 2021;326(10):916–25.

45. Shen L, Lu Z, Wang J, et al. Sintilimab plus chemotherapy versus chemotherapy as first-line therapy in patients with advanced or metastatic esophageal squamous cell cancer: First results of the phase III ORIENT-15 study. Ann Oncol 2021;32(suppl_5): S1283–346.

46. Wang ZX, Cui C, Yao J, et al. Toripalimab plus chemotherapy in treatment-naive, advanced esophageal squamous cell carcinoma (JUPITER-06): A multi-center phase 3 trial. Cancer Cell 2022;40(3): 277–288 e273.

47. Kato K, Cho BC, Takahashi M, et al. Nivolumab versus chemotherapy in patients with advanced oesophageal squamous cell carcinoma refractory or

intolerant to previous chemotherapy (ATTRACTION-3): a multicentre, randomised, open-label, phase 3 trial. Lancet Oncol 2019;20(11):1506–17.

48. Huang J, Xu J, Chen Y, et al. Camrelizumab versus investigator's choice of chemotherapy as second-line therapy for advanced or metastatic oesophageal squamous cell carcinoma (ESCORT): a multicentre, randomised, open-label, phase 3 study. Lancet Oncol 2020;21(6):832–42.

49. Shen L, Kato K, Kim S-B, et al. RATIONALE 302: Randomized, phase 3 study of tislelizumab versus chemotherapy as second-line treatment for advanced unresectable/metastatic esophageal squamous cell carcinoma. J Clin Oncol 2021;39. 15_suppl abstr 4012.

50. van Hagen P, Hulshof MC, van Lanschot JJ, et al. Preoperative chemoradiotherapy for esophageal or junctional cancer. N Engl J Med 2012;366(22): 2074–84.

51. Goodman KA, Ou FS, Hall NC, et al. Randomized phase II Study of PET response-adapted combined modality therapy for esophageal cancer: mature results of the CALGB 80803 (Alliance) trial. J Clin Oncol 2021;39(25):2803–15.

52. Rozeman EA, Menzies AM, van Akkooi ACJ, et al. Identification of the optimal combination dosing schedule of neoadjuvant ipilimumab plus nivolumab in macroscopic stage III melanoma (OpACIN-neo): a multicentre, phase 2, randomised, controlled trial. Lancet Oncol 2019;20(7):948–60.

53. Janjigian YY, Wolchok JD, Ariyan CE. Eradicating micrometastases with immune checkpoint blockade: Strike while the iron is hot. Cancer Cell 2021;39(6):738–42.

54. Klempner SJ, Lee K-W, Metges J-P, et al. Phase 2 study of zolbetuximab plus mFOLFOX6 in claudin 18.2-positive locally advanced or metastatic gastric or gastroesophageal junction adenocarcinoma (G/GEJ): ILUSTRO cohort 2. J Clin Oncol 2021; 39(15):e16063.

55. Deng N, Goh LK, Wang H, et al. A comprehensive survey of genomic alterations in gastric cancer reveals systematic patterns of molecular exclusivity and co-occurrence among distinct therapeutic targets. Gut 2012;61(5):673–84.

56. Klempner SJ, Madison R, Pujara V, et al. FGFR2-Altered Gastroesophageal Adenocarcinomas Are an Uncommon Clinicopathologic Entity with a Distinct Genomic Landscape. Oncologist 2019; 24(11):1462–8.

57. Wainberg ZA, Enzinger PC, Kang Y-K, et al. Randomized double-blind placebo-controlled phase 2 study of bemarituzumab combined with modified FOLFOX6 (mFOLFOX6) in first-line (1L) treatment of advanced gastric/gastroesophageal junction adenocarcinoma (FIGHT). J Clin Oncol 2021;39: 160.

58. Wang KL, Wu TT, Choi IS, et al. Expression of epidermal growth factor receptor in esophageal and esophagogastric junction adenocarcinomas: association with poor outcome. Cancer 2007; 109(4):658–67.

59. Maron SB, Alpert L, Kwak HA, et al. Targeted therapies for targeted populations: anti-EGFR treatment for EGFR-amplified gastroesophageal adenocarcinoma. Cancer Discov 2018;8(6):696–713.

60. Petty RD, Dahle-Smith A, Stevenson DAJ, et al. Gefitinib and EGFR gene copy number aberrations in esophageal cancer. J Clin Oncol 2017;35(20): 2279–87.

61. Lordick F, Kang Y-K, Salman P, et al. Clinical coutcome according to tumor HER2 status and EGFR expression in advanced gastric cancer patients from the EXPAND study. J Clin Oncol 2013;31(15): 4021.

62. Maron SB, Moya S, Morano F, et al. Epidermal growth factor receptor inhibition in epidermal growth factor receptor-amplified gastroesophageal cancer: retrospective global experience. J Clin Oncol 2022;40:2458–67.

63. Sanchez-Vega F, Hechtman JF, Castel P, et al. EGFR and MET amplifications determine response to HER2 inhibition in ERBB2-amplified esophagogastric cancer. Cancer Discov 2019;9(2):199–209.

64. Ott PA, Hodi FS, Buchbinder EI. Inhibition of immune checkpoints and vascular endothelial growth factor as combination therapy for metastatic melanoma: an overview of rationale, preclinical evidence, and initial clinical data. Front Oncol 2015;5:202.

65. Doleschel D, Hoff S, Koletnik S, et al. Regorafenib enhances anti-PD1 immunotherapy efficacy in murine colorectal cancers and their combination prevents tumor regrowth. J Exp Clin Cancer Res 2021;40(1):288.

66. Nakajima TE, Kadowaki S, Minashi K, et al. Multicenter phase I/II study of nivolumab combined with paclitaxel plus ramucirumab as second-line treatment in patients with advanced gastric cancer. Clin Cancer Res 2021;27(4):1029–36.

67. Fukuoka S, Hara H, Takahashi N, et al. Regorafenib plus nivolumab in patients with advanced gastric or colorectal cancer: an open-label, dose-escalation, and dose-expansion phase Ib trial (REGONIVO, EPOC1603). J Clin Oncol 2020;38(18):2053–61.

Endoscopic Management of Esophageal Cancer

Akira Dobashi, MD, PhD[a,1], Darrick K. Li, MD, PhD[b,1], Georgios Mavrogenis, MD[c],
Kavel H. Visrodia, MD[d], Fateh Bazerbachi, MD[e,*]

KEYWORDS

- Esophageal cancer • Endoscopy • Endoscopic submucosal dissection • Stent • Curative
- Palliative

KEY POINTS

- Curative endoscopic resection via endoscopic mucosal resection and endoscopic submucosal dissection are options for mucosal (T1a) and selected submucosal (T1b) esophageal cancers.
- Bleeding and perforation are the most common acute adverse events of endoscopic resection while esophageal stricturing may occur as a late adverse event, particularly with circumferential resections.
- Endoscopic placement of partially covered or fully covered self-expanding metal stents is strongly recommended as first-line palliative therapy for dysphagia in nonresectable malignant esophageal cancers.
- Endoscopic techniques offer palliative options in the management of malnutrition, esophagorespiratory fistulas, and tumor-related bleeding.

INTRODUCTION

In 2018, the GLOBOCAN effort estimated that 3.1% of all worldwide newly diagnosed cancer cases were related to esophageal malignancy, which resulted in more than half a million deaths that year.[1] There are 2 subtypes of esophageal cancer—esophageal squamous cell carcinoma (ESCC) and esophageal adenocarcinoma (EAC) with the former accounting for most cases globally and the latter predominating the West. Although surgery has been the traditional curative approach to esophageal malignancies, the significant morbidity associated with surgical interventions has prompted efforts to identify patients who can be treated with a minimally invasive, endoscopic approach. At the other end of the spectrum, patients with advanced malignancy suffer from adverse events requiring palliative interventions, which can be addressed endoscopically. Given these advances, a pragmatic strategy for curative and palliative esophageal cancer therapy can be optimized in a multidisciplinary environment involving gastroenterologists, thoracic surgeons, oncologists, radiation oncologists, palliative medicine specialists, and shared decision-making with patients, in care delivery. This review will discuss endoscopic treatments for the curative and palliative management of esophageal cancer.

[a] Department of Endoscopy, The Jikei University School of Medicine, 3-Chome-25-8 Nishi Shinbashi, Minato City, Tokyo 105-8461, Japan; [b] Department of Medicine, Section of Digestive Diseases, Yale School of Medicine, 333 Cedar Street, New Haven, CT 06510, USA; [c] Division of Hybrid Interventional Endoscopy, Department of Gastroenterology, Mediterraneo Hospital, 8-12, Ilias St. Glyfada, Athens 16675, Greece; [d] Division of Digestive and Liver Diseases, Department of Medicine, Columbia University Irving Medical Center, 630 West 168th Street, New York, NY 10032, USA; [e] CentraCare, Interventional Endoscopy Program, St Cloud Hospital, 1406 6th Avenue North, St Cloud, MN 56303, USA

[1] [†] Dr. Dobashi and Dr. Li are contributed equally.

* Corresponding author.
E-mail address: bazer001@umn.edu

Thorac Surg Clin 32 (2022) 479–495
https://doi.org/10.1016/j.thorsurg.2022.07.005

Abbreviations	
APC	argon plasma coagulation
BE	Barrett's esophagus
CLE	confocal laser endomicroscopy
EAC	esophageal adenocarcinoma
EMR	endoscopic mucosal resection
ESCC	esophageal squamous cell carcinoma
ESD	endoscopic submucosal dissection
EUS	endoscopic ultrasound
EVAC	Endoluminal vacuum-assisted closure
GI	gastrointestinal
HGD	high-grade dysplasia
IEE	Image-enhanced endoscopy
LGD	low-grade dysplasia
LVI	lymphovascular invasion
ME	magnifying endoscopy
NBI	narrow-band imaging
PDT	photodynamic therapy
RFA	radiofrequency ablation
SEMS	Self-expanding metal stents
SESCC	superficial esophageal squamous cell carcinoma
WLE	white-light endoscopy

CURATIVE MANAGEMENT OF ESOPHAGEAL CANCER
Detection

Given the rarity of lymph node metastasis among superficial (ie, intramucosal) esophageal neoplasms, endoscopic therapy approach should be considered.[2] This is justified by equipoise in the risks of metastatic disease and surgical morbidity and/or mortality, applicable for intramucosal ESCC and EAC. Select patients with more invasive cancers (eg, submucosal [T1b] lesions) may also benefit from this minimally invasive treatment particularly in the setting of poor surgical candidacy because the risk of lymph node metastases may be as high as 25% with deep submucosal invasion. Unfortunately, identifying such patients is challenging, given difficulties in characterizing the accurate depth of malignant involvement.

Under high-definition white-light endoscopy (WLE), superficial esophageal cancer typically presents as a flat, isochromatic lesion, which can be difficult to detect at an early stage (**Fig. 1**A).[3] Image-enhanced endoscopy (IEE), including narrow-band imaging (NBI; **Fig. 1**B,C), provides higher accuracy for superficial ESCC (SESCC), with a sensitivity of more than 90% compared with approximately 50% for WLE in select high-risk groups (ie, patients with a histologically proven ESCC or history of ESCC).[4,5] Lugol chromoendoscopy (**Fig. 1**D) has a high detection rate for

SESCC but it is time-consuming and can cause pain and discomfort.[6,7] Thus, IEE is a useful endoscopic screening method for SESCC.[8]

A randomized clinical trial for superficial EAC patients showed similar detection rates of dysplasia/neoplasia using NBI or high-definition WLE.[9] However, fewer biopsies were required when NBI was implemented. To improve the detection of neoplasia in barrett's esophagus (BE), the American Society for Gastrointestinal Endoscopy recommends targeted biopsies with acetic acid chromoendoscopy, IEE with NBI, or endoscope-based confocal laser endomicroscopy (CLE) in contrast to the commonly applied 4-quadrant biopsies at 1 to 2 cm intervals.[10] NBI is most commonly used.

Tumor Staging and Evaluation of Tumor Margins

Accurate staging is critical to identifying appropriate lesions for endoscopic resection (ER). An accurate and effective framework for the staging of ESCC is the Japan Esophageal Society classification, which involves magnifying endoscopy (ME) under IEE to identify abnormal microvessels.[11] Microvessels are classified as type A, B1, B2, and B3 (**Fig. 2**) with 90% accuracy for predicting the depth of invasion.[11] These classes correspond to noncancer, mucosal neoplasia (T1a) with invasion into the epithelium (T1a-EP) or lamina propria

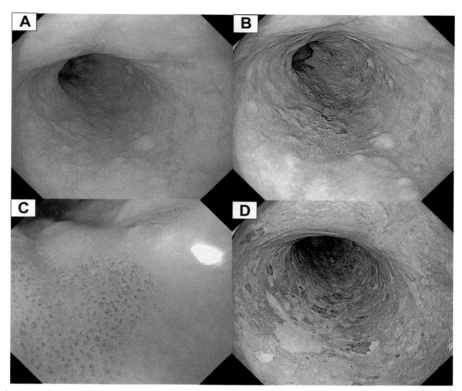

Fig. 1. Endoscopic image of squamous cell carcinoma. (*A*): A slightly reddish lesion was detected at the left wall of the esophagus using WLE. (*B*) NBI demonstrates a well-demarcated brownish area. (*C*) NBI magnification revealed irregular loop-like vessels. Those irregular vessels were classified as type B1. (*D*) Under Lugol chromoendoscopy, the lesion showed an unstained area and turned pinkish in 3 minutes. ESD was performed, and histology showed a T1a-LPM SCC.

(T1a-LPM), T1a lesion with invasion into the muscularis mucosa (T1a-MM) or submucosal neoplasia (T1b) with less than 200 μm submucosal invasion (T1b-SM1), and T1b lesion with more than 200 μm submucosal invasion (T1b-SM2), respectively. It is important to highlight that for EAC, T1b-SM1 implies submucosal neoplasia depth of ≤500 μm, whereas T1b-SM2 is designated when the depth of invasion is >500 μm in the submucosa. Although endoscopic ultrasound (EUS) may, in theory, help improve the assessment of invasion depth,[12] this was not shown in a recent prospective study.[13] May and colleagues reported similar accuracy of invasion depth assessment based on the macroscopic type at 83.4% using WLE and at 79.6% with EUS.[14] Furthermore, a superficial lesion at the esophagogastric junction may be overestimated to involve a deeper extent.[15] Therefore, in the absence of lymph node involvement, EUS may overstage or understage early-stage disease by 20%, and dissuade from a potentially curative ER. In a rare subtype of ESCC (verrucous ESCC), EUS often

overestimated the stage in the assessment of lymph node status possibly due to the heavy inflammatory infiltration seen in this subtype.[16]

CLE or IEE can enhance the demarcation of ESCC tumor margins, and IEE may become an alternative modality for delineating the margin of extent.[17] For EAC, however, IEE with NBI can delineate a clear margin (**Fig. 3**) but some lesions may not show a delineation line because other dysplasia at the margins may coexist and obliterate the demarcation pattern.

Indications for Endoscopic Resection

For ESCC, invasion depth and lateral extension are key factors in determining the appropriate treatment strategy. ER is appropriate for T1a-EP/LPM given the low risk of metastatic disease.[15] Suspected T1a-MM or T1b-SM1 are relative indications for ER given that this strategy will at least serve a diagnostic benefit by providing accurate staging, should the invasion have been underestimated. ER for circumferential lesions increases the

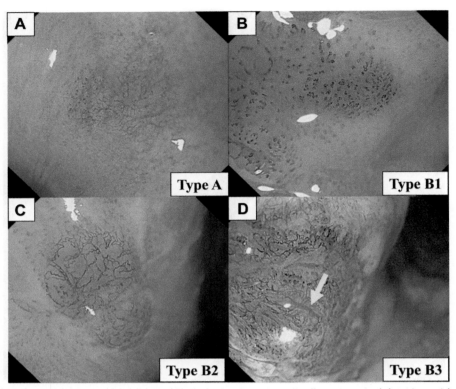

Fig. 2. Magnifying endoscopic classification for superficial squamous cell carcinoma. (*A*) Lesion with abnormal microvessels without severe irregularity classified as type A. (*B*) Lesion with irregular vessels in a loop-like formation classified as type B1. (*C*) Lesion with irregular vessels without a loop-like formation classified as type B2. Pathology with the endoscopically resected lesion showed pT1a-MM. (*D*) Lesion with significantly dilated abnormal vessels (*yellow arrow*) with caliber greater than 3 times that of the B2 vessels classified as type B3 Pathology of the surgically resected lesion showed a pT1b-SM2 SCC.

risk of esophageal stricture formation.[18] Therefore, a longitudinal length of ≤50 mm is recommended, if possible, when ER is prescribed for a circumferential lesion.[15] It is worthy of mentioning that definitive chemoradiation without the risks of esophagectomy is more commonly used in ESCC than EAC.

ER is the first choice for EAC when confined to the mucosa, given the chance of cure with avoidance of esophagectomy. Carefully selected patients with T1b-SM with submucosal EAC, invading < 500 μm, without poor differentiation or lymphovascular invasion (LVI) may be candidates for endoscopic management, with strict close follow-up.[19]

Endoscopic Resection Techniques

Preprocedural considerations

Upper endoscopy can be performed under general anesthesia and endotracheal intubation, conscious sedation, or propofol sedation, depending on the size and extent of the lesion. Carbon dioxide should be used. If available, carbon dioxide is preferred for insufflation to decrease the risk of postprocedural pneumomediastinum.[20]

Endoscopic resection

1. Cap-assisted endoscopic mucosal resection (**Fig. 4**; **Table 1**).

A clear plastic distal attachment (cap) is fitted at the tip of the endoscope.[21] After injection of a lifting agent, a snare is opened and seated inside the cap. The lesion is brought into the cap via continuous suctioning, and the snare is closed around the lesion. High-frequency current is applied to cut the lesion. Although cap-assisted endoscopic mucosal resection (EMR-C) is conceptually simple, seating the snare within the cap can be challenging and may require the use of a snare with a special contour. Moreover, the size of the target lesion is limited by cap diameter.

2. Multiband mucosectomy (**Fig. 5**)

This method uses a modified variceal band ligator that includes a transparent cap with multiple

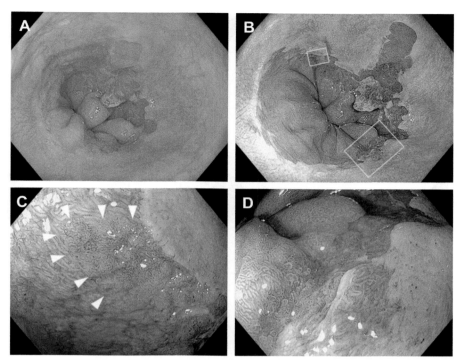

Fig. 3. Endoscopic image of Barrett's adenocarcinoma. (*A*) Under WLE, a slightly depressed lesion was seen at the esophagogastric junction. (*B*) Under NBI, the lesion is seen as a brownish area, (*C, D*) NBI magnification revealed a demarcated line (white arrowheads) between the lesion and surrounding mucosa. Microsurface and microvessels showed irregularity. ESD was performed, and the pathology showed a T1b-SM2 adenocarcinoma.

bands, and a snare passed through the working channel of the endoscope.[22] The target lesion is brought into the cap by continuous suction, and a rubber band is deployed. The rubber band forms a pseudopolyp that is immediately resected, either above or below the rubber band, using a snare with electrocautery. Repeated, overlapping resections can be performed with either cap-assisted or multiband mucosectomy to achieve a wide-field resection. However, the piecemeal nature and risk of esophageal stricturing are disadvantages of these techniques.[23]

3. Endoscopic submucosal dissection (**Fig. 6**)

A single-channel endoscope with a water-jet system (GIF-H290 T or GIF-HQ190, Olympus, Tokyo, Japan) is used. The addition of a distal cap is necessary for scope stability, exerting tension on the submucosal layer, and maintaining a clear view.[24] First, cautery markings are placed a minimum of 2 mm outside the lesion margin. A viscous solution such as glycerol or sodium hyaluronic acid is injected into the submucosal layer to lift the lesion away from the muscularis propria. Next, the initial mucosal incision is initiated, typically beginning from the

gastric (distal) side in a gravity-dependent position. The endoscopist then begins submucosal dissection, by tunneling through the submucosa beneath the lesion. This technique is called the "pocket-creation method"[25] or "tunneling method."[26] Finally, the lesion is completely removed after completing the submucosal circumferential incision.

To achieve optimal dissection, various knives are available and are categorized into 3 types: needle, insulated-tip, and scissors. Some knives provide fluid injection capability. Traction devices enhance the speed and safety of endoscopic submucosal dissection (ESD) particularly during submucosal dissection. This includes the use of a suture or dental floss tied to a hemostatic clip, which is then affixed to the incised edge after deployment of the hemostatic clip (clip-line technique).[27] New innovative approaches, such as magnetic traction, are also being evaluated.[28]

ESD provides a higher rate of *en bloc* resection regardless of size and location, and therefore an accurate histologic assessment.[29] ESD is technically demanding, and the endoscopist should be skilled and have a focused practice to achieve mastery.[30] The rate of delayed bleeding and

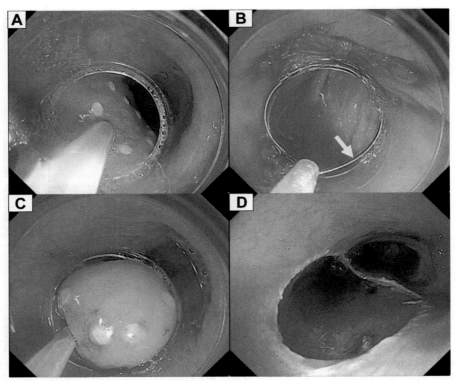

Fig. 4. Endoscopic image of cap-assisted EMR (EMR-C). (*A*) After cautery markings with a needle knife, submucosal injection was performed using an endoscope fitted with a clear oblique cap. (*B*) A snare (*yellow arrow*) was opened inside the cap. (*C*) The lesion was suctioned into the cap, and the snare loop was quickly closed. (*D*) After removing the lesion with a high-frequency current, the mucosal defect was inspected showing no perforation.

stenosis for ESD is reported up to 2% and 17%, respectively, and a meta-analysis showed there was no difference between those for ESD and EMR.[31,32] However, the perforation rate was reported up to 10% with ESD, significantly higher than that of EMR (**Table 2**).

Ablation Therapy

Ablation techniques include argon plasma coagulation (APC),[33] radiofrequency ablation[34] (RFA), and cryotherapy (see **Table 1**). In general, ablative therapy is not first-line for curative treatment of mucosal esophageal cancer but may play a role in select high-risk patients. APC is widely available, with very low postoperative bleeding and perforation rates after ESCC therapy.[33] However, tumor recurrence rates have been reported up to 10%.[33] In contrast, ablation is routinely applied after endoscopic recurrence for EAC as salvage therapy.

RFA involves delivering radiofrequency energy waveforms to destroy target tissues and is the

Table 1
Summary of endoscopic resection and ablation

	Endoscopic Resection	Ablation
Indication	Mucosal cancer Slightly invading submucosal cancer can be a relative indication ($\leq$200 μm for SCC, $\leq$500 μm for EAC)	After ER for LGD/HGD or EAC in BE Frail patients with significant comorbidities
Advantage	Accurate pathology Lower recurrence (Enable R0 resection)	Simple procedure Lower adverse events (perforation)

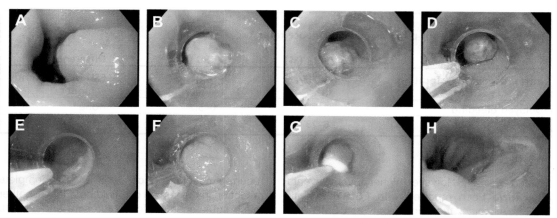

Fig. 5. Endoscopic image of multiband mucosectomy steps (*A-H*).

recommended endoscopic ablative technique for esophageal neoplasia (low-grade dysplasia [LGD], high-grade dysplasia [HGD], and flat intramucosal cancer after visible lesions and nodularity have been endoscopically resected).[35] Cryotherapy ablation (**Fig. 7**) is a more recent application in which an extremely cold gas-filled balloon (eg, liquid nitrogen or carbon dioxide) ablates abnormal tissue while maintaining the extracellular matrix and allowing for an anesthetic effect.[36] This approach potentially permits deeper ablation with a lower rate of stricturing and less discomfort than RFA. Promising cohort data on cryotherapy demonstrate high rates of complete eradication

of intestinal metaplasia and neoplasia.[37] These different therapy modalities offer different penetration depths and thus different profile risks. The cryoablative effect goes beyond the mucosa, unlike RFA. With additional therapy cycles and thus increased penetrative depth, the risk of transmural esophageal injury increases.[38]

Selection of Endoscopic Therapy

1. Endoscopic mucosal resection versus endoscopic submucosal dissection

EMR is associated with a higher local recurrence rate than ESD, estimated for ESCC to be between

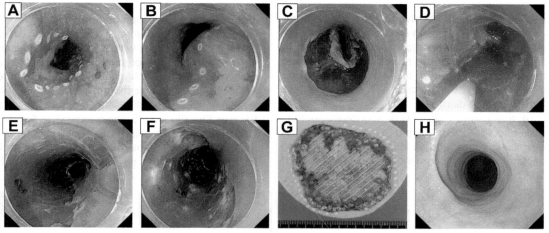

Fig. 6. Endoscopic image of ESD. (*A*) After spraying iodine solution, cautery markings with a needle knife were performed. (*B*) The submucosal injection started from the anal (gastric) side of the lesion. (*C*) A circumferential incision was completed by a needle knife. (*D*) The submucosal injection and submucosal dissection were repeated. (*E*) The mucosal defect was extended almost circumferentially. (*F*) Triamcinolone diluted with normal saline was injected into the remaining submucosal tissue. (*G*) The resected specimen was pinned on the corkboard and contained all markings. After formalin fixation, the lesion was cut into 2 to 3 mm width specimens. Pathology revealed SCC, 48 × 33 mm, 0-IIa, pT1b-SM1 (75 μm), INFb, ly1, v0, pHM0, pVM0, pR0. (*H*) Patient received postresection oral prednisolone and follow-up at 2 months did not show esophageal stricturing.

Table 2
Adverse events in each procedure and incidence rates

	EMR (%)	ESD (%)	Differences
Intraprocedural perforation	0–2.5	0–10	ESD is significantly higher
Delayed bleeding	0.6–11	0–5.2	none
Esophageal stricture	6–23	0–17.2	none

Data from Refs.[31,32,113]

3% and 26%.[29,39] However, higher adverse events rates have been reported with ESD than with EMR.[31] As such, the choice between EMR and ESD should be based on several factors balancing the risks of local recurrence with patient safety, dictated by the size and location of the lesion and local expertise[40] (**Table 3**). According to the European Society of Gastrointestinal Endoscopy, EMR can be an option for ESCC lesions less than 10 mm,[41] whereas ESD should be the first choice for larger lesions. In addition, fibrotic lesions (which may result from previous resection attempts, biopsies, or tumor recurrence) may be better suited for ESD.[42] For EAC, lesions with a bulky component and possible submucosal involvement are better suited for ESD to achieve histopathology staging if not cure.[43]

2. Combined therapies

EMR is limited by the smaller size of the resected specimen and the inability to obtain an accurate margin assessment when piecemeal EMR is performed. Ablative therapy can be combined with EMR, wherein APC or soft coagulation via snare tip or hemostatic forceps is used to ablate the edges of the resection margin. When this technique is added, the local recurrence rate was reported as less than 1% for ESCC less than 20 mm in diameter.[29]

BE associated with HGD or adenocarcinoma in situ should be managed with resection of dysplastic areas and ablation of the remaining background BE segment, given the risk of recurrent dysplasia or cancer even after complete resection in the setting of a field defect.[44] Whether these subsequent lesions represent undetected, metachronous lesions or residual lesions is unclear. However, endoscopic ablative treatment of the remaining BE markedly diminishes the recurrence risk.[34] In addition, a recent study showed the benefit of ablative therapy in patients with BE and LGD to reduce the progression toward HGD or EAC.[45] It is worth mentioning that APC is effective in the eradication of flat BE lesions.[46]

Management of Adverse Events

Bleeding and perforation are the most common acute adverse events of ER. Hemostasis is achieved by applying a coagulation forceps or hemostatic clips. Immediate recognition of perforation during ER is important because it can be addressed with through-the-scope or over-the-scope clips, endoscopic suturing, or esophageal stents. The application of fibrin glue and polyglycolic acids sheets have also been described in addressing postresection perforations.[47]

Postresection stricturing is a late adverse event, and the risk increases with circumferential resections. When the level of stricturing affects greater than 75% of the esophageal circumference after ER for ESCC, local injection of triamcinolone into remaining submucosal tissue immediately after ER (see **Fig. 5**F) is recommended[32] (see **Fig. 6**F). Oral prednisolone has also been used in extensive resections. Oral prednisolone is prescribed at an initial dose of 30 mg on the second day of ER,

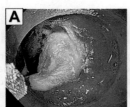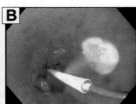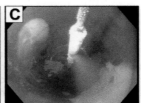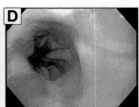

Fig. 7. Endoscopic image of balloon cryotherapy. (*A*) Spray cryotherapy. (*B, C*) Multifocal balloon cryotherapy of residual intestinal metaplasia. (*D*) Cherry-red appearance of mucosa immediately after balloon cryotherapy ablation. (*Courtesy of* Julian A. Abrams, MD, New York, NY.)

Table 3
Summary of endoscopic mucosal resection and endoscopic submucosal dissection

	EMR	ESD
Indication: size	< 10 mm	≥10 mm
Indication: staging	See **Table 1**.	
Advantage	Less technically demanding Shorter-time procedure	Higher *en bloc* resection rate regardless of lesion size Scarred/fibrotic lesions (residual lesion after CRT, near a scar after ER) can be safely removed
Disadvantage	Higher recurrence rate	Demanding technique requiring mastery
Adverse events	Lower	Higher

with a gradual tapering of the dose.[48] Postresection strictures may also be managed with endoscopic balloon dilation and/or radial incision therapies.[49]

Postresection Surveillance

1. Esophageal Squamous Cell Carcinoma

When R0 resection is achieved, and in the absence of LVI, annual endoscopic surveillance is recommended.[15] Metachroncous ESCC lesions were detected in almost 25% of patients within 2 years of ER.[50] Surveillance with IEE or Lugol chromoendoscopy is recommended, given a lower detection rate with WLE alone.[51] Other modalities, including EUS, computed tomography, and tumor markers, can be used to detect metastatic disease in ESCC beyond T1a-MM.

2. Esophageal Adenocarcinoma

After achieving complete eradication of intestinal metaplasia, endoscopic surveillance for patients with HGD or intramucosal carcinoma is recommended every 3 months in the first year, every 6 months in the second year, and annually thereafter.[35]

Recurrence and Management

Local resection failure is defined as residual or recurrent lesion after definitive therapy without lymph node involvement, or distant metastases (cT1N0M0). Repeat ER can be curative in some of these scenarios.[52,53] ER is also offered to nonsurgical candidates who demonstrate recurrent neoplasm with submucosal involvement. However, coexisting fibrosis may increase the adverse events rate, such as perforation.[42] Although with a higher recurrence rate, ablation can become an alternative therapy to avoid deleterious adverse events in these frail patients.[54]

Endoscopic Palliation Techniques in Esophageal Cancer

More than half of all new esophageal cancer cases present with unresectable disease due to invasion depth, distant metastases, or poor patient performance status.[55,56] Moreover, patients experience dysphagia, malnutrition, and may suffer from other adverse events, including gastrointestinal bleeding. Therefore, endoscopic techniques for palliative and supportive facets of esophageal cancer sequelae are important in the care of these patients.

Dysphagia

Self-expanding metal stents
Approximately 75% of patients with esophageal cancer present with dysphagia due to intraluminal obstruction.[57] Self-expanding metal stents (SEMS) are typically made of either nitinol (an alloy of nickel and titanium) or stainless steel and are available in various forms. All stent types can rapidly relieve dysphagia with high technical success.[58] Stent expansion is usually complete within 24 to 48 hours, and patients are allowed to ingest liquids immediately after the procedure, followed by advancement to a low residue diet. Initially, SEMS were developed as uncovered stents but were found to have a significantly higher risk of tumor ingrowth compared with partially (pc) or fully covered (fc) stents (20%–30% vs 3%–4%).[59,60] Given these findings and the relative ease of deployment, placement of pcSEMS or fcSEMS is strongly recommended by multiple international societies as first-line palliative therapy for malignant dysphagia.[61,62]

Stent-related adverse events are common and have been increasing in frequency, in part related to the increasing use of chemoradiotherapy before SEMS placement.[63] Stent-related adverse events can be early (within 4 weeks after stent placement) or delayed (greater than 4 weeks after stent placement).[58] The most frequent immediate adverse events include severe chest pain (2%–35%), which persists for an average of 10 days and typically does not need stent removal.[64] Appropriate stent selection, taking stent diameter/length, expansion force and stricture location into consideration, may help mitigate postprocedural pain. For example, palliative stenting for esophageal cancer is tailored differently than when stenting is needed to seal a perforation. In the latter, using the largest caliber stent is desired, wherein a larger diameter stent may cause significant chest pain without necessarily being conducive to a better quality of life in terms of diet restrictions. Postplacement bleeding in the immediate period can occur but is usually mild and self-limited.

Stent migration is both a common immediate and delayed adverse event and occurs more frequently with covered SEMS (upward of 36%). pcSEMS are uncovered at the flanges, allowing for tissue ingrowth and fixation, reducing migration risk. Antimigration stents, including those with a metal mesh, stent flares, double-layered coverage, and antimigration rings have also been developed, although their clinical efficacy remains in question.[65] Recently, the use of endoscopic suturing[66] or an over-the-scope clip[67] to anchor the stent to the esophageal wall has also been described to decrease migration rates. A recent multicenter study comparing pcSEMS, fcSEMS, and fcSEMS with antimigration fins in patients with malignant dysphagia demonstrated that stent migration occurred less frequently with pcSEMS compared with fcSEMS (25.3% vs 10.9%), and risk of stent migration was increased with stricture negotiability with a 9 mm endoscope or the use of fcSEMS regardless of features.[68]

Tumor ingrowth and recurrent obstruction can complicate SEMS placement, with similar rates seen in fcSEMS and pcSEMS (~20%).[69] Techniques to address recurrent obstruction include overlapping a second stent coaxially, endoscopic clearance of food impaction, and debulking therapies.

Gastroesophageal reflux is a common adverse event, particularly when stenting across the gastroesophageal junction. Symptoms may be refractory to high-dose proton pump inhibitor treatment, and although several antireflux stent designs have been developed, they have been evaluated only in small trials with conflicting results.[70]

For patients who may be candidates for surgical or neoadjuvant chemoradiation, pretreatment SEMS placement is controversial. In a French study where 38 patients with esophageal cancer who underwent SEMS as a bridge to surgery were compared with a propensity-matched control group of 152 patients without stenting. Stented patients had significantly higher morbidity, mortality, lower R0 resections, time to recurrence, and overall survival.[71] SEMS placement in the setting of neoadjuvant therapy was associated with adverse events, including stent migration (30%), chest pain (16%), tumor ingrowth (2%), and esophageal perforation (2%).[72] Moreover, a recent systematic review suggested that SEMS placement in this setting has equivocal effects on nutritional status.[73] Conversely, other studies have shown that SEMS placement effectively relieves dysphagia and improves nutritional status.[74,75] In addition, a recent study of 29 patients with resectable esophageal cancer undergoing SEMS showed that postsurgical mortality and oncological outcomes were not different compared with 71 patients who were only treated with neoadjuvant therapy and esophagectomy.[76] As such, the role of SEMS as a bridge to curative treatment in patients with potentially resectable disease needs to come after a multidisciplinary review involving oncologists, thoracic surgeons, and gastroenterologists.[61]

Endoscopic Brachytherapy

As an alternative to SEMS placement, endoscopic brachytherapy involves direct delivery of high radiation doses with minimal exposure to adjacent healthy tissue. Several trials have demonstrated that while brachytherapy does not result in rapid improvement in dysphagia compared with SEMS, the effect can be quite durable and is associated with a lower risk of serious adverse events.[77,78] However, the use of brachytherapy for the treatment of esophageal cancer has been limited by availability, expertise, and the need for coordination between gastroenterologists and radiation oncologists in the application of treatment.

Recently, irradiation stents preloaded with iodine-125 seeds that aim to combine the benefits of SEMS with intraluminal brachytherapy have been developed. Limited comparative clinical data suggest that irradiation stents are at least as effective as traditional SEMS in palliation of dysphagia but mayimprove overall survival.[79–81] Larger studies in more diverse populations are needed before determining whether these stents will play a more significant role in the endoscopic management of malignant dysphagia.

Debulking Therapies

Various tumor destruction endoscopic techniques can be administered when patients remain symptomatic despite therapy. In this setting, high-energy laser therapy with neodymium-yttrium-aluminum garnet has been the traditional palliative debulking treatment, although it has been supplanted by photodynamic therapy (PDT). In the United States, PDT involves parenteral administration of porfimer sodium, a photosensitizer that accumulates preferentially in tumor cells, followed by exposure of the tumor endoscopically to low power laser, which initiates a photochemical reaction that leads to tumor ischemia and necrosis. PDT and laser therapy offered similar overall efficacy with dysphagia amelioration in a prospective randomized trial, although PDT was associated with fewer perforations and better response for more proximal cancers.[82] The main side effect of PDT is photosensitivity, which has limited its use.

Widely available APC can also play a role in debulking but does not lead to durable symptoms relief. However, it may have a role in combination with other therapies or to manage tumor ingrowth within stents.[83]

Cryotherapy can be used for palliation, where supercooled liquid nitrogen is applied to the tumor and allowed to thaw. The freeze/cool cycles lead to the formation of intracellular and extracellular ice crystals that disrupt cell membranes and lead to the apoptosis of tumor cells. Several studies have suggested that cryotherapy is another technique that is safe and well-tolerated, although prospective comparative studies are still needed to delineate its role in malignant dysphagia management.[84–86]

Malnutrition

Malnutrition is a significant concern in the management of esophageal cancer with important mortality implications.[87,88] In patients with resectable disease, preoperative nutrition optimization is also critical for postsurgical outcomes and quality of life.[88] However, there is little consensus to define the optimal nutritional approach.

When surgery is delayed beyond 4 weeks, endoscopic percutaneous gastrostomy (PEG) placement is often considered, particularly in patients with resectable disease. A prospective study of 86 patients with esophageal cancer comparing SEMS, gastrostomy/jejunostomy, nasogastric tube placement, and oral diet before chemoradiation or surgery found that patients with percutaneous tube feeding had the most improvement in symptoms and quality of life with similar changes in body weight.[89] However, depending on the placement technique, PEG placement in aerodigestive cancer carries a small but serious risk of

tumor seeding to the abdominal wall, and PEG placement using the introducer technique in which the gastrostomy tube does not pass through the oral cavity during placement may avoid stomal tumor seeding.[90] Additional concerns related to preoperative PEG placement include surgical reconstruction, such as the potential disruption of the gastroepiploic artery, which could put the conduit at greater risk for ischemia and postoperative anastomotic leak.[91] These concerns are controversial, and recent retrospective studies have suggested that preoperative PEG placement does not increase postoperative adverse events or increase mortality in patients with esophageal cancer.[92,93]

Esophagorespiratory Fistula

Fistulization from the esophagus to the respiratory tree is a severe adverse event of esophageal cancer that can occur via direct ingrowth by the tumor, tumor necrosis as a result of chemoradiotherapy, or as an adverse event of esophagectomy. This can result in recurrent aspiration pneumonia and weight loss. Multiple endoscopic treatment approaches have been studied, although SEMS placement represents the treatment of choice, with successful fistula closure in up to 90% of patients.[94,95] Adverse events of SEMS placement in this setting include perforation or respiratory compromise due to compression of major airways and/or stent migration, particularly with stents placed in the cervical esophagus.[96] Multidisciplinary management with interventional pulmonology to provide preemptive bronchial prosthesis placement before esophageal stenting may be necessary for patients at high risk of airway compromise. Over-the-scope clips have also been explored as a potential management strategy, although technical failure, likely due to the fibrotic and retracted edges of the fistula, was high.[97]

Endoluminal vacuum-assisted closure (EVAC) is a recent proposed technique, where a negative pressure environment is created while placing a polyurethane sponge in the fistula lumen, which induces the accelerated formation of granulation tissue and closure of the fistula.[98,99] Small case series described the successful treatment of esophagorespiratory fistula with EVAC,[100,101] and larger prospective studies are needed.

It is important to note that fistulization can also be an adverse event of SEMS placement. In a retrospective study of 397 patients undergoing esophageal SEMS placement, 4% of patients developed esophagorespiratory fistulas within a median of 5 months.[102] Risk factors for fistula development included stents in the proximal and mid-esophagus, the use across benign anastomotic strictures, and in patients with prior radiation therapy and higher Charlson comorbidity index score.[102]

Bleeding

Gastrointestinal (GI) tumor bleeding is a challenging and potentially terminal event. Between 2016 and 2018, esophageal cancer bleeding was responsible for at least 2200 hospitalizations in the United States alone.[103] Few studies have investigated the effectiveness of endoscopic hemostasis in patients who experience GI tumor bleeding. Standard injection, thermal and mechanical endoscopic hemostatic techniques including heater probe, bipolar cautery, and mechanical clips have been evaluated in GI tumor bleeding and exhibit varying success rates, ranging from 31% to 100% in initial hemostasis but with very high rebleeding rates.[104,105] Noncontact hemostatic therapies are important due to tumor friability and the frequently diffuse nature of hemorrhage. APC has been evaluated in small case series and which report rates of 75% to 100% for initial hemostasis and recurrent bleeding rates of approximately 30%.[106,107]

Bentonite-based hemostatic spray has also been used to treat GI tumor bleeding.[108,109] In a pilot randomized control trial of 20 patients comparing TC-325 versus standard of care for the management of gastrointestinal tumor bleeding, 90% versus 40% of patients achieved initial hemostasis.[110] Moreover, 20% versus 60% of patients developed recurrent bleeding at 180 days. Although larger trials are needed to confirm these findings, these initial studies suggest that TC-325 can be used effectively to manage GI tumor bleeding. Esophageal stent placement has been described in case reports and small case series for the treatment of refractory gastrointestinal tumor bleeding.[111,112]

CLINICS CARE POINTS

- Staging of ESCC may be assisted by ME under IEE to identify abnormal microvessels.
- ESD leads to higher *en bloc* resection rates compared with endoscopic mucosal resection (EMR) but is limited by expertise as well as a higher risk of adverse events including intraprocedural perforation.

- For circumferential resections, submucosal glucocorticoid injection may help prevent stricturing.
- Stent migration is a common adverse event of SEMS placement and occurs more frequently with covered SEMS. Several endoscopic techniques allow anchoring of stents after placement, and their efficacy is being studied.
- The decision to follow SEMS placement or percutaneous feeding tube placement in patients who are candidates for surgical or neoadjuvant therapy should be determined after a multidisciplinary review between medical, radiation, and surgical oncologists, and interventional endoscopy gastroenterologists.
- EVAC may assist with the management of esophagorespiratory fistulas due to tumor invasion or radiation treatment.
- Tumor bleeding temporary hemostasis can be achieved with the use of hemostatic spray.

DISCLOSURE

The authors have nothing to disclose.

REFERENCES

1. WHO. Cancer Today: data visualization tools for exploring the global cancer burden in 2020. 2020 [cited 2022 1/22/2022]. Available at: https://gco.iarc.fr/today/home.
2. Dunbar KB, Spechler SJ. The risk of lymph node metastases in patients with high grade dysplasia or intramucosal carcinoma in Barrett's esophagus: a systematic review. Am J Gastroenterol 2012; 107(6):850.
3. Goda K, Dobashi A, Tajiri H. Perspectives on narrow-band imaging endoscopy for superficial squamous neoplasms of the orohypopharynx and esophagus. Dig Endosc 2014;26(Suppl 1):1–11.
4. Muto M, Minashi K, Yano T, et al. Early detection of superficial squamous cell carcinoma in the head and neck region and esophagus by narrow band imaging: a multicenter randomized controlled trial. J Clin Oncol 2010;28(9):1566–72.
5. Dobashi A, Goda K, Furuhashi H, et al. Diagnostic efficacy of dual-focus endoscopy with narrow-band imaging using simplified dyad criteria for superficial esophageal squamous cell carcinoma. J Gastroenterol 2019;54(6):501–10.
6. Dubuc J, Legoux J, Winnock M, et al. Endoscopic screening for esophageal squamous-cell carcinoma in high-risk patients: a prospective study conducted in 62 French endoscopy centers. Endoscopy 2006;38(7):690–5.

7. Goda K, Dobashi A, Yoshimura N, et al. Narrow-Band Imaging Magnifying Endoscopy versus Lugol Chromoendoscopy with Pink-Color Sign Assessment in the Diagnosis of Superficial Esophageal Squamous Neoplasms: A Randomised Non-inferiority Trial. Gastroenterol Res Pract 2015;2015: 639462.
8. Morita FH, Bernardo WM, Ide E, et al. Narrow band imaging versus lugol chromoendoscopy to diagnose squamous cell carcinoma of the esophagus: a systematic review and meta-analysis. BMC Cancer 2017;17(1):54.
9. Sharma P, Hawes RH, Bansal A, et al. Standard endoscopy with random biopsies versus narrow band imaging targeted biopsies in Barrett's oesophagus: a prospective, international, randomised controlled trial. Gut 2013;62(1):15–21.
10. Committee AT, Thosani N, Abu Dayyeh BK, et al. ASGE Technology Committee systematic review and meta-analysis assessing the ASGE Preservation and Incorporation of Valuable Endoscopic Innovations thresholds for adopting real-time imaging-assisted endoscopic targeted biopsy during endoscopic surveillance of Barrett's esophagus. Gastrointest Endosc 2016;83(4):684–698 e7.
11. Oyama T, Inoue H, Arima M, et al. Prediction of the invasion depth of superficial squamous cell carcinoma based on microvessel morphology: magnifying endoscopic classification of the Japan Esophageal Society. Esophagus 2017;14(2): 105–12.
12. Mizumoto T, Hiyama T, Oka S, et al. Diagnosis of superficial esophageal squamous cell carcinoma invasion depth before endoscopic submucosal dissection. Dis Esophagus 2018;31(7).
13. Ishihara R, Mizusawa J, Kushima R, et al. Assessment of the Diagnostic Performance of Endoscopic Ultrasonography After Conventional Endoscopy for the Evaluation of Esophageal Squamous Cell Carcinoma Invasion Depth. JAMA Netw Open 2021; 4(9):e2125317.
14. May A, Gunter E, Roth F, et al. Accuracy of staging in early oesophageal cancer using high resolution endoscopy and high resolution endosonography: a comparative, prospective, and blinded trial. Gut 2004;53(5):634–40.
15. Ishihara R, Arima M, Iizuka T, et al. Endoscopic submucosal dissection/endoscopic mucosal resection guidelines for esophageal cancer. Dig Endosc 2020;32(4):452–93.
16. Li DK, Haffar S, Horibe M, et al. Verrucous esophageal carcinoma is a unique indolent subtype of squamous cell carcinoma: a systematic review and individual patient regression analysis. J Gastroenterol 2021;56(1):12–24.
17. Costa-Santos MP, Ferreira AO, Mouradides C, et al. Is Lugol necessary for endoscopic resection of esophageal squamous cell neoplasia? Endosc Int Open 2020;8(10):E1471–7.
18. Miwata T, Oka S, Tanaka S, et al. Risk factors for esophageal stenosis after entire circumferential endoscopic submucosal dissection for superficial esophageal squamous cell carcinoma. Surg Endosc 2016;30(9):4049–56.
19. Ishihara R, Oyama T, Abe S, et al. Risk of metastasis in adenocarcinoma of the esophagus: a multicenter retrospective study in a Japanese population. J Gastroenterol 2017;52(7):800–8.
20. Maeda Y, Hirasawa D, Fujita N, et al. A pilot study to assess mediastinal emphysema after esophageal endoscopic submucosal dissection with carbon dioxide insufflation. Endoscopy 2012;44(6): 565–71.
21. Inoue H, Endo M, Takeshita K, et al. A new simplified technique of endoscopic esophageal mucosal resection using a cap-fitted panendoscope (EMRC). Surg Endosc 1992;6(5):264–5.
22. Alvarez Herrero L, Pouw RE, van Vilsteren FG, et al. Safety and efficacy of multiband mucosectomy in 1060 resections in Barrett's esophagus. Endoscopy 2011;43(3):177–83.
23. Pech O, May A, Manner H, et al. Long-term efficacy and safety of endoscopic resection for patients with mucosal adenocarcinoma of the esophagus. Gastroenterology 2014;146(3):652–660 e1.
24. Oyama T, Tomori A, Hotta K, et al. Endoscopic submucosal dissection of early esophageal cancer. Clin Gastroenterol Hepatol 2005;3(7 Suppl 1): S67–70.
25. Hayashi YSK, Takahashi H. Pocket-creation method of endoscopic submucosal dissection to achieve en bloc resection of giant colorectal subpedunculated neoplastic lesions. Endoscopy 2014;46:E421–2.
26. Sumiyama K, Gostout CJ, Rajan E, et al. Transesophageal mediastinoscopy by submucosal endoscopy with mucosal flap safety valve technique. Gastrointest Endosc 2007;65(4):679–83.
27. Yoshida M, Takizawa K, Suzuki S, et al. Conventional versus traction-assisted endoscopic submucosal dissection for gastric neoplasms: a multicenter, randomized controlled trial (with video). Gastrointest Endosc 2018;87(5):1231–40.
28. Dobashi A, Storm AC, Wong Kee, Song LM, et al. Efficacy and safety of an internal magnet traction device for endoscopic submucosal dissection: ex vivo study in a porcine model (with video). Surg Endosc 2019;33(2):663–8.
29. Kawashima K, Abe S, Koga M, et al. Optimal selection of endoscopic resection in patients with esophageal squamous cell carcinoma: endoscopic mucosal resection versus endoscopic submucosal dissection according to lesion size. Dis Esophagus 2021;34(5):doaa096.

30. Mavrogenis G, Ntourakis D, Wang Z, et al. The learning experience for endoscopic submucosal dissection in a non-academic western hospital: a single operator's untutored, prevalence-based approach. Ann Gastroenterol 2021;34(6):836–44.

31. Han C, Sun Y. Efficacy and safety of endoscopic submucosal dissection versus endoscopic mucosal resection for superficial esophageal carcinoma: a systematic review and meta-analysis. Dis Esophagus 2021;34(4):doaa081.

32. Isomoto H, Yamaguchi N, Minami H, et al. Management of complications associated with endoscopic submucosal dissection/endoscopic mucosal resection for esophageal cancer. Dig Endosc 2013;25(Suppl 1):29–38.

33. Tahara K, Tanabe S, Ishido K, et al. Argon plasma coagulation for superficial esophageal squamous-cell carcinoma in high-risk patients. World J Gastroenterol 2012;18(38):5412–7.

34. Shaheen NJ, Sharma P, Overholt BF, et al. Radiofrequency ablation in Barrett's esophagus with dysplasia. New Engl J Med 2009;360(22):2277–88.

35. Shaheen NJ, Falk GW, Iyer PG, et al. ACG Clinical Guideline: Diagnosis and Management of Barrett's Esophagus. Am J Gastroenterol 2016;111(1):30–50.

36. Mohan BP, Krishnamoorthi R, Ponnada S, et al. Liquid Nitrogen Spray Cryotherapy in Treatment of Barrett's Esophagus, where do we stand? A Systematic Review and Meta-Analysis. Dis Esophagus 2019;32(6):doy130.

37. Tariq R, Enslin S, Hayat M, et al. Efficacy of Cryotherapy as a Primary Endoscopic Ablation Modality for Dysplastic Barrett's Esophagus and Early Esophageal Neoplasia: A Systematic Review and Meta-Analysis. Cancer Control 2020;27(1). 1073274820976668.

38. Ribeiro A, Bejarano P, Livingstone A, et al. Depth of injury caused by liquid nitrogen cryospray: study of human patients undergoing planned esophagectomy. Dig Dis Sci 2014;59(6):1296–301.

39. Pech O, May A, Gossner L, et al. Curative endoscopic therapy in patients with early esophageal squamous-cell carcinoma or high-grade intraepithelial neoplasia. Endoscopy 2007;39(1):30–5.

40. Ishihara R, Iishi H, Takeuchi Y, et al. Local recurrence of large squamous-cell carcinoma of the esophagus after endoscopic resection. Gastrointest Endosc 2008;67(6):799–804.

41. Pimentel-Nunes P, Dinis-Ribeiro M, Ponchon T, et al. Endoscopic submucosal dissection: European society of gastrointestinal endoscopy (ESGE) guideline. Endoscopy 2015;47(09):829–54.

42. Nagami Y, Ominami M, Sakai T, et al. Repeated Endoscopic Submucosal Dissection for Esophageal Neoplasia Located Close to a Previous Endoscopic Submucosal Dissection Scar. Clin Transl Gastroenterol 2020;11(8):e00226.

43. Weusten B, Bisschops R, Coron E, et al. Endoscopic management of Barrett's esophagus: European Society of Gastrointestinal Endoscopy (ESGE) Position Statement. Endoscopy 2017; 49(2):191–8.

44. Pech O, Behrens A, May A, et al. Long-term results and risk factor analysis for recurrence after curative endoscopic therapy in 349 patients with high-grade intraepithelial neoplasia and mucosal adenocarcinoma in Barrett's oesophagus. Gut 2008;57(9):1200–6.

45. Phoa KN, van Vilsteren FG, Weusten BL, et al. Radiofrequency ablation vs endoscopic surveillance for patients with Barrett esophagus and low-grade dysplasia: a randomized clinical trial. JAMA 2014;311(12):1209–17.

46. Knabe M, Beyna T, Rosch T, et al. Hybrid APC in Combination With Resection for the Endoscopic Treatment of Neoplastic Barrett's Esophagus: A Prospective, Multicenter Study. Am J Gastroenterol 2022;117(1):110–9.

47. Seehawong U, Morita Y, Nakano Y, et al. Successful treatment of an esophageal perforation that occurred during endoscopic submucosal dissection for esophageal cancer using polyglycolic acid sheets and fibrin glue. Clin J Gastroenterol 2019;12(1):29–33.

48. Isomoto H, Yamaguchi N, Nakayama T, et al. Management of esophageal stricture after complete circular endoscopic submucosal dissection for superficial esophageal squamous cell carcinoma. BMC Gastroenterol 2011;11:46.

49. Minamino H, Machida H, Tominaga K, et al. Endoscopic radial incision and cutting method for refractory esophageal stricture after endoscopic submucosal dissection of superficial esophageal carcinoma. Dig Endosc 2013;25(2):200–3.

50. Katada C, Yokoyama T, Yano T, et al. Alcohol Consumption and Multiple Dysplastic Lesions Increase Risk of Squamous Cell Carcinoma in the Esophagus, Head, and Neck. Gastroenterology 2016; 151(5):860–869 e7.

51. Ono S, Dobashi A, Furuhashi H, et al. Characteristics of superficial esophageal squamous cell carcinomas undetectable with narrow-band imaging endoscopy. Gastroenterol Rep (Oxf) 2021;9(5):402–7.

52. Tomizawa Y, Friedland S, Hwang JH. Endoscopic submucosal dissection (ESD) for Barrett's esophagus (BE)-related early neoplasia after standard endoscopic management is feasible and safe. Endosc Int Open 2020;8(4):E498–505.

53. Kinoshita S, Nishizawa T, Ochiai Y, et al. Salvage endoscopic submucosal dissection for incompletely resected esophageal or gastric neoplasms (case series). Endosc Int Open 2020;8(1):E20–4.

54. Frederiks CN, van de Water JMW, Ebrahimi G, et al. Cryoballoon ablation as salvage therapy after

nonradical resection of a high-risk T1b esophageal adenocarcinoma: a case report. Eur J Gastroenterol Hepatol 2021.

55. Smyth EC, Lagergren J, Fitzgerald RC, et al. Oesophageal cancer. Nat Rev Dis Primers 2017;3: 17048.

56. van Rossum PSN, Mohammad NH, Vleggaar FP, et al. Treatment for unresectable or metastatic oesophageal cancer: current evidence and trends. Nat Rev Gastroenterol Hepatol 2018;15(4): 235–49.

57. Daly JM, Fry WA, Little AG, et al. Esophageal cancer: results of an American College of Surgeons Patient Care Evaluation Study. J Am Coll Surg 2000;190(5):562–72 [discussion: 72-3].

58. Kang HW, Kim SG. Upper Gastrointestinal Stent Insertion in Malignant and Benign Disorders. Clin Endosc 2015;48(3):187–93.

59. Telford JJ, Carr-Locke DL, Baron TH, et al. A randomized trial comparing uncovered and partially covered self-expandable metal stents in the palliation of distal malignant biliary obstruction. Gastrointest Endosc 2010;72(5):907–14.

60. Vakil N, Morris AI, Marcon N, et al. A prospective, randomized, controlled trial of covered expandable metal stents in the palliation of malignant esophageal obstruction at the gastroesophageal junction. Am J Gastroenterol 2001;96(6):1791–6.

61. Ahmed O, Lee JH, Thompson CC, et al. AGA Clinical Practice Update on the Optimal Management of the Malignant Alimentary Tract Obstruction: Expert Review. Clin Gastroenterol Hepatol 2021; 19(9):1780–8.

62. Spaander MCW, van der Bogt RD, Baron TH, et al. Esophageal stenting for benign and malignant disease: European Society of Gastrointestinal Endoscopy (ESGE) Guideline - Update 2021. Endoscopy 2021;53(7):751–62.

63. Reijm AN, Didden P, Schelling SJC, et al. Self-expandable metal stent placement for malignant esophageal strictures - changes in clinical outcomes over time. Endoscopy 2019;51(1):18–29.

64. Spaander MC, Baron TH, Siersema PD, et al. Esophageal stenting for benign and malignant disease: European Society of Gastrointestinal Endoscopy (ESGE) Clinical Guideline. Endoscopy 2016; 48(10):939–48.

65. Uitdehaag MJ, Siersema PD, Spaander MC, et al. A new fully covered stent with antimigration properties for the palliation of malignant dysphagia: a prospective cohort study. Gastrointest Endosc 2010; 71(3):600–5.

66. Law R, Prabhu A, Fujii-Lau L, et al. Stent migration following endoscopic suture fixation of esophageal self-expandable metal stents: a systematic review and meta-analysis. Surg Endosc 2018;32(2): 675–81.

67. Diana M, Swanstrom LL, Halvax P, et al. Esophageal covered stent fixation using an endoscopic over-the-scope clip. Mechanical proof of the concept and first clinical experience. Surg Endosc 2015;29(11):3367–72.

68. Das KK, Hasak S, Elhanafi S, et al. Performance and Predictors of Migration of Partially and Fully Covered Esophageal Self-Expanding Metal Stents for Malignant Dysphagia. Clin Gastroenterol Hepatol 2021;19(12):2656–26563 e2.

69. Didden P, Reijm AN, Erler NS, et al. Fully vs. partially covered selfexpandable metal stent for palliation of malignant esophageal strictures: a randomized trial (the COPAC study). Endoscopy 2018;50(10):961–71.

70. Pandit S, Samant H, Morris J, et al. Efficacy and safety of standard and anti-reflux self-expanding metal stent: A systematic review and meta-analysis of randomized controlled trials. World J Gastrointest Endosc 2019;11(4):271–80.

71. Mariette C, Gronnier C, Duhamel A, et al. Self-expanding covered metallic stent as a bridge to surgery in esophageal cancer: impact on oncologic outcomes. J Am Coll Surg 2015;220(3):287–96.

72. Huddy JR, Huddy FMS, Markar SR, et al. Nutritional optimization during neoadjuvant therapy prior to surgical resection of esophageal cancer-a narrative review. Dis Esophagus 2018;31(1):1–11.

73. Ahmed O, Bolger JC, O'Neill B, et al. Use of esophageal stents to relieve dysphagia during neoadjuvant therapy prior to esophageal resection: a systematic review. Dis Esophagus 2020;33(1).

74. Siddiqui AA, Sarkar A, Beltz S, et al. Placement of fully covered self-expandable metal stents in patients with locally advanced esophageal cancer before neoadjuvant therapy. Gastrointest Endosc 2012;76(1):44–51.

75. Yang J, Siddiqui AA, Kowalski TE, et al. Esophageal stent fixation with endoscopic suturing device improves clinical outcomes and reduces complications in patients with locally advanced esophageal cancer prior to neoadjuvant therapy: a large multicenter experience. Surg Endosc 2017;31(3): 1414–9.

76. Rodrigues-Pinto E, Ferreira-Silva J, Sousa-Pinto B, et al. Self-expandable metal stents in esophageal cancer before preoperative neoadjuvant therapy: efficacy, safety, and long-term outcomes. Surg Endosc 2021;35(9):5130–9.

77. Homs MY, Steyerberg EW, Eijkenboom WM, et al. Single-dose brachytherapy versus metal stent placement for the palliation of dysphagia from oesophageal cancer: multicentre randomised trial. Lancet 2004;364(9444):1497–504.

78. Fuccio L, Mandolesi D, Farioli A, et al. Brachytherapy for the palliation of dysphagia owing to esophageal cancer: A systematic review and meta-analysis

of prospective studies. Radiother Oncol 2017; 122(3):332–9.

79. Zhongmin W, Xunbo H, Jun C, et al. Intraluminal radioactive stent compared with covered stent alone for the treatment of malignant esophageal stricture. Cardiovasc Intervent Radiol 2012;35(2): 351–8.

80. Li LF, Lv LL, Xu YS, et al. Case Control Study on Radioactive Stents Versus Conventional Stents for Inoperable Esophageal Squamous Cell Carcinoma. Surg Laparosc Endosc Percutan Tech 2020;30(4):312–6.

81. Zhu HD, Guo JH, Mao AW, et al. Conventional stents versus stents loaded with (125)iodine seeds for the treatment of unresectable oesophageal cancer: a multicentre, randomised phase 3 trial. Lancet Oncol 2014;15(6):612–9.

82. Lightdale CJ, Heier SK, Marcon NE, et al. Photodynamic therapy with porfimer sodium versus thermal ablation therapy with Nd:YAG laser for palliation of esophageal cancer: a multicenter randomized trial. Gastrointest Endosc 1995;42(6):507–12.

83. Rupinski M, Zagorowicz E, Regula J, et al. Randomized comparison of three palliative regimens including brachytherapy, photodynamic therapy, and APC in patients with malignant dysphagia (CONSORT 1a) (Revised II). Am J Gastroenterol 2011;106(9):1612–20.

84. Tsai FC, Ghorbani S, Greenwald BD, et al. Safety and efficacy of endoscopic spray cryotherapy for esophageal cancer. Dis Esophagus 2017;30(11): 1–7.

85. Greenwald BD, Dumot JA, Abrams JA, et al. Endoscopic spray cryotherapy for esophageal cancer: safety and efficacy. Gastrointest Endosc 2010; 71(4):686–93.

86. Kachaamy T, Prakash R, Kundranda M, et al. Liquid nitrogen spray cryotherapy for dysphagia palliation in patients with inoperable esophageal cancer. Gastrointest Endosc 2018;88(3):447–55.

87. Bower MR, Martin RC 2nd. Nutritional management during neoadjuvant therapy for esophageal cancer. J Surg Oncol 2009;100(1):82–7.

88. Steenhagen E. Preoperative nutritional optimization of esophageal cancer patients. J Thorac Dis 2019; 11(Suppl 5):S645–53.

89. Yu FJ, Shih HY, Wu CY, et al. Enteral nutrition and quality of life in patients undergoing chemoradiotherapy for esophageal carcinoma: a comparison of nasogastric tube, esophageal stent, and ostomy tube feeding. Gastrointest Endosc 2018;88(1): 21–31 e4.

90. Toh Yoon EW, Yoneda K, Nakamura S, et al. Percutaneous endoscopic gastrostomy (PEG) using a novel large-caliber introducer technique kit: a retrospective analysis. Endosc Int Open 2016;4(9): E990–6.

91. Wormuth JK, Heitmiller RF. Esophageal conduit necrosis. Thorac Surg Clin 2006;16(1):11–22.

92. Matsumoto A, Yuda M, Tanaka Y, et al. Efficacy of Percutaneous Endoscopic Gastrostomy for Patients With Esophageal Cancer During Preoperative Therapy. Anticancer Res 2019;39(8): 4243–8.

93. Siddique MZ, Mehmood S, Ismail M, et al. Preoperative percutaneous endoscopic gastrostomy tube placement does not increase post-operative complications or mortality in oesophageal cancer. J Gastrointest Oncol 2019;10(3):492–8.

94. Silon B, Siddiqui AA, Taylor LJ, et al. Endoscopic Management of Esophagorespiratory Fistulas: A Multicenter Retrospective Study of Techniques and Outcomes. Dig Dis Sci 2017;62(2):424–31.

95. Ramai D, Bivona A, Latson W, et al. Endoscopic management of tracheoesophageal fistulas. Ann Gastroenterol 2019;32(1):24–9.

96. Herth FJ, Peter S, Baty F, et al. Combined airway and oesophageal stenting in malignant airway-oesophageal fistulas: a prospective study. Eur Respir J 2010;36(6):1370–4.

97. Haito-Chavez Y, Law JK, Kratt T, et al. International multicenter experience with an over-the-scope clipping device for endoscopic management of GI defects (with video). Gastrointest Endosc 2014;80(4): 610–22.

98. Pines G, Bar I, Elami A, et al. Modified Endoscopic Vacuum Therapy for Nonhealing Esophageal Anastomotic Leak: Technique Description and Review of Literature. J Laparoendosc Adv Surg Tech A 2018; 28(1):33–40.

99. Archid R, Bazerbachi F, Thomas MC, et al. Endoscopic negative pressure therapy for upper gastrointestinal leaks: description of a fashioned device allowing simultaneous enteral feeding. VideoGIE 2021;6(2):58.

100. Rubicondo C, Lovece A, Pinelli D, et al. Endoluminal vacuum-assisted closure (E-Vac) therapy for postoperative esophageal fistula: successful case series and literature review. World J Surg Oncol 2020;18(1):301.

101. Kuckelman J, Bryan D, Wiener D. Endoluminal vacuum therapy for definitive management of an Esophagobronchial fistula. Ann Thorac Surg 2021.

102. Bick BL, Song LM, Buttar NS, et al. Stent-associated esophagorespiratory fistulas: incidence and risk factors. Gastrointest Endosc 2013;77(2): 181–9.

103. Minhem MA, Nakshabandi A, Mirza R, et al. Gastrointestinal hemorrhage in the setting of gastrointestinal cancer: Anatomical prevalence, predictors, and interventions. World J Gastrointest Endosc 2021;13(9):391–406.

104. Savides TJ, Jensen DM, Cohen J, et al. Severe upper gastrointestinal tumor bleeding: endoscopic

findings, treatment, and outcome. Endoscopy 1996;28(2):244–8.

105. Sheibani S, Kim JJ, Chen B, et al. Natural history of acute upper GI bleeding due to tumours: short-term success and long-term recurrence with or without endoscopic therapy. Aliment Pharmacol Ther 2013;38(2):144–50.

106. Martins BC, Wodak S, Gusmon CC, et al. Argon plasma coagulation for the endoscopic treatment of gastrointestinal tumor bleeding: A retrospective comparison with a non-treated historical cohort. United Eur Gastroenterol J 2016;4(1):49–54.

107. Thosani N, Rao B, Ghouri Y, et al. Role of argon plasma coagulation in management of bleeding GI tumors: evaluating outcomes and survival. Turk J Gastroenterol 2014;25(Suppl 1):38–42.

108. Arena M, Masci E, Eusebi LH, et al. Hemospray for treatment of acute bleeding due to upper gastrointestinal tumours. Dig Liver Dis 2017;49(5):514–7.

109. Pittayanon R, Prueksapanich P, Rerknimitr R. The efficacy of Hemospray in patients with upper gastrointestinal bleeding from tumor. Endosc Int Open 2016;4(9):E933–6.

110. Chen YI, Wyse J, Lu Y, et al. TC-325 hemostatic powder versus current standard of care in managing malignant GI bleeding: a pilot randomized clinical trial. Gastrointest Endosc 2020;91(2):321–328 e1.

111. Bilal S, Saeed SM, Siddique MZ, et al. Salvage therapy of bleeding esophageal tumor by fully covered self-expandable metallic stent: A case report. SAGE Open Med Case Rep 2021;9. 2050313X21997198.

112. Zhou Y, Huo J, Wang X, et al. Covered self-expanding metal stents for the treatment of refractory esophageal nonvariceal bleeding: a case series. J Laparoendosc Adv Surg Tech A 2014; 24(10):713–7.

113. Namasivayam V, Wang KK, Prasad GA. Endoscopic mucosal resection in the management of esophageal neoplasia: current status and future directions. Clin Gastroenterol Hepatol 2010;8(9): 743–54.

Lymph Node Dissection for Esophageal Squamous Cell Carcinoma

Po-Kuei Hsu, MD, PhD[a],*, Yi-Ying Lee, MD[a], Lin-Chi Chuang, BS[b], Yu-Chung Wu, MD[c]

KEYWORDS

- Esophageal cancer • Intraoperative neural monitoring • Lymphadenectomy
- Recurrent laryngeal nerve • Squamous cell carcinoma • Thoracic duct resection

KEY POINTS

- The upper mediastinum is the most common region of lymph node metastasis in esophageal squamous cell carcinoma, irrespective of the location of the primary tumor.
- The lack of randomized controlled trials comparing the outcomes of recurrent laryngeal nerve lymphadenectomy is frequently cited as a criticism of recurrent laryngeal nerve lymphadenectomy in esophageal squamous cell carcinoma.
- Three-field lymph node dissection provides the most accurate lymph node staging and complete locoregional disease control. However, a recent randomized clinical trial showed that the three-field dissection did not improve survival for patients with middle and lower thoracic esophageal cancer compared with two-field dissection.
- The prognostic impact of thoracic duct resection in esophageal squamous cell carcinoma is another controversial issue. There is no consensus on whether thoracic duct resection helps to improve survival in patients with earlier or more advanced esophageal squamous cell carcinoma.

INTRODUCTION

Esophageal squamous cell carcinoma (ESCC) is a highly aggressive malignancy with a dismal prognosis even after multimodality treatment. Even after curative resection, the survival of patients with lymph node metastases is disappointing. It is well accepted that lymph node metastasis is an important prognostic factor in ESCC, and there are a number of studies that provide evidential proof that the number of metastatic nodes, the ratio of involved nodes to total nodes sampled, and even the total number of resected nodes, are of prognostic significance.[1–3] The aim of this article is to review the role of lymph node dissection in esophageal cancer. We specifically address several controversies regarding lymph node dissection in ESCC.

THE EXTENT OF LYMPH NODE DISTRIBUTION

Esophageal cancer is characterized by a unique pattern of spread of cancer cells via the lymphatic system. Anatomically, the esophagus is located in three body compartments. The lymph fluid from the esophagus is drained upward and downward by the abundant longitudinal submucosal lymphatic plexus; it then passes through the muscular coat into the lymph nodes. Anatomical studies of the esophagus have shown that

[a] Division of Thoracic Surgery, Department of Surgery, Taipei Veterans General Hospital and School of Medicine, National Yang Ming Chiao Tung University, Taipei, Taiwan; [b] Department of Nursing, Taipei Veterans General Hospital, Taipei, Taiwan; [c] Division of Thoracic Surgery, Department of Surgery, Taipei Medical University Hospital and Department of Surgery, School of Medicine, College of Medicine, Taipei Medical University, Taipei, Taiwan
* Corresponding author.
E-mail address: hsupokuei@yahoo.com.tw

Thorac Surg Clin 32 (2022) 497–510
https://doi.org/10.1016/j.thorsurg.2022.07.001
1547-4127/22/© 2022 Elsevier Inc. All rights reserved.

submucosal longitudinal lymphatic vessels connect to the superior mediastinal and the paracardial lymphatics, whereas the intermuscular lymphatic routes eventually drain into the periesophageal nodes.[4,5] Therefore, for esophageal cancers, lymph node involvement may occur in the abdominal, thoracic, or cervical nodes regardless of whether the primary tumor is located at the gastroesophageal junction, distal, mid, or upper esophagus.

In an analysis of 1562 patients who underwent esophagectomy for ESCC at a Chinese center, the regions demonstrating the most frequent lymph node metastasis were paratracheal (34.5%) and left supraclavicular (12.6%) in patients with tumors in the upper esophagus, middle periesophagus (18.8%), and paratracheal (17.5%) in patients with tumors in the middle esophagus, and lower periesophagus (21.1%), and pericardial (18.9%) in patients with tumors in the lower esophagus. Although there was an association between tumor location and the region of lymph node metastasis, the upper mediastinum was the most common region of lymph node metastasis, regardless of the tumor location.[6] The same group subsequently reported the prevalence of lymph node metastases in superficial ESCC.[7] For upper and middle submucosal cancers, lymph node metastases were common in the upper mediastinum and abdomen. For lower submucosal cancers, lymph node metastases were common in the lower mediastinum and abdomen. Overall, paratracheal lymph nodes were the most frequently involved (12.0%), followed by the lesser curvature (10.6%), middle periesophageal (5.6%), and pericardial nodes (5.6%). In another study, Akutsu and colleagues[8] reviewed ESCC patients who were recruited to a prospective multi-institutional randomized trial (JCOG0502) and investigated the distribution of metastatic lymph nodes in clinical T1bN0 esophageal cancer. Whereas the upper mediastinal and mediastinal/abdominal regions were frequent sites of lymph node metastases in patients with tumors in the upper and lower esophagus, respectively, nodal involvement was observed in many fields (neck, mediastinal, and abdominal regions) in patients with tumors in the middle esophagus. In addition, they reported an overall skip lymph node metastasis frequency of 36.7%. To compare the distribution of lymph node metastasis in patients with different tumor invasion depths, Tachimori and colleagues[9] reviewed 356 consecutive patients with ESCC who underwent esophagectomy with three-field lymph node dissection (3FD). Patients with pT1 tumors located in the upper esophagus most frequently showed lymph node metastasis in the upper mediastinum (54.5%). In patients with tumors located in the mid-esophagus, node metastasis was more frequent in the upper mediastinum (22.4%) and perigastric area (23.9%) than in the mid-mediastinum (6.0%) or lower mediastinum (9.0%). Even in patients with tumors located in the lower esophagus, node metastasis was more frequent in the upper mediastinum (13.2%) and perigastric area (39.5%) than in the mid-mediastinum (5.3%) or lower mediastinum (5.3%). In patients with tumors invading or penetrating the muscle layer (pT2-4), node metastasis in the mid- and lower mediastinum increased dramatically but was still less frequent than in the upper mediastinum or the perigastric area.

In brief, the aforementioned studies reported a high incidence rate of lymph node metastasis, even during the early stages of the disease. Most importantly, almost all studies have observed that the upper mediastinum is the most frequently involved region in ESCC, irrespective of the location of the primary tumor.

THE EXTENT OF LYMPHADENECTOMY

Despite evidence showing the widespread occurrence of lymph node metastasis in ESCC, whether a more extended lymph node dissection is needed remains unclear. Whether lymphadenectomy is of therapeutic value or whether increased lymph node harvest simply allows better staging has been a long-standing controversy. Many surgeons believe that lymphadenectomy is an essential part of surgical treatment and that more radical surgery with extensive lymph node dissection is necessary to ensure oncological completeness and can provide benefits of locoregional disease control and longer survival.[10,11] However, there are surgeons who contend that esophageal cancer is associated with a high rate of nodal and distant metastasis even in the early stages and that lymphatic spread is merely a marker of systemic disease and lymphadenectomy alone is not expected to confer a survival benefit or cure the disease. Moreover, the morbidity associated with extensive lymphadenectomy should be weighed against the potential impact on survival.[12,13] For example, a population-based cohort study in Sweden in which 52.98% of patients had squamous cell carcinoma demonstrated that there was no influence of the "number of resected lymph nodes" analyzed as a continuous variable or categorical analysis on overall survival, suggesting that a more extensive lymphadenectomy does not improve survival after surgery for esophageal cancer.[14]

The role of lymph node dissection in patients after neoadjuvant chemoradiotherapy (nCRT) is also controversial. Hamai and colleagues[15] reported that, despite the fact that approximately 50% of patients who were clinically positive for lymph node metastasis before treatment were downstaged by nCRT, lymph node metastases were frequent and extensively disseminated from the cervical, through mediastinal, to upper abdominal laryngeal nerve (LN) stations. Moreover, a substantial number (91.5%) of lymph node metastases were found within the radiation field, indicating that radiotherapy could not eradicate many lymph node metastases. Therefore, the administration of nCRT is not a sufficient reason to minimize the extent of lymphadenectomy in ESCC. In a secondary analysis of a prospective trial by Guo and colleagues[16] that compared "nCRT followed by surgery" versus "surgery alone" for locally advanced ESCC, the extent of lymphadenectomy (<20 versus $\geq$ 20 total number of resected nodes) was significantly associated with overall survival, local recurrence, and total recurrence rates in the nCRT group. Therefore, systemic lymphadenectomy should still be considered as an integrated part of surgery in patients with post-nCRT ESCC.

Although the extent of lymph node dissection is still under debate, most studies on ESCC histology have favored the importance of lymphadenectomy in esophagectomy, even after neoadjuvant treatments. However, the extent of lymph node dissection should be determined according to the location, size, and depth of invasion of the main lesion.

THE EFFICACY OF LYMPHADENECTOMY

To evaluate the effectiveness and importance of lymph node dissection in each region, Japanese surgeons use the efficacy index (EI), which is defined as the incidence of metastasis to a region (%), multiplied by the 5-year-survival rate (%) of patients with metastasis to that region, and divided by 100, as a surrogate measure for the therapeutic value of lymph node dissection.[17] Udagawa and colleagues[18] had reported that the lymph node regions with the highest EI were the right recurrent laryngeal nerve (RLN) and right cervical paraesophageal regions in upper esophageal tumors; bilateral RLN, left cardiac, and lesser curvature regions in middle esophageal tumors; and cardiac, lesser curvature, and left gastric artery regions in lower esophageal tumors. Based on the Japanese nationwide registry, Tachimori and colleagues[19] further reported that the EI was high in supraclavicular and upper mediastinal zones in patients with upper esophageal tumors, highest in upper mediastinal zone followed by

supraclavicular and perigastric zones in patients with middle esophageal tumors, and highest in the perigastric zone followed by upper and lower mediastinal zones in patients with lower esophageal tumors. According to their analysis, it is suggested that supraclavicular dissection is indispensable for patients with upper esophageal tumors and recommended for patients with middle esophageal tumors, whereas the upper mediastinal dissection is recommended for all patients with thoracic ESCC, irrespective of the location. In patients who received neoadjuvant chemotherapy followed by surgery, Miyata and colleagues[20] showed that for tumors located in the upper thoracic esophagus, EI was high in the cervical and upper mediastinal regions. For tumors located in the middle thoracic esophagus, EI was approximately similar between cervical, thoracic, and abdominal regions. In tumors located in the lower thoracic esophagus, EI was high in the perigastric lymph nodes and in the middle and lower thoracic periesophageal regions. Taken together, the cardiac and RLN regions showed the highest EI, irrespective of tumor location. Their results suggested that preoperative therapy did not affect the therapeutic value of lymph node dissection, and minimizing the extent of lymphadenectomy after neoadjuvant treatments may be inappropriate.

THE RECURRENT LARYNGEAL NERVE LYMPH NODE DISSECTION

As the frequency of metastasis in lymph nodes along the RLN has been reported to be as high as 50% regardless of the location of the tumor in the thoracic esophagus, and as bilateral RLN nodes have the highest EI, the clinical value of RLN dissection cannot be overemphasized.[18–25] Anatomically, both RLNs ascend from the superior mediastinum through the root of the neck, and lymph nodes around the nerves in the mediastinum also continue to the deep cervical group as cervicothoracic nodes.[26] In a single-institution cohort that included 567 patients, Hong and colleagues[24] reported that patients with T1N0 ESCC who had sufficient harvested RLN nodes showed significantly superior 5-year-recurrence-free survival (89.1% versus 74.8%, $P < 0.001$). Adequate RLN node dissection during surgery may reduce the risk of recurrence and enhance the accuracy of nodal staging in early-stage ESCC. However, not all studies have the same opinions. Yu and colleagues[27] compared 204 patients who underwent esophagectomy with bilateral RLN node dissection and 107 patients who did not undergo RLN node dissection. There were no survival differences between the dissection and control groups.

They developed a scoring system based on age, tumor length, tumor location, and macroscopic tumor type to predict RLN metastasis. As the rate of RLN node metastases was 0% in the low-risk subgroup, it was suggested that RLN lymphadenectomy may be safely omitted for such patients. Chao and colleagues[28] evaluated the impact of resection of upper mediastinal lymph nodes located along the bilateral RLN in patients with clinically negative RLN nodes following nCRT. The survival curves showed no significant intergroup differences with regard to 3-year disease-specific and overall survival. Although the upper mediastinal nodal recurrence rate was higher in the standard dissection group (no RLN dissection, 21.4%) than in the total dissection group (with RLN dissection, 6.5%), the difference was not statistically significant ($P = 0.134$). Recently, Pai and colleagues[29] also reported no significant differences in 3-year overall and disease-free survival between patients with and without RLN node dissection. However, RLN node dissection was associated with better outcomes in a subgroup of patients with pretreatment radiological evidence of RLN lymph node involvement.

Given the high incidence of RLN node metastasis and the wealth of data demonstrating its prognostic value, RLN lymphadenectomy has been routinely performed by most esophageal surgeons in Asia. However, only retrospective studies have compared the outcomes between patients with and without RLN dissection (**Table 1**). The lack of well-conducted randomized controlled trials comparing the outcomes of RLN lymphadenectomy is often the criticism that hampers the determination of its oncological value.

TECHNIQUES AND TECHNOLOGIES IN RECURRENT LARYNGEAL NERVE LYMPH NODE DISSECTION

The RLN is very fragile, and dissection of the RLN node may inevitably increase the risk of RLN injury due to traction, compression, thermal damage, and reduced blood supply. Subsequent vocal cord paresis or paralysis can not only cause serious morbidities, such as postoperative aspiration and pneumonia but also have sequelae, such as hoarseness, that affect patients' long-term quality of life.[30,31] Lymphadenectomy adjacent to the RLN is technically demanding. Even in experienced surgeons, the incidence of RLN injury could be as high as 40%.[31–33] Therefore, new concepts of surgical anatomy of the upper mediastinum, technical details, and technologies for RLN dissection have been proposed.

Osugi and colleagues[34] proposed a microanatomy-based supracarinal dissection of the esophagus and lymphadenectomy. The magnified view obtained by positioning the camera in close vicinity to the dissection can demonstrate the layer structure of the upper mediastinum and enables the dissection following this layer structure. Anatomically, the visceral sheath wraps the esophagus, trachea, and meso-esophagus containing lymph nodes around the RLN. In contrast, the vascular sheath wraps surrounding vessels and nerves. Anatomical knowledge is crucial during the mesenteric excision of the upper esophagus.[35–37] In addition to identifying the overlying shiny thin layer of connective tissue, Otsuka and colleagues[36] proposed the "native tissue preservation technique" to prevent RLN injury; it is based on the premise that by not actually touching the nerve, traction and injury to the RLN are limited and the normal anatomical position of the RLN is maintained. To make RLN lymphadenectomy easier, safer, and more feasible during thoracoscopic esophagectomy, Oshikiri and colleagues[32,38] introduced the following methods of lymphadenectomy along the bilateral RLN. On the left side, the tissue that includes the left RLN and lymph nodes is not released from the divided esophagus proximally. Using a traction suture, the proximal portion of the divided esophagus is drawn and the tissue that includes the left RLN and the lymph nodes is also drawn through so that a membrane similar to the "esophageal mesenteriolum" could be more easily recognized. They named it the "Bascule method."[32] On the right side, a two-dimensional membrane that includes the right RLN, lymph nodes along the right RLN, and the primary esophageal artery is exfoliated from the trachea toward the neck to prepare for lymphadenectomy along the right RLN. Lymphadenectomy along the right RLN is possible from the inner and outer sides of the two-dimensional membrane. Oshikiri and colleagues[38] named it the "Pincers maneuver."

In addition to surgical techniques, there are technologies that facilitate RLN node dissection. Near-infrared (NIR)/indocyanine-green (ICG) imaging has emerged as a safe and promising intraoperative technology for sentinel lymph node identification and lymphatic mapping, which could guide the tailored extent of the lymphadenectomy in patients undergoing cancer surgery.[39] For example, ICG visualization at regions, including lower mediastinum, celiac, and left gastric artery has been used in patients with tumors at the distal esophagus and esophagogastric junction.[40,41] Similarly, NIR image-guided lymphatic mapping can be used for the identification of nodal

Table 1
Studies comparing outcomes between patients with and without recurrent laryngeal nerve lymph node dissection

Authors	Patients	LN Dissections	N	RLN LN (+) (%)	RLNP (%)	OS (%)	P
Hong [2021]	pT1N0	RLND (s)	428	-	13	89 (5 yr RFS)	<0.001
		RLND (i)	139		11	75 (5 yr RFS)	
Tan [2014]	Thoracic EC	RLND (+)	254[a]	26	6	51 (5 yr)	<0.001
		RLND (−)	254[a]		4	35 (5 yr)	
Yu [2016]	pT1-2 EC	RLND (+)	204	14	19	46 (5 yr)	0.255
		RLND (−)	107		9	33 (5 yr)	
Chao [2020]	ycN-RLN(−)	RLND (+)	33	21	9	59 (3 yr)	0.233
		RLND (−)	85		13	48 (3 yr)	
Pai [2021]	Thoracic EC	RLND (+)	53	15	26	57 (3 yr)	0.329
		RLND (−)	258		18	52 (3 yr)	
	In cN-RLN (+)	RLND (+)	21	-	-	62 (3 yr)	0.029
	subgroup	RLND (−)	73			33 (3 yr)	

Abbreviations: EC, esophageal cancer; i, insufficient; LN, lymph node; N, patient number; OS, overall survival; RFS, recurrence-free survival; RLN, recurrent laryngeal nerve; RLND, recurrent laryngeal nerve lymph node dissection; RLNP, recurrent laryngeal nerve palsy; s, sufficient.
[a] Propensity score-matched patients.

metastasis along bilateral RLNs and to avoid unnecessary radical lymphadenectomy along bilateral RLNs in patients with ESCC (**Fig. 1**A, B).[42–45] Park and colleagues[43] reported a protocol of injection of 0.5 mL of ICG solution (0.5 mg/mL) at four quadrants of the tumor by esophagogastroendoscopy, 1 day before the operation, in patients with cT1 ESCC. The negative predictive value in the detection of nodal metastasis was 100% for the right RLN chain and 98.2% for the left RLN chain. Thus, NIR image-guided lymphatic mapping was not only used to identify clinically undetectable nodal metastasis but also to avoid complications that may result from unnecessary radical lymphadenectomy for ESCC. In a study conducted in China, Li's protocol was to endoscopically inject 1.6 mL of ICG solution (1.25 mg/mL) into the esophageal submucosa at the four quadrants around the tumor, after positioning for thoracotomy.[44] False-negative results were noted in 2/9 (22.2%) patients with lymph node metastasis. The negative predictive value was 100% for pT1/T2 diseases and 71.4% for pT3 diseases, respectively. In another study conducted in China, 4 mL (1.25 mg/mL) of ICG was injected into the four quadrants of the superior and inferior tumor edges within 2 cm (0.5 mL per quadrant), 30 min before the operation.[45] The retrieved lymph nodes were divided according to NIR status and the presence of metastasis. The positive predictive values at the right RLN and left RLN were 12.7 and 7.4%, respectively; the negative predictive values were 98.3% and 95.5%, respectively.

Another progress in RLN dissection is the utilization of intraoperative neural monitoring (IONM) during esophagectomy (**Fig. 1**C–E). Certain studies have shown that IONM may facilitate RLN identification, decrease the incidence of RLN injury, and improve the efficiency of lymphadenectomy.[46–51] In a study on patients without notable RLN injury during the operation, postoperative RLN injury was identified in 9.8% of patients without monitoring, whereas none of the patients that was monitored had postoperative hoarseness.[48] Moreover, the patients that were monitored had a significantly higher number of dissected lymph nodes. In another study, the incidence of RLN palsy was lower in the IONM group than in the control group (6.0% versus 21.2%, $P = 0.02$). The rate of RLN palsy recovery within 6 months was also significantly higher in the IONM group.[49] Similarly, Zhao and colleagues[50] reported that the postoperative RLN palsy rate in the IONM group was significantly lower than that in the control group (8.6% versus 21.3%, respectively, $P = 0.032$). Besides, the number of RLN lymph nodes harvested in the IONM group was higher than that in the control group (13.74 ± 5.77 versus 11.03 ± 5.78, respectively, $P = 0.005$). Furthermore, whereas all patients with IONM abnormality developed postoperative vocal cord palsy, 66.7% of patients with a reduction in signal (decreasing waveform amplitude of more than 50% after dissection around the RLN) showed transient palsy (returned to normal within 6 months) and 100% with a loss of signal (failure to detect waveform amplitude after dissection) showed permanent vocal cord palsy. Therefore, IONM also predicts the development and recovery of postoperative vocal cord palsy. Recently, the

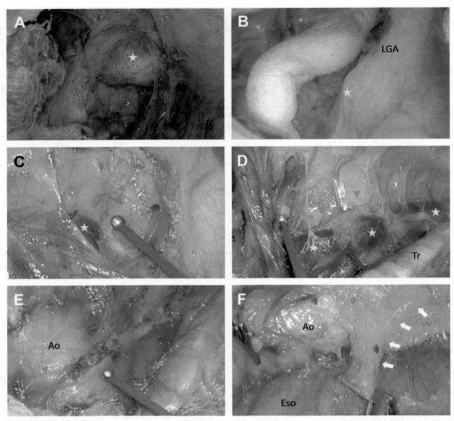

Fig. 1. (*A*) Near-infrared (NIR) image-guided identification of upper mediastinal lymph node (*yellow star*) close to the right recurrent laryngeal nerve. (*B*) NIR image-guided identification of intra-abdominal lymph node (*yellow star*) at the root of left gastric artery (LGA). (*C*) Intraoperative neural monitoring to confirm the integrity of the right recurrent laryngeal nerve (*blue triangles*) during lymph node (*yellow star*) dissection. (*D*) Left recurrent laryngeal nerve (*red triangles*) labeling by the signal from intraoperative neural monitoring before lymph node (*yellow star*) dissection. Tr: trachea. (*E*) The integrity of left recurrent laryngeal nerve (*red triangles*) was confirmed by intraoperative neural monitoring at the end of dissection. Ao: aortic arch. (*F*) The thoracic duct (*white arrows*) was clipped and the thoracic duct and lymph node were divided from the descending aorta (Ao). Eso: esophagus.

Hong Kong group reported a novel technique, combined nerve monitoring (CNM), which included periodic stimulation of the left vagal electrode and intermittent nerve monitoring to identify the RLN.[51] In this technique, the patient is first positioned in a supine manner and a 2-mm nerve electrode is applied onto the left vagus nerve through a cervical incision. The results showed that the CNM group had a higher number of harvested RLN nodes and a lower rate of vocal cord palsy.

In addition, the application of robotic-assisted surgery can provide greater flexibility in the narrow space of the superior mediastinum and improve the quality of RLN dissection. Robotic-assisted minimally invasive esophagectomy has been shown to yield more left RLN lymph nodes than conventional video-assisted esophagectomy;

furthermore, the incidence of RLN injury is decreased.[52,53] A recent multicenter randomized controlled trial robot-assisted minimally invasive esophagectomy (RAMIE) provided evidence for the superiority of robotic-assisted esophagectomy with regard to improved efficiency of thoracic lymph node dissection, especially in the dissection along the left RLN and in patients following neoadjuvant therapy.[54] However, evidence for how this improved RLN dissection technique can translate to improved long-term survival is awaited.

THE ROLE OF CERVICAL LYMPHADENECTOMY

In addition to RLN dissection, cervical lymphadenectomy for ESCC is another controversial topic.

Although proper lymph node dissection is important during radical esophagectomy, the optimal extent of lymph node dissection is not well defined. Several studies have shown that the occurrence rate of cervical lymph node metastasis is more than 40% in patients with upper thoracic ESCC and approximately 30% in patients with middle or lower thoracic ESCC[21,55–57]; Japanese surgeons developed the 3FD in 1980. It is assumed that removing all potentially positive lymph nodes from the cervical and mediastinal to the abdominal regions would eliminate occult metastases, improve local control, and possibly achieve more favorable results, especially in patients with upper thoracic esophageal cancer. Many nonrandomized comparative studies have demonstrated the oncologic advantages of 3FD over the 2FD groups.[21,55,58–61] As 3FD has been accepted worldwide, Altorki and colleagues[62] reported 80 patients who underwent an esophagectomy with 3FD, of which 36% of the participants had clinically unsuspected metastases to the cervicothoracic nodes. Lerut and colleagues[63] reviewed 192 patients who underwent esophagectomy with 3FD and reported low mortality (1.2%), acceptable morbidity, and high prevalence of involved cervical nodes (23% of patients with adenocarcinoma and 25% of patients with ESCC). There is no doubt that such extended lymphadenectomy can guarantee accurate staging; however, the debate on the survival benefit of 3FD in comparison to 2FD persists because of the conflicting results.[13,64,65] Retrospective studies from Korea and China have shown no significance in the overall survival and disease-free survival between the 2FD and 3FD groups.[64,65] The overall recurrence rate and incidence of cervical nodal recurrence were not significantly different between the two groups. In a prospective randomized control trial that supported 3FL, the 5-year-survival rates were 66.2% and 48.0% in the 3FD and conventional lymphadenectomy groups, respectively. While the prognosis appeared to be somewhat better in the 3FD group, the difference was not statistically significant ($P = 0.192$).[66] The recent randomized clinical trial which compares 3FD with 2FD for middle and lower thoracic ESCC has shown comparable outcomes between the two arms.[67] Although 3FD offered more accurate tumor staging with a 21.5% rate of unforeseen cervical lymphatic metastasis, it did not improve survival for patients with middle and lower thoracic esophageal cancer compared with 2FD. The cumulative 5-year overall survival rate was 63% in the 3 FD arm, compared with 63% in the 2FD arm; 5-year-disease-free survival was 59% and 53%, respectively (**Table 2**).

At the same time, it has been argued that more extended lymph node dissection may increase surgical morbidity, including higher rates of RLN paralysis, anastomotic leakage, tracheobronchial ulcer, pulmonary complications, longer duration of systemic inflammatory response syndrome, and postoperative hospital stays compared with 2 FL.[13,65,68–72] Moreover, Nakamura and colleagues[73] reported that postoperative gastrointestinal dysfunction was significantly increased in patients who had undergone 3FD. The 3FD group had a higher frequency of decreased physical activity, symptoms of reflux, dumping-like syndrome, nausea and vomiting, and passage dysfunction.

Strategies have been established to identify patients that may need cervical lymph node dissection. For example, Igaki and colleagues[57] studied the outcomes in patients with ESCC of the lower thoracic esophagus. The 5-year-survival rate for patients with lymph node metastases in the upper and/or middle mediastinum was 23.3%. Among them, the 5-year-survival rates after 2FD and 3FD were 5.6% and 30.0%, respectively, indicating that the 3-field approach for extensive lymph node dissection provides better survival benefit for patients with ESCC of the lower thoracic esophagus when lymph node metastases are present in the upper and/or middle mediastinum. In addition, many authors have hypothesized that the RLN lymph nodes are the sentinel lymph nodes for cervical lymph node metastasis and the status of the RLN lymph nodes can be an indicator of cervical lymphadenectomy.[74–77] Data have shown that the incidence of cervical lymph node metastasis was similar regardless of RLN chain node metastasis in patients with upper thoracic esophageal cancer; however, cervical lymph node metastases were significantly more common in patients with positive rather than negative RLN lymph nodes in patients with middle/lower thoracic ESCC (50.8% versus 28.2% in Li's study; 51.6% versus 11.6% in Shiozaki's study).[76,77]

With recent improvements in surgical techniques and multimodal treatments, the clinical value of cervical lymph node dissection has been further challenged. Magnified views of the microstructure of the lymph node, artery, and nerve under thoracoscopic vision have improved the anatomical understanding and quality of lymph node dissection along the RLN and in the superior mediastinum. Adequate dissection of cervical paraesophageal lymph nodes in continuation with the nodes surrounding the RLN as an en bloc resection has been shown to be feasible during thoracoscopic esophagectomy.[78] In a retrospective study, including 294 patients who underwent thoracoscopic esophagectomy, Koterazawa and colleagues[71] reported no overall survival difference

Table 2
Randomized studies comparing 2-field and 3-field lymph node dissection

Authors	Patients	LN Dissections	N	Total Resected LNs	RLNP (%)	Hospital Mortalities (%)	OS (%)	P
Nishihara [1998]	Thoracic EC	2FD	30	43 (mean)	30	7	48 (5 yr)	0.192
		3FD	32	82 (mean)	56	3	66 (5 yr)	
Li [2020]	Middle and Lower thoracic EC	2FD	200	24 (median)	12	0.5	63 (5 yr)	0.912
		3FD	200	37 (median)	11	0	63 (5 yr)	

Abbreviations: EC, esophageal cancer; LN, lymph node; N, patient number; OS, overall survival; RLNP, recurrent laryngeal nerve palsy.

between the 3FD and 2FD groups. Therefore, prophylactic cervical lymph node dissection in thoracoscopic esophagectomy provides no additional survival benefit and can be omitted for patients without evident metastasis. As neoadjuvant treatment followed by esophagectomy is currently considered the standard treatment worldwide, Mine and colleagues[79] investigated the outcome of patients who did or did not undergo cervical lymphadenectomy with esophagectomy after nCRT. Although the prevalence of pathologically confirmed cervical metastasis in clinically negative nodes was 10.3%, there was no statistically significant difference in relapse-free or overall survival between patients with or without cervical lymphadenectomy. Therefore, prophylactic cervical lymphadenectomy in patients with clinically negative lymph nodes may be omitted when neoadjuvant treatment has been administered.

Although 3FD provides the most accurate lymph node staging and complete locoregional disease control, the oncological advantages should be weighed against the associated morbidity. Furthermore, the role of radical 3FD in an era of minimally invasive surgery and neoadjuvant therapy needs to be redefined.

THORACIC DUCT RESECTION AS PART OF LYMPHADENECTOMY

Another issue with lymphadenectomy for ESCC is thoracic duct (TD) resection (**Fig. 1**F). The TD originates in the cisterna chyli, and ascends along the thoracic descending aorta entering the posterior mediastinum, crosses from right to left in the upper mediastinum, and empties into the left subclavian veins.[80] Whereas prophylactic TD ligation has been advocated to avoid post-esophagectomy chylothorax,[81] TD resection has been recommended as part of extended lymphadenectomy because there are some mediastinal TD lymph nodes (TDLN) lying within the adipose tissue surrounding the TD, located between the thoracic

esophagus and the descending aorta. Previously, Udagawa and colleagues[82] showed that the incidence of metastasis in the nodes along the TD was 2.2% in pT1/T2, and 10.0% in pT3/T4 stage ESCC. A subsequent study by Matsuda and colleagues[83] reported similar incidences. The overall rate of positive TDLNs was 11%, and it was 4% and 26% in patients with pT1/2 and pT3/4 diseases, respectively. This reported incidence of metastatic TDLNs in patients with ESCC, mainly from Asian studies, was confirmed in a European cohort. A recent observational study demonstrated that TDLNs were present in 52% of patients with esophageal cancer. Metastatic TDLNs were observed in 3% and 10% of pT3 stage ESCCs and adenocarcinomas, respectively.[84]

Although there are reports about the frequency of metastasis to TDLNs, few have studied its prognostic impact (**Table 3**). Besides, TD ligation/resection has been reported to have negative effects on circulatory dynamics, immune function, and nutritional status.[85–88] As a result, TD resection during esophagectomy remains a controversial topic. In a two-institutional study, Oshikiri and colleagues[89] reported the effect of TD resection on postoperative complications and survival. The TD was clipped behind the lower thoracic esophagus and resected above the diaphragm and at the level of the thoracic inlet. The TDLNs were then divided from the descending aorta. Such extended lymphadenectomy was associated with higher rates of chylothorax (2.5%) and left RLN palsy (29.8%). However, there was a nonsignificant difference in the 5-year overall survival rate between the TD-resected group (49%) and the TD-preserved group (60%). No significant differences in locoregional recurrence patterns were observed between the two groups. Oshikiri and colleagues subsequently performed a multicenter cohort study investigating 12,237 esophagectomies in Japan. Among 1638 pair propensity score-matched patients, the 5-year overall survival and cause-specific survival rates were 57.5% and 55.2% in the TD-resected group

Table 3
Studies comparing outcome between patients with and without thoracic duct resection during esophagectomy

Authors	Patients	TD Resections	N	Outcomes (%)	P
Matsuda [2016]	cStage I	(+)	34	90 (5 yr RFS)	0.055
		(−)	36	67 (5 yr RFS)	
	cStage II-IV	(+)	36	RFS	0.575
		(−)	45		
Oshikiri [2019]	All stages	(+)	122[a]	49 (5 yr OS)	0.08
		(−)	122[a]	60 (5 yr OS)	
Yoshida [2019]	cStage I	(+)	25	OS	0.154
		(−)	190		
	cStage II	(+)	24	OS	0.251
		(−)	62		
	cStage III	(+)	79	OS	0.655
		(−)	81		
	cStage IV	(+)	13	OS	0.538
		(−)	13		
Matsuda [2020]	cT1N0	(+)	79	96 (3 yr RFS)	0.002
		(−)	14	71 (3 yr RFS)	
	Stage II	(+)	42	RFS	0.535
		(−)	14		
	Stage III/IV	(+)	55	RFS	0.632
		(−)	8		
Tanaka [2021]	All stages	(+)	642[a]	58 (5 yr OS)	0.008
		(−)	642[a]	49 (5 yr OS)	
Oshikiri [2022]	All stages	(+)	1638[a]	58 (5 yr OS)	0.367
		(−)	1638[a]	55 (5 yr OS)	

Abbreviations: N, patient number; OS, overall survival; RFS, recurrence-free survival; TD, thoracic duct.
[a] Propensity score-matched patients.

and 65.6% and 63.4% in the TD-preserved group, respectively, without significant differences.[90] Similarly, Yoshida and colleagues[91] showed that TD resection was an independent risk factor for pulmonary morbidity in the multivariate analysis. Although the nutritional parameters at 1 year after surgery were equivalent irrespective of TD procedure, the long-term overall survival was also equivalent irrespective of the TD procedure. However, among patients with clinical stage I esophageal cancer, the overall survival in the TD-resected group seemed to be better than that in the TD-preserved group, although the difference was not statistically significant ($P = 0.154$). In concordance with the aforementioned reports, Matsuda and colleagues[83,92] reported that TD resection had a favorable impact on recurrence-free survival in patients with clinical stage I disease and cT1N0 ESCC, whereas no significant difference was found for the other disease stages. One possible explanation is that surgery with lymph node dissection is generally effective in early-stage cancers; once cancer has advanced systemically, the usefulness of more aggressive local treatments decreases. The positive effect of TD resection on prognosis was demonstrated by a

six-institutional study with 2269 ESC patients.[85] Tanaka and colleagues reported that the TD-resected group had a 5-year overall survival of 57.7%, which was significantly higher than the corresponding rates of 48.7% in the TD-preserved group ($P = 0.0078$). Interestingly, when comparing the survival between the TD-preserved and TD-resected groups, survival was significantly higher in the TD-resected group for patients with cStage 3 or 4 (not cStage 1 or 2), cT3–4 (not cT1-2), cN1-3 (not cN0), cM0 (not cM1) diseases, tumor location in the lower thoracic and abdominal esophagus, and a history of preoperative treatments. A consistent conclusion was drawn by Ohkura's analysis, which demonstrated that the significance of TD resection was low in T0-2 diseases due to the low metastatic rate but became evident in cases with invasion depth of T3-4.[93]

The efficacy of TD resection is still under debate. Although TD is indispensable for immune and nutritional status, studies have shown no negative impact on nutritional status at 1 year after surgery. With regard to survival, the prognostic impact of TD resection is not consistent in the literature. Moreover, there is no consensus on whether TD resection may help to improve survival in patients with earlier or more advanced ESCC.

SUMMARY

There is no doubt that lymphadenectomy is an essential part of radical esophagectomy. From the analysis of the pattern of lymph node metastases and therapeutic value of lymph node dissection, mediastinal lymphadenectomy including bilateral RLN lymph nodes and lower cervical paraesophageal lymph nodes, through a transthoracic approach, is recommended for most thoracic ESCC cases. A new concept of surgical anatomy and technologies has been proposed to facilitate RLN dissection and decrease morbidity. However, controversy persists regarding whether a more extended lymphadenectomy, such as prophylactic cervical lymphadenectomy and TD resection, is necessary. More comparative studies are needed to clarify the oncological value of lymph node dissection for ESCC.

CLINICS CARE POINTS

- Whether lymphadenectomy in esophageal squamous cell carcinoma (ESCC) is of therapeutic value or simply allows better staging has long been controversial; the extent of lymph node dissection is still under debate.

- The upper mediastinum is the most frequent region of lymph node metastasis in ESCC, irrespective of the location of the primary tumor.

- Although recurrent laryngeal nerve (RLN) lymphadenectomy is thought to have a high therapeutic value in ESCC, the lack of randomized controlled trials comparing the outcomes of RLN lymphadenectomy is frequently cited as a barrier to determining its oncological value. Near-infrared/indocyanine-green imaging and intraoperative neural monitoring are technologies that facilitate RLN lymphadenectomy during esophagectomy.

- Three-field lymph node dissection (3FD) provides the most accurate lymph node staging and complete locoregional disease control. However, a recent randomized clinical trial showed that the 3FD did not improve survival for patients with middle and lower thoracic esophageal cancer compared with 2FD.

- The prognostic impact of thoracic duct (TD) resection in ESCC is controversial. There is no consensus on whether TD resection helps to improve survival in patients with earlier or more advanced ESCC.

DISCLOSURE

The authors have nothing to disclose.

REFERENCES

1. Mariette C, Piessen G, Briez N, et al. The number of metastatic lymph nodes and the ratio between metastatic and examined lymph nodes are independent prognostic factors in esophageal cancer regardless of neoadjuvant chemoradiation or lymphadenectomy extent. Ann Surg 2008;247:365–71.

2. Hsu WH, Hsu PK, Hsieh CC, et al. The metastatic lymph node number and ratio are independent prognostic factors in esophageal cancer. J Gastrointest Surg 2009;13:1913–20.

3. Chein HC, Chen HS, Wu SC, et al. The prognostic value of metastatic lymph node number and ratio in esophageal squamous cell carcinoma patients with or without neoadjuvant chemoradiation. Eur J Cardiothorac Surg 2016;50:337–43.

4. Kuge K, Murakami G, Mizobuchi S, et al. Submucosal territory of the direct lymphatic drainage system to the thoracic duct in the human esophagus. J Thorac Cardiovasc Surg 2003;125:1343–9.

5. Wang Y, Zhu L, Xia W, et al. Anatomy of lymphatic drainage of the esophagus and lymph node metastasis of thoracic esophageal cancer. Cancer Manag Res 2018;26(10):6295–303.

6. Li B, Chen H, Xiang J, et al. Pattern of lymphatic spread in thoracic esophageal squamous cell carcinoma: a single-institution experience. J Thorac Cardiovasc Surg 2012;144:778–85.

7. Li B, Chen H, Xiang J, et al. Prevalence of lymph node metastases in superficial esophageal squamous cell carcinoma. J Thorac Cardiovasc Surg 2013;146:1198–203.

8. Akutsu Y, Kato K, Igaki H, et al. The prevalence of overall and initial lymph node metastases in clinical t1n0 thoracic esophageal cancer: from the results of JCOG0502, a Prospective Multicenter Study. Ann Surg 2016;264:1009–15.

9. Tachimori Y, Nagai Y, Kanamori N, et al. Pattern of lymph node metastases of esophageal squamous cell carcinoma based on the anatomical lymphatic drainage system. Dis Esophagus 2011;24:33–8.

10. Peyre CG, Hagen JA, DeMeester SR, et al. The number of lymph nodes removed predicts survival in esophageal cancer: an international study on the impact of extent of surgical resection. Ann Surg 2008;248:549–56.

11. Rizk NP, Ishwaran H, Rice TW, et al. Optimum lymphadenectomy for esophageal cancer. Ann Surg 2010;251:46–50.

12. Koen Talsma A, Shapiro J, Looman CW, et al. Lymph node retrieval during esophagectomy with and without neoadjuvant chemoradiotherapy: prognostic

and therapeutic impact on survival. Ann Surg 2014; 260:786–92.

13. Wang J, Yang Y, Shafiulla Shaik M, et al. Three-field versus two-field lymphadenectomy for esophageal squamous cell carcinoma: a meta-analysis. J Surg Res 2020;255:195–204.

14. van der Schaaf M, Johar A, Wijnhoven B, et al. Extent of lymph node removal during esophageal cancer surgery and survival. J Natl Cancer Inst 2015;107:djv043.

15. Hamai Y, Emi M, Ibuki Y, et al. Distribution of lymph node metastasis in esophageal squamous cell carcinoma after trimodal therapy. Ann Surg Oncol 2021;28:1798–807.

16. Guo X, Wang Z, Yang H, et al. Impact of lymph node dissection on survival after neoadjuvant chemoradiotherapy for locally advanced esophageal squamous cell carcinoma: from the results of NEOCRTEC5010, a Randomized Multicenter Study. Ann Surg 2021. https://doi.org/10.1097/SLA.0000000000004798.

17. Sasako M, McCulloch P, Kinoshita T, et al. New method to evaluate the therapeutic value of lymph node dissection for gastric cancer. Br J Surg 1995; 82:346–51.

18. Udagawa H, Ueno M, Shinohara H, et al. The importance of grouping of lymph node stations and rationale of three-field lymphoadenectomy for thoracic esophageal cancer. J Surg Oncol 2012; 106:742–7.

19. Tachimori Y, Ozawa S, Numasaki H, et al. Efficacy of lymph node dissection by node zones according to tumor location for esophageal squamous cell carcinoma. Esophagus 2016;13:1–7.

20. Miyata H, Yamasaki M, Makino T, et al. Therapeutic value of lymph node dissection for esophageal squamous cell carcinoma after neoadjuvant chemotherapy. J Surg Oncol 2015;112:60–5.

21. Akiyama H, Tsurumaru M, Udagawa H, et al. Radical lymph node dissection for cancer of the thoracic esophagus. Ann Surg 1994;220:364–72.

22. Ma L, Xiang J, Zhang Y, et al. Characteristics and clinical significance of recurrent laryngeal nerve lymph node metastasis in esophageal squamous cell carcinoma. J BUON 2017;22:1533–9.

23. Ye K, Xu JH, Sun YF, et al. Characteristics and clinical significance of lymph node metastases near the recurrent laryngeal nerve from thoracic esophageal carcinoma. Genet Mol Res 2014;13:6411–9.

24. Hong TH, Kim HK, Lee G, et al. Role of recurrent laryngeal nerve lymph node dissection in surgery of early-stage esophageal squamous cell carcinoma. Ann Surg Oncol 2022;29:627–39.

25. Tan Z, Ma G, Zhao J, et al. Impact of thoracic recurrent laryngeal node dissection: 508 patients with triincisional esophagectomy. J Gastrointest Surg 2014;18:187–93.

26. Krasna MJ, Forti G. Nerve injury: injury to the recurrent laryngeal, phrenic, vagus, long thoracic, and sympathetic nerves during thoracic surgery. Thorac Surg Clin 2006;16:267–75.

27. Yu S, Lin J, Chen C, et al. Recurrent laryngeal nerve lymph node dissection may not be suitable for all early stage esophageal squamous cell carcinoma patients: an 8-year experience. J Thorac Dis 2016; 8:2803–12.

28. Chao YK, Chiu CH, Liu YH. Safety and oncological efficacy of bilateral re- current laryngeal nerve lymph-node dissection after neoadjuvant chemodiotherapy in esophageal squamous cell carcinoma: a propensity- matched analysis. Esophagus 2020; 17:33–40.

29. Pai CP, Hsu PK, Chien LI, et al. Clinical outcome of patients after recurrent laryngeal nerve lymph node dissection for oesophageal squamous cell carcinoma. Interact CardioVasc Thorac Surg 2021. https://doi.org/10.1093/icvts/ivab293.

30. Wang X, Guo H, Hu Q, et al. Efficacy of intraoperative recurrent laryngeal nerve monitoring during thoracoscopic esophagectomy for esophageal cancer: a systematic review and meta-analysis. Front Surg 2021;8:773579.

31. Taniyama Y, Miyata G, Kamei T, et al. Complications following recurrent laryngeal nerve lymph node dissection in oesophageal cancer surgery. Interact Cardiovasc Thorac Surg 2015;20:41–6.

32. Oshikiri T, Yasuda T, Harada H, et al. A new method (the "Bascule method") for lymphadenectomy along the left recurrent laryngeal nerve during prone esophagectomy for esophageal cancer. Surg Endosc 2015;29:2442–50.

33. Jang HJ, Lee HS, Kim MS, et al. Patterns of lymph node metastasis and survival for upper esophageal squamous cell carcinoma. Ann Thorac Surg 2011; 92:1091–7.

34. Osugi H, Narumiya K, Kudou K. Supracarinal dissection of the oesophagus and lymphadenectomy by MIE. J Thorac Dis 2017;9:S741–50.

35. Shirakawa Y, Noma K, Maeda N, et al. Microanatomy-based standardization of left upper mediastinal lymph node dissection in thoracoscopic esophagectomy in the prone position. Surg Endosc 2021;35:349–57.

36. Otsuka K, Murakami M, Goto S, et al. Minimally invasive esophagectomy and radical lymph node dissection without recurrent laryngeal nerve paralysis. Surg Endosc 2020;34:2749–57.

37. Tsunoda S, Shinohara H, Kanaya S, et al. Mesenteric excision of upper esophagus: a concept for rational anatomical lymphadenectomy of the recurrent laryngeal nodes in thoracoscopic esophagectomy. Surg Endosc 2020;34:133–41.

38. Oshikiri T, Nakamura T, Miura Y, et al. A new method (the "Pincers maneuver") for lymphadenectomy

along the right recurrent laryngeal nerve during thoracoscopic esophagectomy in the prone position for esophageal cancer. Surg Endosc 2017;31: 1496–504.

39. Chandler P, Wiesel O, Sherwinter DA. Fluorescence-guided surgery of the esophagus. Ann Transl Med 2021;9:908.

40. Hachey KJ, Gilmore DM, Armstrong KW, et al. Safety and feasibility of near-infrared image-guided lymphatic mapping of regional lymph nodes in esophageal cancer. J Thorac Cardiovasc Surg 2016;152:546–54.

41. Helminen O, Mrena J, Sihvo E. Near-infrared image-guided lymphatic mapping in minimally invasive oesophagectomy of distal oesophageal cancer. Eur J Cardiothorac Surg 2017;52:952–7.

42. Hosogi H, Yagi D, Sakaguchi M, et al. Upper mediastinal lymph node dissection based on mesenteric excision in esophageal cancer surgery: confirmation by near-infrared image-guided lymphatic mapping and the impact on locoregional control. Esophagus 2021;18:219–27.

43. Park SY, Suh JW, Kim DJ, et al. Near-infrared lymphatic mapping of the recurrent laryngeal nerve nodes in T1 esophageal cancer. Ann Thorac Surg 2018;105:1613–20.

44. Jiang H, Teng H, Sun Y, et al. Near-infrared fluorescent image-guided lymphatic mapping in esophageal squamous cell carcinoma. Ann Surg Oncol 2020;27:3799–807.

45. Wang X, Hu Y, Wu X, et al. Near-infrared fluorescence imaging-guided lymphatic mapping in thoracic esophageal cancer surgery. Surg Endosc 2021. https://doi.org/10.1007/s00464-021-08720-7.

46. Kobayashi H, Kondo M, Mizumoto M, et al. Technique and surgical outcomes of mesenterization and intra-operative neural monitoring to reduce recurrent laryngeal nerve paralysis after thoracoscopic esophagectomy: a cohort study. Int J Surg 2018;56:301–6.

47. Hikage M, Kamei T, Nakano T, et al. Impact of routine recurrent laryngeal nerve monitoring in prone esophagectomy with mediastinal lymph node dissection. Surg Endosc 2017;31:2986–96.

48. Zhong D, Zhou Y, Li Y, et al. Intraoperative recurrent laryngeal nerve monitoring: a useful method for patients with esophageal cancer. Dis Esophagus 2014;27:444–51.

49. Takeda S, Iida M, Kanekiyo S, et al. Efficacy of intra-operative recurrent laryngeal neuromonitoring during surgery for esophageal cancer. Ann Gastroenterol Surg 2021;5:83–92.

50. Zhao L, He J, Qin Y, et al. Application of intraoperative nerve monitoring for recurrent laryngeal nerves in minimally invasive McKeown esophagectomy. Dis Esophagus 2021. https://doi.org/10.1093/dote/doab080.

51. Wong IYH, Zhang RQ, Tsang RKY, et al. Improving outcome of superior mediastinal lymph node dissection during esophagectomy: a novel approach combining continuous and intermittent recurrent laryngeal nerve monitoring. Ann Surg 2021;274: 736–42.

52. Deng HY, Luo J, Li SX, et al. Does robot-assisted minimally invasive esophagectomy really have the advantage of lymphadenectomy over video-assisted minimally invasive esophagectomy in treating esophageal squamous cell carcinoma? A propensity score-matched analysis based on short-term outcomes. Dis Esophagus 2019;32:doy110.

53. Duan X, Yue J, Chen C, et al. Lymph node dissection around left recurrent laryngeal nerve: robot-assisted vs. video-assisted McKeown esophagectomy for esophageal squamous cell carcinoma. Surg Endosc 2021;35:6108–16.

54. Yang Y, Li B, Yi J, et al. Robot-assisted versus conventional minimally invasive esophagectomy for resectable esophageal squamous cell carcinoma: early results of a multicenter randomized controlled trial: the RAMIE trial. Ann Surg 2021. https://doi.org/10.1097/SLA.0000000000005023.

55. Isono K, Sato H, Nakayama K. Results of a nationwide study on the three-field lymph node dissection of esophageal cancer. Oncology 1991;48:411–20.

56. Li H, Zhang Y, Cai H, et al. Pattern of lymph node metastases in patients with squamous cell carcinoma of the thoracic esophagus who underwent three-field lymphadenectomy. Eur Surg Res 2007; 39:1–6.

57. Igaki H, Tachimori Y, Kato H. Improved survival for patients with upper and/or middle mediastinal lymph node metastasis of squamous cell carcinoma of the lower thoracic esophagus treated with 3-field dissection. Ann Surg 2004;239:483–90.

58. Kato H, Watanabe H, Tachimori Y, et al. Evaluation of neck lymph node dissection for thoracic esophageal carcinoma. Ann Thorac Surg 1991;51:931–5.

59. Fujita H, Kakegawa T, Yamana H, et al. Cervico-thoraco- abdominal (3-field) lymph node dissection for carcinoma in the thoracic esophagus. Kurume Med J 1992;39:167–74.

60. Noguchi T, Wada S, Takeno S, et al. Two-step three-field lymph node dissection is beneficial for thoracic esophageal carcinoma. Dis Esophagus 2004;17: 27–31.

61. Tabira Y, Kitamura N, Yoshioka M, et al. Significance of three-field lymphadenectomy for carcinoma of the thoracic esophagus based on depth of tumor infiltration, lymph nodal involvement and survival rate. J Cardiovasc Surg (Torino) 1999;40:737–40.

62. Altorki N, Kent M, Ferrara C, et al. Three-field lymph node dissection for squamous cell and adenocarcinoma of the esophagus. Ann Surg 2002;236: 177–83.

63. Lerut T, Nafteux P, Moons J, et al. Three-field lymphadenectomy for carcinoma of the esophagus and gastroesophageal junction in 174 R0 resections: impact on staging, disease-free survival, and outcome: a plea for adaptation of TNM classification in upper-half esophageal carcinoma. Ann Surg 2004;240:962–72.

64. Shim YM, Kim HK, Kim K. Comparison of survival and recurrence pattern between two-field and three-field lymph node dissections for upper thoracic esophageal squamous cell carcinoma. J Thorac Oncol 2010;5:707–12.

65. Fan N, Yang H, Zheng J, et al. Comparison of short- and long-term outcomes between 3-field and modern 2-field lymph node dissections for thoracic oesophageal squamous cell carcinoma: a propensity score matching analysis. Interact CardioVasc Thorac Surg 2019;29:434–41.

66. Nishihira T, Hirayama K, Mori S. A prospective randomized trial of extended cervical and superior mediastinal lymphadenectomy for carcinoma of the thoracic esophagus. Am J Surg 1998;175:47–51.

67. Li B, Zhang Y, Miao L, et al. Esophagectomy with three-field versus two-field lymphadenectomy for middle and lower thoracic esophageal cancer: long-term outcomes of a randomized clinical trial. J Thorac Oncol 2021;16:310–7.

68. Fujita H, Kakegawa T, Yamana H, et al. Mortality and morbidity rates, postoperative course, quality of life, and prognosis after extended radical lymphadenectomy for esophageal cancer. Comparison of three-field lymphadenectomy with two-field lymphadenectomy. Ann Surg 1995;222:654–62.

69. Ma GW, Situ DR, Ma QL, et al. Three-field vs two-field lymph node dissection for esophageal cancer: a meta-analysis. World J Gastroenterol 2014;20:18022–30.

70. Ye T, Sun Y, Zhang Y, et al. Three-field or two-field resection for thoracic esophageal cancer: a meta-analysis. Ann Thorac Surg 2013;96:1933–41.

71. Koterazawa Y, Oshikiri T, Takiguchi G, et al. Prophylactic cervical lymph node dissection in thoracoscopic esophagectomy for esophageal cancer increases postoperative complications and does not improve survival. Ann Surg Oncol 2019;26:2899–904.

72. Yamashita K, Makino T, Yamasaki M, et al. Comparison of short-term outcomes between 2- and 3-field lymph node dissection for esophageal cancer. Dis Esophagus 2017;30:1–8.

73. Nakamura M, Kido Y, Hosoya Y, et al. Postoperative gastrointestinal dysfunction after 2-field versus 3-field lymph node dissection in patients with esophageal cancer. Surg Today 2007;37:379–82.

74. Ueda Y, Shiozaki A, Itoi H, et al. Intraoperative pathological investigation of recurrent nerve nodal metastasis can guide the decision whether to perform cervical lymph node dissection in thoracic esophageal cancer. Oncol Rep 2006;16:1061–6.

75. Taniyama Y, Nakamura T, Mitamura A, et al. A strategy for supraclavicular lymph node dissection using recurrent laryngeal nerve lymph node status in thoracic esophageal squamous cell carcinoma. Ann Thorac Surg 2013;95:1930–7.

76. Li H, Yang S, Zhang Y, et al. Thoracic recurrent laryngeal lymph node metastases predict cervical node metastases and benefit from three-field dissection in selected patients with thoracic esophageal squamous cell carcinoma. J Surg Oncol 2012;105:548–52.

77. Shiozaki H, Yano M, Tsujinaka T, et al. Lymph node metastasis along the recurrent nerve chain is an indication for cervical lymph node dissection in thoracic esophageal cancer. Dis Esophagus 2001;14:191–6.

78. Yagi D, Hosogi H, Akagawa S, et al. Is complete right cervical paraesophageal lymph node dissection possible in the prone position during thoracoscopic esophagectomy? Esophagus 2019;16:324–9.

79. Mine S, Watanabe M, Kumagai K, et al. Oesophagectomy with or without supraclavicular lymphadenectomy after neoadjuvant treatment for squamous cell carcinoma of the oesophagus. Br J Surg 2018;105:1793–8.

80. Brotons ML, Bolca C, Fréchette E, et al. Anatomy and physiology of the thoracic lymphatic system. Thorac Surg Clin 2012;22:139–53.

81. Chen JY, Liu QW, Zhang SS, et al. Prophylactic thoracic duct ligation is associated with poor prognosis and regional lymph node relapse in esophageal squamous cell carcinoma. J Surg Oncol 2020;122:336–43.

82. Udagawa H, Ueno M, Shinohara H, et al. Should lymph nodes along the thoracic duct be dissected routinely in radical esophagectomy? Esophagus 2014;11:204–10.

83. Matsuda S, Takeuchi H, Kawakubo H, et al. Clinical outcome of transthoracic esophagectomy with thoracic duct resection: Number of dissected lymph node and distribution of lymph node metastasis around the thoracic duct. Medicine (Baltimore) 2016;95:e3839.

84. Defize IL, Gorgels SMC, Mazza E, et al. The presence of metastatic thoracic duct lymph nodes in western esophageal cancer patients: a multinational observational study. Ann Thorac Surg 2022;113:429–35.

85. Tanaka K, Yamasaki M, Sugimura K, et al. Thoracic duct resection has a favorable impact on prognosis by preventing hematogenous spread of esophageal cancer cells: a multi-institutional analysis of 2269 patients. Ann Surg Oncol 2021;28:4402–10.

86. Imamura M, Shimada Y, Kanda T, et al. Hemodynamic changes after resection of thoracic duct for

en bloc resection of esophageal cancer. Surg Today 1992;22:226–32.

87. Yang RF, Liu TT, Wang P, et al. Ligation of thoracic duct during thoracoscopic esophagectomy can lead to decrease of T lymphocyte. J Cancer Res Ther 2018;14:1535-9.

88. Aiko S, Yoshizumi Y, Matsuyama T, et al. Influences of thoracic duct blockage on early enteral nutrition for patients who underwent esophageal cancer surgery. Jpn J Thorac Cardiovasc Surg 2003;51: 263–71.

89. Oshikiri T, Takiguchi G, Miura S, et al. Thoracic duct resection during esophagectomy does not contribute to improved prognosis in esophageal squamous cell carcinoma: a propensity score matched-cohort study. Ann Surg Oncol 2019;26: 4053–61.

90. Oshikiri T, Numasaki H, Oguma J, et al. Prognosis of patients with esophageal carcinoma following routine thoracic duct resection: a propensity-matched analysis of 12,237 patients based on the Comprehensive Registry of Esophageal Cancer in Japan. Ann Surg 2021. https://doi.org/10.1097/SLA.0000000000005340.

91. Yoshida N, Nagai Y, Baba Y, et al. Effect of resection of the thoracic duct and surrounding lymph nodes on short- and long-term and nutritional outcomes after esophagectomy for esophageal cancer. Ann Surg Oncol 2019;26:1893–900.

92. Matsuda S, Kawakubo H, Takeuchi H, et al. Minimally invasive oesophagectomy with extended lymph node dissection and thoracic duct resection for early-stage oesophageal squamous cell carcinoma. Br J Surg 2020;107:705–11.

93. Ohkura Y, Ueno M, Iizuka T, et al. Effectiveness of lymphadenectomy along the thoracic duct for radical esophagectomy. Esophagus 2022;19:85–94.

Colon Interposition for Esophageal Cancer

Manuel Villa Sanchez, MD[a], Evan T. Alicuben, MD[b], James D. Luketich, MD[c], Inderpal S. Sarkaria, MD, MBA[d],*

KEYWORDS

• Colon interposition • Esophagectomy • Esophageal cancer

KEY POINTS

• There is significant operative technical variation in colon interposition, including choice of route and colonic segment used.
• Perioperative and long-term functional outcomes after colon interposition are generally good.
• Revisional surgery after colon interposition may be required for complications significantly impacting functional outcomes.

INTRODUCTION

Colon is a reliable and versatile conduit for esophageal replacement when the stomach is not available. Described initially but with few reported cases during the first half of the 20th century,[1–4] the procedure was popularized by Belsey[5] and Skinner[6] and then refined by Demeester.[7] Right, transverse, and left colon have been used with blood supply from the right colic, middle colic and left colic arteries; most commonly esophago-colonic anastomosis is performed in the neck but could also be in the chest. Routes used are retrosternal and posterior mediastinal. The isoperistaltic left colon interposition pedicled on the ascending branch of the left colic artery is favored, but several variations are possible. Stomach is the most common first choice for esophageal replacement after work by Akiyama,[8] with colonic interposition representing the most common alternative when the stomach is not available. It is a procedure that should be within the armamentarium of esophageal surgeons and can carry significant morbidity and mortality even in experienced centers. In a recent meta-analysis of over 1849 patients, Brown and colleagues[9] found mortality of 7.8%, morbidity of 13.6%, and an 11% leak rate. Colonic interposition requires careful planning, and a multidisciplinary team approach is highly recommended. Depending upon the individual experience of the thoracic surgeon, involving surgical colleagues from ENT for complex caustic injuries and neck dissection, plastics microvascular surgeons for occasional need of supercharged conduits, and colorectal surgical colleagues can be critical to the outcome of the patient. We present here technical details for the procedure, a review of the largest published studies, long-term results, and indications and outcomes for revisional surgery.

Surgical Considerations

The surgical technique has been described extensively. Midline laparotomy, complete mobilization of the colon, using transillumination of the mesentery, the vessels of interest are dissected and temporarily clamped to assess collateral

[a] Staten Island University Hospital, 501 Seaview Avenue, Suite 202, Staten Island, NY 10305, USA; [b] Department of Cardiothoracic Surgery, University of Pittsburgh Medical Center and University of Pittsburgh School of Medicine, UPMC Presbyterian, 200 Lothrop Street, Suite C-800, Pittsburgh, PA 15213, USA; [c] Division of Thoracic and Foregut Surgery, Department of Cardiothoracic Surgery, University of Pittsburgh Medical Center and University of Pittsburgh School of Medicine, UPMC Presbyterian, 200 Lothrop Street, Suite C-800, Pittsburgh, PA 15213, USA; [d] Clinical Affairs, University of Pittsburgh Medical Center and University of Pittsburgh School of Medicine, Shadyside Medical Building, 5200 Centre Avenue, Suite 715, Pittsburgh, PA 15232, USA
* Corresponding author.
E-mail address: sarkariais@upmc.edu

Thorac Surg Clin 32 (2022) 511–527
https://doi.org/10.1016/j.thorsurg.2022.07.006
1547-4127/22/© 2022 Published by Elsevier Inc.

circulation via the marginal artery of Drummond. Colon is then divided and used to replace the esophagus. Clear understanding of the vascular anatomy and variations, awareness of functional implications according to the segment of colon used, route used for the conduit, and conduit orientation are necessary for optimal outcomes.

Pertinent Vascular Anatomy

Initial works by Sonneland[10] and Ventemiglia[11] facilitated the understanding of the colonic circulation as applied to colon interposition. The vascular anatomy of the colon is shown in **Fig. 1**. Peters and colleagues[12] reported on 25 patients that underwent colonic interposition and who had mesenteric angiography before the procedure. 12% had multiple middle colic arteries, 96% had an ascending branch of the left colic artery, and 48% had an absence of anastomosis between branches of the IMA and SMA. When using the left colic artery as blood supply for the conduit, the vascular anatomy of the splenic flexure is always a concern because of the described avascular area, or Griffith's point,[13] present in 7% to 12% of cases. Murono and colleagues[14] conducted a literature review of studies from 1990 to 2020 describing the vascular supply to the splenic flexure. Studies included cadaver dissection, intraoperative findings, angiography, and three-dimensional computed tomography (CT) angiography. An absence of left colic artery (LCA) was reported at 2.8% to 7.5%; although the LCA typically divides in ascending and descending branches multiple branches are often seen. Michels[15] reported a middle branch in up to 38% of cases. The middle colic artery, originating from the anterior surface of the SMA at the level of the first jejunal artery, usually continues into the right and left branches. In 8.9% to 33.3% of cases, these two branches originate separately from the SMA,[10] which can be particularly important when a long colon conduit is required. The right middle colic vein drains into the gastrocolic trunk of Henle and the left middle colic veins into the SMV. The accessory right middle colic artery reported in 6.7% to 48.9% of cases, originates proximal to the middle colic artery (MCA), sometimes called accessory left colic artery.[10,16] The accompanying vein usually drains into the IMV. The Riolan arch, present in 7.5% to 27.8% of cases, usually runs medially to the marginal artery of Drummond. The artery of Moskowitz is another SMA-IMA communication, and usually is present medial to the arch of Riolan.[17] These additional communications are especially important in the collateral circulation for colonic conduits based on the left

colic artery. Bruzzi and colleagues[18] reviewed the literature from 1913 to 2018 for right colon blood supply originating typically from the right branches of the SMA. The inferior colic artery (ICA), the most constant branch, was found in 99.8% of cases and is the terminal branch of the SMA. It runs posterior to the SMV in 57% and anterior in 43% of cases,[19] the ascending branch of the ICA gives origin to the marginal artery. The right colic artery (RCA) is present in 60% to 80% of individuals[20,21] and its origin is variable with 40% to 70% from the SMA, 12% to 14% from ICA, and 15% to 30% from the MCA. Its course is anterior to the SMV. The communication between the RCA and ICA is absent at 5%.[22] The Marginal Artery of Drummond runs 2.5 cm from the mesocolic side of the colon, gives off perpendicular arteries to the colon, and in 5% of the cases is discontinuous between the cecum and the ascending colon.[22]

Colonic Conduit Motility

Once the colon is transposed for esophageal replacement, its role, and functioning condition changes. It faces a different environment that requires a long-term adaptation. Being pedicled, hormonal factors may still play a role in motor function, but it is the enteric nervous system and the intrinsic properties of the colon that exert most of the local control and determine the motility pattern. Electromyography (EMG), fluoroscopy, and manometry have been used to assess the motor behavior of colonic conduits with many contradictory reports.

Benages[23] and Dantas[24] found that wet versus dry swallows elicit some motility activity in the colonic conduit, suggesting that it is the bolus distention that generates a colonic conduit response. Acidic quality of the wet swallow increases the colonic response as well. Propulsive contraction elicited by wet swallow has been reported by others.[25,26]

Prabhu and colleagues[27] performed high-resolution manometry of colonic conduits at 3 and 6 months post-colonic interposition and found absent peristalsis. They also biopsied the colonic conduit and did not find any change in the colonic mucosal pattern. Kotsis[28] reported changes in the nature of secretion of the transposed colonic mucosa: increased mucus production, hyperproduction of neutral mucopolysaccharide in Lieberkuhn glands and on the mucosal surface, he compared 15 isoperistaltic to 4 anti-peristaltic conduits; longer passage time in cineradiography and inflammatory mucosal changes were noted in the anti-peristaltic colonic conduits.

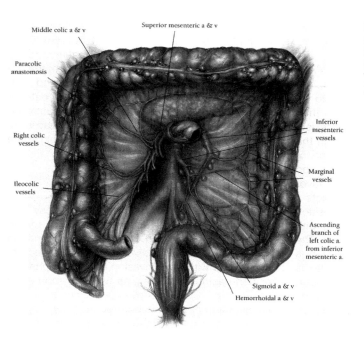

Middle colic a & v

Superior mesenteric a & v

Paracolic anastomosis

Right colic vessels

Ileocolic vessels

Inferior mesenteric vessels

Marginal vessels

Ascending branch of left colic a. from inferior mesenteric a.

Sigmoid a & v

Hemorrhoidal a & v

Fig. 1. Typical vascular arterial and venous anatomy of the colon. (*From* SR DeMeester. Colon Interposition for Benign Disease. Operative Techniques in Thoracic and Cardiovascular Surgery. 2006;11(3):P232-249.)

DeMeester[7] performed fluoroscopic assessment on patients after isoperistaltic colonic interposition compared with normal controls. Transit time for both liquid and solids was delayed in colonic interposition patients. The authors surmised that transport was primarily due to gravity, given that very occasional colonic contraction was observed. Straight conduits emptied faster than redundant ones.

Peppas and colleagues[29] performed continuous manometry over an 8-h period, and reported the colonic conduit behaved mostly similar to in situ,[30] with some increased propulsive rate, but still significantly weaker when compared with esophageal function. Acidic content has been shown to also increases motility[7,23] likely secondary to local irritation.

It is generally accepted that the motility of the proximal esophagus combined with gravity and the quality of meals most determines the colonic conduit transit time and associated sensation of dysphagia after colonic interposition.

Conduit Orientation

The orientation of the colonic conduit has also been studied to identify differences between isoperistaltic and antiperistaltic orientation and its effects on the functional outcome.

Dreuw and colleagues[31] compared motility in isoperistaltic and anti-peristaltic colonic segments in dogs in both fasting and feeding conditions. In fasting conditions, isoperistaltic colons showed mostly (77%) peristaltic contractions and no anti-peristaltic activity. Anti-peristaltic colons had 35% anti-peristaltic, 39% mixed and only 22% peristaltic activity. In feeding status, 100% of isoperistaltic segments presented peristaltic activity, whereas anti-peristaltic segments presented only segmental activity. Emptying was delayed in antiperistaltic segments when compared with peristaltic segments. In a dog model, Predescu[32] et al. reported disorganized electrical activity within the colon segments, and non-specific changes in amplitude and frequency of contraction for both iso and anti-peristaltic segments.

A few groups have reported comparable functional results with anti-peristaltic interpositions[33] but in general most of the groups favor an isoperistaltic orientation.

Isolauri[34] et al. reported their experience in 248 patients, 59% of which were anti-peristaltic, and found no difference in functional outcomes. The authors[35] also reported manometry on 22 patients (17 anti-peristaltic, 5 iso-peristaltic), and found no manometric response in either group.

Right Versus Left Colon

The left colon is favored for its more reliable blood supply and size match to the esophagus, although some groups have shown similar outcomes using the right colon as conduit.[34,36,37] Furst[38] favored a right colonic conduit depending on the left colic artery after ligating right and middle colic arteries. A recent meta-analysis[9] reported a morbidity and mortality of 18.7% and 10.1% for right colon conduits against 15.7% and 6.5% for left colon conduits. The anastomotic leak rate was 15.2% for right colon and 13% for left colon operations.

Route

The retrosternal route is generally thought to be associated with less morbidity and mortality than the posterior mediastinum, although there exists equipoise in the reported evidence. Although the main concern has been that the recognition of conduit ischemia or anastomotic leak may be delayed, the functional outcome seems to favor the posterior mediastinum route. **Fig. 2** depicts a colon conduit in the posterior mediastinal position after hybrid robotic-assisted esophagectomy with linear stapled colo-esophageal anastomosis. The subcutaneous route is associated in most reports with the highest risk. The transpleural route is described but used rarely. A recent meta-analysis found the retrosternal route to have the lowest morbidity and mortality.[9] **Fig. 3** depicts colon conduits in the retrosternal position.

Gawad and colleagues,[39] in a prospective randomized study in 26 patients that underwent esophagectomy with a gastric conduit, assessed the postoperative function and quality of life between 14 patients with retrosternal and 12 patients with posterior mediastinum reconstruction. They found increased morbidity and mortality in the retrosternal route. Esophageal transit was delayed for both liquids and solids in the retrosternal conduit compared with the posterior mediastinal conduit. There were no differences in QOL.

Oida and colleagues,[40] in a retrospective study on 30 patients using isoperistaltic right colon pedicled from the middle colic artery, compared 15 posterior mediastinal and 15 subcutaneous conduits. More cases in the subcutaneous group required supercharging due to ischemia and had more anastomotic leak. The authors suggest the shortest route could be associated with improved perfusion and less tension with an associated lower risk of ischemia and anastomotic leak. Yasuda and colleagues[41] in 112 Japanese patients, measured the distance from the superior border of the duodenum to the cricoid cartilage and found the retrosternal route was the shortest. Measured distances were 34.7 ± 2.37 cm via posterior mediastinum, 32.4 ± 2.24 cm via retrosternal route, and 36.3 ± 2.27 cm for subcutaneous route. However, other studies differ in findings based on the initial reference points including celiac axis, gastroduodenal artery, duodenum, and pylorus. Hu and colleagues[42] in 20 cadavers found the posterior mediastinal route shorter if the celiac axis reference point was used and retrosternal shorter if the reference point was the gastroduodenal

artery or pylorus. Of note, the true difference in length between the groups was 1 to 2 cm. Chen and colleagues[43] in a study of 60 patients found the retrosternal route shorter by 3 cm from the pyloric ring to cricoid cartilage. Coral and colleagues[44] in 50 cadavers found the posterior mediastinum shorter by 2.5 cm from the gastroduodenal artery and by 5 cm from the celiac axis. Orringer[45] found the posterior mediastinal route to be shorter.

Preoperative Assessment

Upper endoscopy is performed for biopsy and diagnosis, and to assess the extent of tumor. Endoscopic ultrasound is useful to understand the depth of tumor involvement, the presence of T4 disease with local invasion of peri-esophageal or peri-gastric structures, as well as lymph node assessment. Colonoscopy is performed to assess the segment of colon to be used as a conduit and ensure no primary pathology is present. A CT-mesenteric angiogram can be useful to examine blood supply to the colon, and should be obtained at minimum when patients have a history of major abdominal vascular surgery or if the extensive vascular disease is evident in CT. For long colonic conduits, the need for supercharging should be considered with anticipation and a microvascular surgeon to be available during the procedure. A contrasted CT scan of the chest, abdomen, and pelvis is routine to help assess the anatomy and the presence of metastatic or other pathology. PET/CT and other routine cancer staging (if performed for primary malignancy) should also be obtained. Staging laparoscopy should be strongly considered for primary gastric malignancy to assess the extent of intra-abdominal peritoneal or visceral disease.

Surgical Technique

Careful planning and meticulous surgical technique are required to minimize the short-term most feared complications: colonic conduit ischemia, anastomotic leak, and long-term poor functional outcome most commonly due to anastomotic stricture and colonic conduit redundancy. The most commonly performed procedures use isoperistaltic left colon with blood supply from the ascending branch of the left colic artery via the posterior mediastinal route.

The surgical technique for colonic interposition has not changed significantly and follows basic principles of surgery: clean dissection with en-bloc resection to negative margins (if for cancer), and creation of a technically sound and tension-

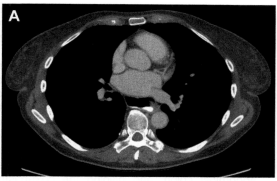
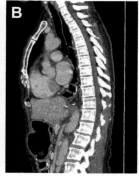
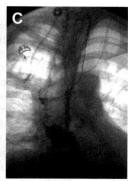

Fig. 2. (*A*). Colon conduit in the posterior mediastinal position after robotic assisted esophagectomy and creation of linear stapled esophago-colic anastomosis. (*B*). Sagittal view of same patient. (*C*). Barium esophagram of same patient.

free anastomosis with adequate vascular perfusion.

A few technical details specific to harvest and creation of the colonic conduit are considered fundamental, including complete colonic mobilization and methodical assessment of blood supply using temporary selective arterial isolation of the segment to be used. Before colonic division and harvest, transillumination of the colonic mesentery, palpation of arterial pulses, selective clamping and isolation of colonic vascular supply, visual assessment of ischemia, Doppler examination, and other intraoperative imaging techniques such as perfusion assessment with near-infrared fluorescence imaging, are all used to assess the viability of the proposed conduit. It is the intraoperative assessment that will determine the segment to be used.

As mentioned, most groups report a preference for isoperistaltic left colon with blood supply from ascending branch of the left colic artery and then the right colon if this segment is not available or useable after intraoperative assessment of blood supply. When considering colonic segment to be used, possibilities include isoperistaltic right colon with middle colic pedicle, isoperistaltic right colon with left colic artery, antiperistaltic right colon with ICA and RCA, isoperistaltic left and transverse colon with left colic artery, and antiperistaltic left colon with MCA.

Preserving the marginal artery at the distal colonic transection site allows additional blood supply from the IMA and venous drainage through the hemorrhoidal veins into the inferior vena cava (IVC). In addition to adequate arterial blood supply, a commonly cited cause of ischemia is venous obstruction, which may be more vulnerable to compromise given lower flow pressures. Therefore, it is of utmost importance to ensure the vascular pedicle is not potentially compromised by undue tension, compression at the hiatus or thoracic inlet, or twisting or kinking. Special

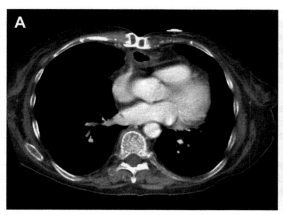
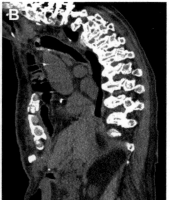

Fig. 3. (*A*). Colon conduit in the substernal position. (*B*). Substernal colon conduit in a patient with severe kyphosis.

attention not to spiral or twisting the conduit when traversing to the chest or neck is critical to prevent venous outflow obstruction in the immediate post-operative period and poor functional outcome in the long-term. In cases of foreshortened and thick colonic mesentery, excision of a short segment of colon has been described to release tension on the vascular pedicle.[37] When using the posterior mediastinal route, suturing the conduit to the dia-phragmatic hiatus after verifying the colonic posi-tion is straight is recommended to prevent conduit or para-conduit herniation and redun-dancy. Similarly, a prevertebral fascial stitch when the anastomosis is in the neck can help maintain straight conduit orientation as well.

The substernal route is commonly used when the posterior mediastinum is not available such as for staged esophagectomy operations with delayed reconstruction including caustic injuries, gastric conduit necrosis, traumatic perforation with sepsis, or other urgent conditions where reconstruction may not have been performed at the index case. Some additional technical details have been described when using the substernal route. Generous dissection of a wide retro-sternal passage may help prevent conduit compression from loss of the domain. This is especially important for patients with larger or bulkier colonic segments or excessive peri-colonic fat. Fat may also be excised to optimize any conduit-to-path size mismatch. Partial peri-cardiotomy may be helpful to smooth the angle of conduit entry in transition from the abdomen to the chest.[7] Takedown of the hepatic ligament and releasing/dropping the left lobe of the liver can similarly be useful to facilitate straighter pas-sage of the conduit. Excision of the sternoclavicu-lar joint or portion of the manubrium, and/or clavicle, sternum, and first rib[37,46,47] to widen the anterior thoracic inlet may help prevent obstruc-tion and potential ischemia due to undue compression. Some have advised full sternotomy in cases with loss of domain and possible exces-sive compression of the conduit, in particular if concern for disadvantageous conduit-to-path size mismatch and potential for vascular compres-sion/congestion. This may be of particular concern in patients for whom the colon may be the conduit of last resort after previous failed operations and/or lack of other viable conduit options. In these pa-tients, delayed closure of the sternum may be advisable. Delayed pectoralis muscle graft and secondary closure may also be considered or necessary if loss of domain and excessive pres-sure on the conduit when attempting to close the sternum is of concern. In these cases, it should be considered that preservation of the conduit is

the primary concern impacting the long-term outcome of these patients. Similarly, leaving the upper part of the abdominal fascia open to prevent tension on the conduit has been described.[36]

A few other technical points deserve mention. Colonic conditioning, introduced by Bar-Maor and Nissan 1970,[48] has not been widely used. Popovici[37] reported this method in 33 patients and found that the resulting abundant collateral vascularity made the interposition procedure more challenging. When performing the distal reconstruction, leaving 10 to 12 cm of the intra-abdominal colon, and placing the colo-gastric anastomosis in the posterior aspect of the stom-ach may help prevent colo-gastric reflux. No consensus exists on routine pyloroplasty.

The MCA may be divided at its origin/trunk for long grafts (preserving left and right branches), and at the left branch divided for short left/descending colon grafts. DeMeester[7] described occasional resection/creation of a button of the superior mesenteric artery (SMA) to preserve a common trunk to the right and left branches for long grafts.

Reported Series of Colon Interposition

Interest in colonic interposition in the modern era was sparked by the personal series from Belsey[5] in 1964, in which 105 cases were reported with a mortality of 4.8%. In 1979, Skinner[6] reported on 33 patients, all of them were isoperistaltic left co-lon with a 9% mortality. Three patients developed graft necrosis one of whom died, the author attrib-uted it to venous obstruction. There was a 3% anastomotic leak rate. Wilkins Jr. in 1980 pre-sented outcomes in 100 patients with a mortality of 9%. The reports by DeMeester[7] and Isolauri[34] consolidated colonic interposition as a potential primary conduit of choice for esophageal replace-ment. DeMeester[7] reported detailed technical points that refined the technique, Isolauri[34] with one of the largest series to date had similar out-comes with differences in approach, did not favor preoperative angiography and 59% of conduits were placed anisoperistaltic with good functional outcomes.

Table 1 summarizes some of the most repre-sentative reports and associated rates of overall complications, anastomotic leak, conduit necro-sis, and mortality. Although most of the authors favored the left colon, there are large series using the right colon with similar outcomes including Iso-lauri,[34] Mansour,[49] Furst,[49] Popovici37, and Chir-ica.[36] Preoperative testing including use of computed tomography, selective angiography, and colonoscopy varied significantly between the

Table 1
Anastomotic leak and conduit necrosis rates in reported series of colon interposition with greater than 25 cases

Author	Period	Number	Complications	Anastomotic Leak	Conduit Necrosis	Mortality
Isolauri,[34,35] 1987	1965–1984	248	37%	5%	3%	16%
DeMeester,et al[7] 1988	1971–1988	92	24%	1.50%	7.60%	9%
Cerfolio,et al[50] 1995	1985–1993	32	24%	3.10%	6.30%	9%
Thomas,et al[51] 1997	1985–1995	60	65%	10%	5%	8.30%
Mansour[49] 1997	1972–1996	107	38%	14.80%	3%	5.90%
Wain[82] 1999	1956–1997	52	17.30%	5.80%	9%	4%
Furst[83] 2001	1997–2000	53	60%	16%	1.60%	9.40%
Popovici,et al[37] 2003	1973–2002	347	NR	7%	2%	4.60%
Han[84] 2004	1971–2001	63	25%	14.20%	NR	0
Knezevic,et al[69] 2007	1964–2004	336	26.50%	9.20%	2.40%	4.16%
Motoyama[85] 2007	1989–2006	34	35%	9%	0	0
Bothereau[86] 2007	1995–2005	81	NR	31%	7%	4%
Mine[87] 2009	1990–2008	95	64%	13%	0	3.20%
Chirica,et al[36] 2010	1987–2006	246	56%	14.20%	2%	3.70%
Klink,et al[33] 2010	1986–2006	43	61%	30%	9%	16%
Boukerrouche[57] 2014	1999–2011	70	40%	20%	2.80%	2.80%
Lee[88] 2018	2000–2013	67	54%	16.40%	NR	6%
Reslinger[89] 2016	2004–2014	28	86%	NR	14%	14%
Zeng[90] 2019	2005–2017	119	NR	4.20%	0	0
Coevoet,et al[81] 2019	2002–2016	80	80%	37.50%	NR	4 (5%)
Sert[54] 2021	1984–2018	268	NR	3.40%	1.50%	NR

reported series (when described). Technical descriptions vary significantly between the reports, including use of right or left colon, widening of the thoracic inlet, use of pyloroplasty, and route of conduit transit. Overall complication rates range from 40% to 60%, with the majority of mortality below 10%. Comparisons in outcomes need to consider the etiology of the primary disease, with cancer patients associated with poorer outcomes compared with patients undergoing esophagectomy for benign conditions. Also, the scope of functional outcomes (in particular dysphagia) differs by the nature of disease, such as caustic injuries or for extensive esophageal injury with prior abnormal deglutition. The left colic vascular pedicle is the most used likely for its reliable and less variable vascular supply. For one-stage operations, the posterior mediastinum or retrosternal routes are most used, and the retrosternal route for two-stage operations when the posterior mediastinal route is preferentially avoided due to prior surgical intervention.

Cerfolio[50] reported 9/19 patients with the sternoclavicular joint (SCJ) resected to enlarge the thoracic outlet. 3 patients had necrosis of the conduit necrosis, and 2 died. Selective angiography was used to determine perfusion of the conduits. Thomas[51] reported 66% good and 18.5% fair alimentary function (poor in 14.8%) in 60 patients undergoing colon interposition. Of note, selective angiography was not used, and all patients received preoperative colonoscopy. Postoperative sequelae of regurgitation, early fullness, and diarrhea were also reported (20%, 16%, and 16%). Reslinger and colleagues reported one intraoperative graft ischemia, ischemia from 1 previously damaged marginal vascular arch. Preoperative CT and colonoscopy were routinely obtained. Lee and colleagues performed angiography, CT, and colonoscopy in a series of 67 patients. The authors reported 35.2% dysphagia, 23% reflux, 14.9% diarrhea, dumping in 6%. Popovici and colleagues preferred ileocecum with a long ileal loop and preservation of the ileocecal valve. The authors reported 4 gastrocolic ulcers, and 80% oral alimentation rate, 13% of patients with mild symptoms, and 7% with poor quality of life (QOL). Mansour and colleagues used selective angiography routinely, whereas Bothereu and colleagues and Isolauri and colleagues did not obtain preoperative angiography. Mine and colleagues reported on 95 patients with cancer from 1990 to 2008 and cited 40% dysphagia, 24% reflux, 39% diarrhea, 24% dumping in these patients after surgery. Isolauri and colleagues reported on 248 patients of which 8 developed conduit necrosis, 6 of whom died. Pyloroplasty was routinely used, and no preoperative angiography was obtained. The authors reported no dysphagia in 76% of patients at 1 year after surgery. One stricture developed out of 10 patients with the anastomotic leak.

Supercharged Conduits

Although not used routinely, supercharging colonic conduits have been reported mostly for extra-long conduits and when there is intraoperative evidence of ischemia. Both arterial and venous supercharging is usually performed but on occasion only venous (superdrainage). Recipient vessels frequently used: transverse cervical artery, IMA, superior thyroid artery, external jugular vein, internal jugular vein (IJV), and inferior mesenteric vein (IMV). **Table 2** summarizes the case series of supercharged colonic conduits.

Introduced by Longmire[52] in 1946, it was not until O'Rourke[53] published in 1985 a series of 14 supercharged colonic conduits for esophageal replacement, all using the subcutaneous route, with no anastomotic leak and no conduit ischemia that supercharging became the most widely used. Most of the published studies show a low incidence of conduit ischemia with supercharging but the number of patients is too small to drive definitive conclusions. Recently, the largest series to date from Sert[54] presented a 1% leak rate and 1% conduit ischemia rate in 104 patients with supercharged colonic conduit. The authors reported no significant difference for graft necrosis and leak, but less stricture in supercharged conduits (1% vs 6.7%). Awsakulsutthi and colleagues[55] compared 11 supercharged with 15 non-supercharged colonic interpositions and found a trend toward lower anastomotic leak rated in supercharged conduits (9% vs 35%). Fujita and colleagues[56] reported a 7% incidence of anastomotic leak in 29 supercharged conduits versus 54% in 24 non-supercharged (most of the conduits were subcutaneous). In general, most of the surgical groups use supercharged colonic conduits on a patient-by-patient basis when there is intraoperative evidence of ischemia and for long colonic conduits. Mansour and colleagues[49] reported on 107 patients with 1 intraoperative conduit ischemia (stomach was used to

reconstruct) and 1 in the immediate postoperative period requiring takedown and free jejunal graft. They reported 14.8% anastomotic leak and 5.9% mortality rates. The authors favored right colon (85 cases), and less frequently left colon (18 cases) and transverse colon (4 cases).

Postoperative Complications

Anastomotic leak is commonly associated with ischemia and comorbid conditions.[57] In a meta-analysis by Brown and colleagues[9] right colon conduit and posterior mediastinum route were associated with higher leak rates. Tsutsui[58] found the retrosternal route to be a risk factor for anastomotic leak. DeMeester[7] associated ischemia with right colon conduits using the middle colic artery.

Conduit necrosis has an incidence of 0% to 13%. Systemic Inflammatory Response Syndrome (SIRS), anastomotic leak, bloody nasogastric tube (NGT) output, enteric-looking output from drains, lactic acidosis, and frank sepsis[59,60] are all possible findings that should alert the surgeon to investigate viability of the conduit. Conduit necrosis is associated with high mortality, with some series reporting death rates as high as 60% to 70%.

A recent meta-analysis[61] reported that anastomotic leakage and graft necrosis decreased for esophagectomy with gastric conduit when using advanced imaging with near-infrared fluorescence imaging with indocyanine green. There was a 25% change in management after assessment with indocyanine green (ICG). Despite shown benefit, it is a subjective process and there are ongoing attempts to quantify the assessment of perfusion with ICG and similar imaging technologies, and make it more objective such as the "90 sec rule"[62] and time-fluorescence intensity curves.[63,64] Some groups have reported its use to assess colonic conduit perfusion, particularly in supercharged conduits.[65,66]

Venous obstruction has been reported as a significant cause of ischemia[5,7,57] due to excessive traction, graft torsion, or kinking of the vascular pedicle. Venous return abnormalities can also lead to congestion and subacute ischemia of the conduit resulting acute graft failure, and/or longer-term fibrosis and diffuse stricturing as end-stage of the process.[36]

Early endoscopic assessment of ischemia is safe and useful. Different degrees of ischemia based on mucosal discoloration,[67,68] venous congestion and hemorrhagic infarction, and mucosal bleeding are all findings in conduit ischemia. Bedside exploration of the neck wound is helpful to assess the conduit and anastomosis,

Table 2
Supercharged conduit case series

Author	Period	Number	Conduit Left colon	Conduit Right colon	Pedicle Left colic	Pedicle Middle colic	Pedicle Right colic	Conduit perfusion	Supercharge Arterial and venous	Supercharge venous	Route PM	Route RS	Route SC	AL	CI	Mortality
O'Rourke[53] 1986	1979–1985	14	iso 8, aniso 4	2 aniso	8	1	5	NR	14	0	0	0	14	0	0	1 (7%)
Fujita,et al[56] 1997	1981–1996	29	17 iso	12 iso	29	0	0	NR	29	0	0	NR	NR	2 (7%)	0	2 (7%)
Shirakawa[91] 2006	1998–2004	41	0	41 iso	0	41	0	NR	41	0	0	0	41	4 (7.8%)	0	0
Doki[92] 2008	1998–2005	28	0	28 iso	0	28	0	NR	28	0	0	0	28	13 (24%)	0	1
Oida,et al[40] 2012	1989–2008	10	0	10, iso	0	10	0	Doppler	10	0	4	0	6	4 (40%)	NR	0
Saeki[93] 2013	2004–2009	21	0	21 iso	0	21	0	NR	7	14	0	0	21	5 (23.8%)	0	1 (4.8%)
Kesler,et al[65] 2013	2005–2012	11	iso 2	iso 9	2	9	0	ICG and Spy in 2 patients	11	0	0	11	0	1 (9%)	0	1 (9%)
Awsakulsutthi[55] 2015	2004–2012	11	9 iso	2 aniso	9	2	0	direct inspection	11	0	0	11	0	1 (9%)	0	0
Charalabopoulos, et al[66] 2021	2016–2018	5	5 iso	0	5	0	0	ICG and Spy system	3	2	3	2	0	0	0	1 (20%)
Sert[54] 2021	1984–2018	104	mostly iso left	NR	most NR	NR	NR	NR	104	0	0	104	0	1%	1%	0

as well as potential thoracoscopy/thoracotomy if needed to assess the conduit's viability.

DeMeester described three patients with reflux gastritis/colitis treated with bile diversion. In 3/15 with no pyloroplasty, a subsequent drainage procedure for delayed gastric emptying was required. 4 patients required surgical treatment for anastomotic stricture (two esophago-colonic and two colo-gastric). Twenty-four patients showed delayed conduit transit times for both liquids and solids and took longer and smaller meals when compared with normal controls.

Knezevic and colleagues[69] endorsed selective enlargement of the thoracic inlet, but still reported seven patients (2.08%) with thoracic outlet compression. Fifteen (4.46%) patients developed cervical anastomotic stricture, 13 required surgical resection, and 2 improved with dilation. Four (1.19%) developed peptic ulceration of the distal colon proximal to the colo-gastric anastomosis requiring segmental colonic resection in two patients. Most graft necroses were due to poor venous drainage, although the authors did not elaborate. Fourteen patients (4.17%) developed colon redundancy.

Late Complications

Anastomotic stricture

Anastomotic stricture with associated dysphagia and colonic redundancy with regurgitation and aspiration pneumonia is the most common late complications; colo-gastric reflux, pyloric obstruction, and thoracic inlet obstruction are also often described but less frequently presented.

Chirica and colleagues[36] reported in 223 patients with a median follow-up of 5 years after colonic interposition for caustic injury, 55% incidence of late complications: stenosis 36%, reflux 11%, redundancy 5%. Anastomotic stenosis was responsible for 80% of graft dysfunction. Colonic redundancy up to 25% Renzulli, Knezevic,[69] Jeyasingham and colleagues[70] described different types of redundancy: supra-aortic, supra-diaphragmatic, and sub-diaphragmatic.

Anastomotic stricture is generally associated with anastomotic leak and conduit ischemia, it is also more frequently seen in caustic injuries, Chirica and colleagues[36] found higher incidence if reconstruction is undertaken less than 6 months after the caustic insult. They also reported that the incidence decreased from 29% to 12% once thoracic inlet widening was performed routinely. Briel and colleagues[71] reported a 22% incidence of stricture, 48% of ischemic conduits developed stricture as well as 47% of the anastomotic leak patients, other factors associated with stenosis

were comorbid conditions and increasing weight. Kotsis[28] reported the development of cervical pseudodiverticulum as a consequence of anastomotic stenosis.

The initial treatment is endoscopic dilation but if unsuccessful then surgical revision, Chirica and colleagues[36] reported a 55% success ratio with endoscopic dilation in 58 patients, if more than three dilations were required the success ratio dropped to 35%. Revision in 29 patients with a 76% success ratio. Five patients required a second revision for recurrent stenosis. Endoscopic dilation and surgery had a combined success ratio of 83%. Stricturoplasty and resection and re-anastomosis are the most used surgical techniques Kotsis[28]

Diffuse conduit stricture has been described and thought to result from subacute ischemia of the conduit due to venous return abnormalities with multi-focal fibrosis as the end stage of the process. Chirica[36] reported 8 cases and Cheng[72] reported the radiographic findings in 3 patients represented by loss of haustral folds and thumb-printing on initial barium swallow and followed by extensive structuring.

Conduit redundancy

With a reported incidence up to 25%, conduit redundancy is associated with dysphagia, retrosternal fullness, postprandial regurgitation, chest pain, aspiration pneumonia and, postprandial cervical bulging.[70,73–76] **Fig. 4** depicts a posterior mediastinal colon conduit with mild redundancy. A few factors have been suggested as favoring redundancy including the structure and length of the colon with length longer than the vascular arcade potentially favoring/creating conduit redundancy. The presence of areas of extrinsic compression including the thoracic inlet and diaphragmatic hiatus, as well as pressure differences

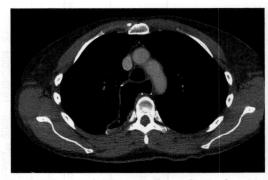

Fig. 4. Colon conduit in posterior mediastinal position with mild redundancy of the conduit in a patient with otherwise good functional outcome.

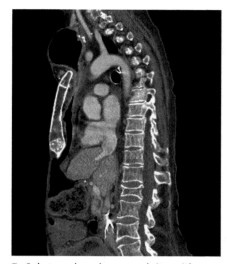

Fig. 5. Substernal colon conduit with proximal obstruction at thoracic inlet resulting in partial obstruction and dilation. Patient required reoperation with sternotomy, partial manubriectomy, resection of sterno-clavicular joint, and revision of anastomosis.

between the abdomen and chest are considered predisposing factors to conduit redundancy. Careful surgical techniques including straightening of the conduit, fixation to the diaphragmatic hiatus, widening of thoracic inlet and hiatus, and obtaining an appropriate length of the conduit may also decrease the incidence of conduit redundancy. The described techniques for surgical treatment of colonic redundancy are resection and anastomosis, side-to-side bypass, and strengthening and anchoring without resection (less effective).

Reflux

Left colon, anastomosis in the anterior wall of stomach and anisoperistaltic conduit have been described as risk factors by DeMeester,[7] deDelva.[77] Chirica found coloduodenal anastomosis as a risk factor. The role of pyloroplasty is not clear in etiology of reflux.

Pyloric obstruction

Pyloric obstruction requiring pyloroplasty have been reported but there is no consensus regarding routine pyloroplasty, DeMeester 3/15 patients with no pyloroplasty developed symptomatic gastric outlet obstruction and required pyloroplasty, Kotsis[28] reported two patients that required pyloroplasty.

Obstruction at the thoracic inlet

The thoracic inlet has been reported as natural area of narrowing that predisposes to obstruction due to extrinsic compression. **Fig. 5** depicts a

patient with obstruction of a retrosternal colon conduit at the thoracic inlet. Anastomotic stricture and development of cervical pseudodiverticulum are associated with a narrow thoracic inlet. DeMeester[71] reported one patient before adopting routine enlargement of thoracic inlet for substernal route. Jeyasingham and colleagues[70] presented two patients with thoracic inlet delay in posterior mediastinum route in children with atresia. Chirica[36] reported absence of widening of thoracic inlet a risk factor for long-term cervical anastomotic stricture. Kotsis[28] who did not enlarge the thoracic inlet as routine reported 5 cases of cervical pseudodiverticulum, he treated with closure of esophageal stump or end-to-end re-anastomosis.

Functional outcomes

When functional outcomes are considered, it is necessary to differentiate according to level of anastomosis and etiology, caustic injuries are associated with significant pharynx and larynx injury and affect deglutition. Nocturnal regurgitation, gurgling and early satiety were the most reported long-term side effects of colonic interposition.

Irino and colleagues[78] in a systematic review of the literature compared the long-term functional outcomes after esophageal replacement irrespective of the conduit used, gastric, colonic or jejunal. Up to 10% suffered from dysphagia, 3% to 19% regurgitation, a decrease in 14.3% in body weight from baseline at a median follow-up of 6 years.

DeMeester[7] on 34 patients, 88% had an unrestricted diet with 50% reported able to tolerate a steak dinner. 35% reported requiring liquids with meals and 53% were last to finish meal. Chirica and colleagues[36] reported a 77% functional success ratio in 223 patients with median follow-up of 5 years. Greene[79] reported on 63 patients 10 or more years after colonic interposition, 45 with cancer and 18 with benign disease; on 59 patients the posterior mediastinal route was used and a retrosternal conduit in 4. Most common reported symptoms were: 40% early satiety, diarrhea 35%, heartburn 19%, and 16% regurgitation. 40% of the patients endorsed at least one episode of aspiration and in 7% aspiration required hospitalization. The QOL score was higher when compared with gastric tubes. Cense[80] studied 36 patients of whom 14 were followed up to 7 to 97 months after colonic interposition. Left colon anti-peristaltic in 11 and right colon in 3. The subcutaneous route was used in 8, the posterior mediastinum in 5 and, the retrosternal route in 1. The author found a better QOL for posterior mediastinal or retrosternal routes compared with the subcutaneous route. He also found a lower quality of life when compared with

Table 3
Indications for revisional surgery

Author	DeMeester, et al[7] 1988	Jeyasingham[7] 1999	Domreis, et al[75] 2002	Kotsis, et al[28] 2002	Popovici, et al[37] 2003	Knezevic, et al[69] 2007	deDelva, et al[77] 2008	Chirica, et al[36] 2010	Boukerrouche[57] 2014
Period	1971–1988	1961–1990	NR	1962–1990	1973–2002	1964–2004	1965–2005	1987–2006	1999–2011
Number of patients	13	24	6	19	39	29	35	96	4
Colonic redundancy	3	17	4	5	3	14	13	19	2
Gastro-colonic reflux	3	0	3		4	2	4	8	
Anastomotic stenosis	4	4	0	7	22	13	11	33	2
Diaphragmatic hernia		2	0					3	
Chronic fistula			0				5	0	
Colon cancer		3	0					0	
Colobronchial fistula		2	1						
Thoracic inlet delay	1	2	0						
Cervical pseudodiverticulum			0	5					
Pyloric obstruction	3		0	2					
Others	3	0	0	0	10	0	20	13	

gastric tubes. Coevoet[81] studied 80 patients and found a similar QOL to gastric tubes, he did not compare the route used. 56% of patients complained of dysphagia and 47% of reflux.

Revisional surgery

Table 3 summarizes reported rates of indications for revisional surgery after colon interposition. 15% to 37.5% of patients after colonic interposition will need revisional surgery. with Chirica and colleagues[36] and Strauss and colleagues[76] citing anastomotic stricture and conduit redundancy as the most common reasons for revision.

Persistent anastomotic stricture despite serial dilation is better dealt with resection and anastomosis. In cases of substernal conduits, thoracic inlet/outlet widening is recommended if not performed during the initial reconstruction. Combined sternotomy and laparotomy may be required to create a tension free anastomosis and avoid venous congestion within the relatively confined sub-sternal space.

Conduit redundancy treatment is challenging, in particular for conduits located in the posterior mediastinum. A combination of thoracotomy and laparotomy is generally required, and possible sequential thoracotomy-laparotomy-thoracotomy is necessary to address the redundant conduit.

Side-to-side colo-colonic anastomosis has also been reported as a less radical treatment for conduit redundancy.

Roux-en-Y colo-jejunostomy is the most effective treatment for colo-gastric reflux. To prevent this potential complication DeMeester,[7] Peters[12] recommended a generous proximal gastrectomy. Belsey[5] described gastro-colonic anastomosis in the posterior stomach to prevent reflux.

Chirica and colleagues[36] reported a 65% success ratio in revisional surgery for stenosis in 63 patients and 89% success for redundancy in 13 patients mostly treated with resection and anastomosis. The authors also reported a 75% success ratio on 8 patients with severe colo-gastric reflux treated with Roux-n-Y reconstruction.

Revisional surgery is challenging technically and need for more than one intervention is not infrequent. De Delva[77] reported that out of 35 patients that underwent revision 9 patients required more than one operation and Chirica reported five patients that underwent a second revision for recurrent anastomotic stricture.

SUMMARY

Esophagectomy and colon interposition in the adult patient, either for primary alimentary reconstruction or as secondary replacement after initial resection/ reconstruction, remains a valuable tool in the thoracic surgeon's armamentarium. It is important for surgeons to remain versed in the complexities of the operation, including preoperative preparation and decision making, operative procedural and technical variations, and recognition and timely treatment of postoperative complications. In our high-volume center, we have found colon interposition to result in favorable functional and quality of life outcomes in appropriately selected patients.

CLINICS CARE POINTS

- Colon interposition is the conduit of choice when the stomach is not available for esophageal replacement

- Isoperistaltic left colonic interposition is the most used configuration for esophageal replacement

- The segment of colon to be used as conduit is determined in the intraoperative instance after methodical assessment of the colonic blood supply

- The posterior mediastinum for one-stage procedures and substernal position for staged reconstruction are the most used locations for the colonic conduit

- Use of indocyanine green provides useful information in the assessment of the perfusion of the conduit

- The need for supercharging the colonic conduit should be planned for long conduits and considered anytime that there is intraoperative evidence of less-than-optimal conduit perfusion

- Careful measurement of the length of the conduit is important to prevent redundancy and poor long-term functional outcome

- Venous outflow obstruction is commonly cited as a cause of ischemia, therefore special attention to avoid kinking or conduit twisting along the mediastinal tract is recommended

- For substernal conduit, excision of the left sternoclavicular joint and first rib prevents obstruction and decreases risk of anastomotic leak

- High clinical suspicion and early endoscopic assessment has proven useful for detection and treatment of postoperative conduit ischemia

- Revisional surgery is challenging technically and frequently, the patients require more than one intervention.

DISCLOSURE

Dr I.S. Sarkaria has education, speaking, and/or consulting disclosures with Intuitive Surgical, Stryker, CMR, On Target Laboratories, and AMSI. There are no relevant financial disclosures for all other authors related to the content of this article.

REFERENCES

1. Oesophagoplastik GK. mit hilfe des Quercolons. Zentralbl Chir 1911;38:1209–12.
2. De I HV. 'oesophagoplastie et de ses diverses modifications. Semaine Med 1911;31:529–34.
3. Uber VVH. Oesophagoplastik in allgemeinen under uber den ersatz der speiserohre durch antethorakle hautdickdarmschlauchbildung im bensonderen. Arch Klin Chir 1914;105:973–1018.
4. Orsoni P, Lemaire M. [Esophagoplasty technique using the transverse and descending colon]. J Chir (Paris) 1951;67(6–7):491–505. Technique des oesophagoplasties par le côlon transverse et descendant.
5. Belsey R. RECONSTRUCTION OF THE ESOPHAGUS WITH LEFT COLON. J Thorac Cardiovasc Surg 1965;49:33–55.
6. Skinner DB. Esophageal reconstruction. Am J Surg 1980;139(6):810–4.
7. DeMeester TR, Johansson KE, Franze I, et al. Indications, surgical technique, and long-term functional results of colon interposition or bypass. Ann Surg 1988;208(4):460–74.
8. Akiyama H, Miyazono H, Tsurumaru M, et al. Use of the stomach as an esophageal substitute. Ann Surg 1978;188(5):606–10.
9. Brown J, Lewis WG, Foliaki A, et al. Colonic Interposition After Adult Oesophagectomy: Systematic Review and Meta-analysis of Conduit Choice and Outcome. J Gastrointest Surg 2018;22(6):1104–11.
10. Sonneland J, Anson BJ, Beaton LE. Surgical anatomy of the arterial supply to the colon from the superior mesenteric artery based upon a study of 600 specimens. Surg Gynecol Obstet 1958;106(4):385–98.
11. Ventemiglia R, Khalil KG, Frazier OH, et al. The role of preoperative mesenteric arteriography in colon interposition. J Thorac Cardiovasc Surg 1977;74(1):98–104.
12. Peters JH, Kronson JW, Katz M, et al. Arterial anatomic considerations in colon interposition for esophageal replacement. Arch Surg 1995;130(8):858–62. ; discussion 862-3.
13. Griffiths JD. Surgical anatomy of the blood supply of the distal colon. Ann R Coll Surg Engl 1956;19(4):241–56.
14. Murono K, Nozawa H, Kawai K, et al. Vascular anatomy of the splenic flexure: a review of the literature.

Surg Today 2021. https://doi.org/10.1007/s00595-021-02328-z.
15. Michels NA, Siddharth P, Kornblith PL, et al. THE VARIANT BLOOD SUPPLY TO THE DESCENDING COLON, RECTOSIGMOID AND RECTUM BASED ON 400 DISSECTIONS. ITS IMPORTANCE IN REGIONAL RESECTIONS: A REVIEW OF MEDICAL LITERATURE. Dis Colon Rectum 1965;8:251–78.
16. Miyake H, Murono K, Kawai K, et al. Evaluation of the vascular anatomy of the left-sided colon focused on the accessory middle colic artery: a single-centre study of 734 patients. Colorectal Dis 2018;20(11):1041–6.
17. Garcia-Granero A, Sánchez-Guillén L, Carreño O, et al. Importance of the Moskowitz artery in the laparoscopic medial approach to splenic flexure mobilization: a cadaveric study. Tech Coloproctol 2017;21(7):567–72.
18. Bruzzi M, M'Harzi L, Poghosyan T, et al. Arterial vascularization of the right colon with implications for surgery. Surg Radiol Anat 2020;42(4):429–35.
19. Negoi I, Beuran M, Hostiuc S, et al. Surgical Anatomy of the Superior Mesenteric Vessels Related to Colon and Pancreatic Surgery: A Systematic Review and Meta-Analysis. Sci Rep 2018;8(1):4184.
20. Haywood M, Molyneux C, Mahadevan V, et al. The right colic artery: An anatomical demonstration and its relevance in the laparoscopic era. Ann R Coll Surg Engl 2016;98(8):560–3.
21. Kuzu MA, İsmail E, Çelik S, et al. Variations in the Vascular Anatomy of the Right Colon and Implications for Right-Sided Colon Surgery. Dis Colon Rectum 2017;60(3):290–8.
22. Sakorafas GH, Zouros E, Peros G. Applied vascular anatomy of the colon and rectum: clinical implications for the surgical oncologist. Surg Oncol 2006;15(4):243–55. https://doi.org/10.1016/j.suronc.2007.03.002.
23. Benages A, Moreno-Ossett E, Paris F, et al. Motor activity after colon replacement of esophagus. Manometric evaluation. J Thorac Cardiovasc Surg 1981;82(3):335–40.
24. Dantas RO, Mamede RC. Motility of the transverse colon used for esophageal replacement. J Clin Gastroenterol 2002;34(3):225–8.
25. Moreno-Osset E, Tomas-Ridocci M, Paris F, et al. Motor activity of esophageal substitute (stomach, jejunal, and colon segments). Ann Thorac Surg 1986;41(5):515–9.
26. Myers JC, Mathew G, Watson DI, et al. Peristalsis in an interposed colonic segment immediately following total oesophagogastrectomy. Aust N Z J Surg 1998;68(4):278–80.
27. Prabhu R, Kantharia C, Bapat R, et al. Morphological and functional changes in colon after coloplasty for management of corrosive esophageal strictures. Indian J Gastroenterol 2013;32(3):165–71.

28. Kotsis L, Krisár Z, Orbán K, et al. Late complications of coloesophagoplasty and long-term features of adaptation. Eur J Cardiothorac Surg 2002;21(1):79–83.

29. Peppas G, Payne HR, Jeyasingham K. Ambulatory motility patterns of the transposed short segment colon. Gut 1993;34(11):1572–5.

30. Narducci F, Bassotti G, Gaburri M, et al. Twenty four hour manometric recording of colonic motor activity in healthy man. Gut 1987;28(1):17–25. https://doi.org/10.1136/gut.28.1.17.

31. Dreuw B, Fass J, Titkova S, et al. Colon interposition for esophageal replacement: isoperistaltic or antiperistaltic? Experimental results. Ann Thorac Surg 2001;71(1):303–8.

32. Predescu D, Predescu I, Boeriu M, et al. Motor criteria evaluation of iso-anisoperistaltic graft in oesophageal reconstruction – an experimental study of isolated colic graft motility pattern in dogs. Chirurgia (Bucur) 2014;109(2):213–7.

33. Klink CD, Binnebösel M, Schneider M, et al. Operative outcome of colon interposition in the treatment of esophageal cancer: a 20-year experience. Surgery 2010;147(4):491–6.

34. Isolauri J, Markkula H, Autio V. Colon interposition in the treatment of carcinoma of the esophagus and gastric cardia. Ann Thorac Surg 1987;43(4):420–4.

35. Isolauri J, Reinikainen P, Markkula H. Functional evaluation of interposed colon in esophagus. Manometric and 24-hour pH observations. Acta Chir Scand 1987;153(1):21–4.

36. Chirica M, Veyrie N, Munoz-Bongrand N, et al. Late morbidity after colon interposition for corrosive esophageal injury: risk factors, management, and outcome. A 20-years experience. Ann Surg 2010; 252(2):271–80.

37. Popovici Z. A new philosophy in esophageal reconstruction with colon. Thirty-years experience. Dis Esophagus 2003;16(4):323–7. https://doi.org/10.1111/j.1442-2050.2003.00358.x.

38. Fürst H, Hartl WH, Löhe F, et al. Colon interposition for esophageal replacement: an alternative technique based on the use of the right colon. Ann Surg 2000;231(2):173–8.

39. Gawad KA, Hosch SB, Bumann D, et al. How important is the route of reconstruction after esophagectomy: a prospective randomized study. Am J Gastroenterol 1999;94(6):1490–6.

40. Oida T, Mimatsu K, Kano H, et al. Anterior vs. posterior mediastinal routes in colon interposition after esophagectomy. Hepatogastroenterology 2012; 59(118):1832–4. https://doi.org/10.5754/hge10213.

41. Yasuda T, Shiraishi O, Kato H, et al. A comparative study of the lengths of different reconstruction routes used after thoracic esophagectomy. Esophagus 2021;18(3):468–74.

42. Hu H, Ye T, Tan D, et al. Is anterior mediastinum route a shorter choice for esophageal reconstruction? A comparative anatomic study. Eur J Cardiothorac Surg 2011;40(6):1466–9.

43. Chen H, Lu JJ, Zhou J, et al. Anterior versus posterior routes of reconstruction after esophagectomy: a comparative anatomic study. Ann Thorac Surg 2009; 87(2):400–4.

44. Coral RP, Constant-Neto M, Silva IS, et al. Comparative anatomical study of the anterior and posterior mediastinum as access routes after esophagectomy. Dis Esophagus 2003;16(3):236–8.

45. Orringer MB, Sloan H. Substernal gastric bypass of the excluded thoracic esophagus for palliation of esophageal carcinoma. J Thorac Cardiovasc Surg 1975;70(5):836–51.

46. Mine S, Watanabe M, Okamura A, et al. Superior Thoracic Aperture Size is Significantly Associated with Cervical Anastomotic Leakage After Esophagectomy. World J Surg 2017;41(10):2598–604.

47. Sato S, Nakatani E, Higashizono K, et al. Size of the thoracic inlet predicts cervical anastomotic leak after retrosternal reconstruction after esophagectomy for esophageal cancer. Surgery 2020;168(3): 558–66.

48. Bar-Maor JA, Nissan S. Improved vascularization of transplanted colon for esophageal replacement. Surg Gynecol Obstet 1970;131(4):755–6.

49. Mansour KA, Bryan FC, Carlson GW. Bowel interposition for esophageal replacement: twenty-five-year experience. Ann Thorac Surg 1997;64(3):752–6.

50. Cerfolio RJ, Allen MS, Deschamps C, et al. Esophageal replacement by colon interposition. Ann Thorac Surg 1995;59(6):1382–4.

51. Thomas P, Fuentes P, Giudicelli R, et al. Colon interposition for esophageal replacement: current indications and long-term function. Ann Thorac Surg 1997; 64(3):757–64. https://doi.org/10.1016/s0003-4975(97)00678-4.

52. Longmire WP Jr. A modification of the Roux technique for antethoracic esophageal reconstruction. Surgery 1947;22(1):94–100.

53. O'Rourke IC, Threlfall GN. Colonic interposition for oesophageal reconstruction with special reference to microvascular reinforcement of graft circulation. Aust N Z J Surg 1986;56(10):767–71. https://doi.org/10.1111/j.1445-2197.1986.tb02323.x.

54. Sert G, Chen SH, Chen HC. How to ensure immediate and long-term good blood supply by the careful dissection of the marginal artery and supercharge with neck vessels in esophageal reconstruction with the colon segment interposition: 35 years of experience. J Plast Reconstr Aesthet Surg 2021; 74(1):101–7. https://doi.org/10.1016/j.bjps.2020.08.013.

55. Awsakulsutthi S, Havanond C. A retrospective study of anastomotic leakage between patients with and without vascular enhancement of esophageal reconstructions with colon interposition: Thammasat

University Hospital experience. Asian J Surg 2015; 38(3):145–9. https://doi.org/10.1016/j.asjsur.2015.01.005.

56. Fujita H, Yamana H, Sueyoshi S, et al. Impact on outcome of additional microvascular anastomosis–supercharge–on colon interposition for esophageal replacement: comparative and multivariate analysis. World J Surg 1997;21(9):998–1003. https://doi.org/10.1007/s002689900339.

57. Boukerrouche A. Isoperistaltic left colic graft interposition via a retrosternal approach for esophageal reconstruction in patients with a caustic stricture: mortality, morbidity, and functional results. Surg Today 2014;44(5):827–33. https://doi.org/10.1007/s00595-013-0758-3.

58. Tsutsui S, Moriguchi S, Morita M, et al. Multivariate analysis of postoperative complications after esophageal resection. Ann Thorac Surg 1992;53(6):1052–6. https://doi.org/10.1016/0003-4975(92)90388-k.

59. Wormuth JK, Heitmiller RF. Esophageal conduit necrosis. Thorac Surg Clin 2006;16(1):11–22. https://doi.org/10.1016/j.thorsurg.2006.01.003.

60. Athanasiou A, Hennessy M, Spartalis E, et al. Conduit necrosis following esophagectomy: An up-to-date literature review. World J Gastrointest Surg 2019;11(3):155–68. https://doi.org/10.4240/wjgs.v11.i3.155.

61. Slooter MD, Eshuis WJ, Cuesta MA, et al. Fluorescent imaging using indocyanine green during esophagectomy to prevent surgical morbidity: a systematic review and meta-analysis. J Thorac Dis 2019;11(Suppl 5):S755–65. https://doi.org/10.21037/jtd.2019.01.30.

62. Kumagai Y, Hatano S, Sobajima J, et al. Indocyanine green fluorescence angiography of the reconstructed gastric tube during esophagectomy: efficacy of the 90-second rule. Dis Esophagus 2018;(12):31. https://doi.org/10.1093/dote/doy052.

63. Ishige F, Nabeya Y, Hoshino I, et al. Quantitative Assessment of the Blood Perfusion of the Gastric Conduit by Indocyanine Green Imaging. *J Surg Res* Feb 2019;234:303–10. https://doi.org/10.1016/j.jss.2018.08.056.

64. Yukaya T, Saeki H, Kasagi Y, et al. Indocyanine Green Fluorescence Angiography for Quantitative Evaluation of Gastric Tube Perfusion in Patients Undergoing Esophagectomy. J Am Coll Surg 2015;221(2):e37–42. https://doi.org/10.1016/j.jamcollsurg.2015.04.022.

65. Kesler KA, Pillai ST, Birdas TJ, et al. Supercharged" isoperistaltic colon interposition for long-segment esophageal reconstruction. Ann Thorac Surg 2013;95(4):1162–8. https://doi.org/10.1016/j.athoracsur.2013.01.006. ; discussion 1168-9.

66. Charalabopoulos A, Davakis S, Syllaios A, et al. Microvascular grafting to enhance perfusion in colonic long-segment oesophageal reconstruction. Langenbecks Arch Surg 2021;406(7):2507–13. https://doi.org/10.1007/s00423-020-01988-8.

67. Oezcelik A, Banki F, Ayazi S, et al. Detection of gastric conduit ischemia or anastomotic breakdown after cervical esophagogastrostomy: the use of computed tomography scan versus early endoscopy. Surg Endosc 2010;24(8):1948–51. https://doi.org/10.1007/s00464-010-0884-6.

68. Maish MS, DeMeester SR, Choustoulakis E, et al. The safety and usefulness of endoscopy for evaluation of the graft and anastomosis early after esophagectomy and reconstruction. Surg Endosc 2005;19(8):1093–102. https://doi.org/10.1007/s00464-004-8816-y.

69. Knezević JD, Radovanović NS, Simić AP, et al. Colon interposition in the treatment of esophageal caustic strictures: 40 years of experience. Dis Esophagus 2007;20(6):530–4. https://doi.org/10.1111/j.1442-2050.2007.00694.x.

70. Jeyasingham K, Lerut T, Belsey RH. Revisional surgery after colon interposition for benign oesophageal disease. Dis Esophagus 1999;12(1):7–9. https://doi.org/10.1046/j.1442-2050.1999.00004.x.

71. Briel JW, Tamhankar AP, Hagen JA, et al. Prevalence and risk factors for ischemia, leak, and stricture of esophageal anastomosis: gastric pull-up versus colon interposition. J Am Coll Surg 2004;198(4):536–41. https://doi.org/10.1016/j.jamcollsurg.2003.11.026. ; discussion 541-2.

72. Cheng W, Heitmiller RF, Jones B. Subacute ischemia of the colon esophageal interposition. Ann Thorac Surg 1994;57(4):899–903.

73. Schein M, Conlan AA, Hatchuel MD. Surgical management of the redundant transposed colon. Am J Surg 1990;160(5):529–30.

74. Bonavina L, Chella B, Segalin A, et al. Surgical treatment of the redundant interposed colon after retrosternal esophagoplasty. Ann Thorac Surg 1998;65(5):1446–8.

75. Domreis JS, Jobe BA, Aye RW, et al. Management of long-term failure after colon interposition for benign disease. Am J Surg 2002;183(5):544–6.

76. Strauss DC, Forshaw MJ, Tandon RC, et al. Surgical management of colonic redundancy following esophageal replacement. Dis Esophagus 2008;21(3):E1–5. https://doi.org/10.1111/j.1442-2050.2007.00708.x.

77. de Delva PE, Morse CR, Austen WG Jr, et al. Surgical management of failed colon interposition. Eur J Cardiothorac Surg 2008;34(2):432–7. https://doi.org/10.1016/j.ejcts.2008.04.008. ; discussion 437.

78. Irino T, Tsekrekos A, Coppola A, et al. Long-term functional outcomes after replacement of the esophagus with gastric, colonic, or jejunal conduits: a systematic literature review. Dis Esophagus 2017;30(12):1–11. https://doi.org/10.1093/dote/dox083.

79. Greene CL, DeMeester SR, Augustin F, et al. Long-term quality of life and alimentary satisfaction after esophagectomy with colon interposition. Ann Thorac Surg 2014;98(5):1713–9. https://doi.org/10.1016/j.athoracsur.2014.06.088. ; discussion 1719-20.

80. Cense HA, Visser MR, van Sandick JW, et al. Quality of life after colon interposition by necessity for esophageal cancer replacement. J Surg Oncol 2004;88(1):32–8. https://doi.org/10.1002/jso.20132.

81. Coevoet D, Van Daele E, Willaert W, et al. Quality of life of patients with a colonic interposition postoesophagectomy. Eur J Cardiothorac Surg 2019;55(6):1113–20. https://doi.org/10.1093/ejcts/ezy398.

82. Wain JC, Wright CD, Kuo EY, et al. Long-segment colon interposition for acquired esophageal disease. Ann Thorac Surg 1999;67(2):313–7. https://doi.org/10.1016/s0003-4975(99)00029-6 [discussion: 317–8].

83. Fürst H, Hüttl TP, Löhe F, et al. German experience with colon interposition grafting as an esophageal substitute. Dis Esophagus 2001;14(2):131–4. https://doi.org/10.1046/j.1442-2050.2001.00170.x.

84. Han Y, Cheng QS, Li XF, et al. Surgical management of esophageal strictures after caustic burns: a 30 years of experience. World J Gastroenterol 2004;10(19):2846–9. https://doi.org/10.3748/wjg.v10.i19.2846.

85. Motoyama S, Kitamura M, Saito R, et al. Surgical outcome of colon interposition by the posterior mediastinal route for thoracic esophageal cancer. Ann Thorac Surg 2007;83(4):1273–8. https://doi.org/10.1016/j.athoracsur.2006.11.049.

86. Bothereau H, Munoz-Bongrand N, Lambert B, et al. Esophageal reconstruction after caustic injury: is there still a place for right coloplasty? Am J Surg 2007;193(6):660–4. https://doi.org/10.1016/j.amjsurg.2006.08.074.

87. Mine S, Udagawa H, Tsutsumi K, et al. Colon interposition after esophagectomy with extended lymphadenectomy for esophageal cancer. Ann Thorac Surg 2009;88(5):1647–53. https://doi.org/10.1016/j.athoracsur.2009.05.081.

88. Lee K, Kim HR, Park SI, et al. Surgical outcome of colon interposition in esophageal cancer surgery: analysis of risk factors for conduit-related morbidity. Thorac Cardiovasc Surg 2018;66(5):384–9. https://doi.org/10.1055/s-0037-1606828.

89. Reslinger V, Tranchart H, D'Annunzio E, et al. Esophageal reconstruction by colon interposition after esophagectomy for cancer analysis of current indications, operative outcomes, and long-term survival. J Surg Oncol 2016;113(2):159–64. https://doi.org/10.1002/jso.24118.

90. Zeng WH, Jiang WL, Kang GJ, et al. Colon interposition for corrosive esophageal stricture: single institution experience with 119 cases. Curr Med Sci 2019;39(3):415–8. https://doi.org/10.1007/s11596-019-2052-0.

91. Shirakawa Y, Naomoto Y, Noma K, et al. Colonic interposition and supercharge for esophageal reconstruction. Langenbecks Arch Surg 2006;391(1):19–23. https://doi.org/10.1007/s00423-005-0010-8.

92. Doki Y, Okada K, Miyata H, et al. Long-term and short-term evaluation of esophageal reconstruction using the colon or the jejunum in esophageal cancer patients after gastrectomy. Dis Esophagus 2008;21(2):132–8. https://doi.org/10.1111/j.1442-2050.2007.00738.x.

93. Saeki H, Morita M, Harada N, et al. Esophageal replacement by colon interposition with microvascular surgery for patients with thoracic esophageal cancer: the utility of superdrainage. Dis Esophagus 2013;26(1):50–6. https://doi.org/10.1111/j.1442-2050.2012.01327.x.

Supercharged Jejunal Interposition

Anita T. Mohan, MBBS, PhD[a], Samir Mardini, MD[a], Shanda H. Blackmon, MD, MPH[b],*

KEYWORDS

- Supercharged jejunum • Jejunum • Interposition • Esophageal reconstruction
- Supercharged pedicled jejunum • Esophageal cancer

KEY POINTS

- Complex esophageal reconstruction is challenging and is associated with high morbidity. .
- Root cause analysis of complications after SPJ has led to the development of targeted modifications to reduce adverse outcomes.
- A systematic checklist approach, dedicated pathway, and multidisciplinary aligned teams are essential to continue to optimize outcomes.
- Targeted modifications can improve recovery, length of hospital stay, surgical outcomes, and long-term (>12 months) patient-reported outcomes such as dumping GI symptoms.
- Patient-reported outcomes (PRO) are important and can identify patients reporting severe symptoms and can assist in the monitoring of symptoms postoperatively and create targeted actions to address symptoms. This can potentially allow the comparison of variable techniques.

BACKGROUND

Esophageal reconstructive options can be limited when a gastric conduit is not available. Alternative sources for reconstruction need to be considered. Salvage or secondary surgery to reestablish gastrointestinal continuity can be extremely challenging in the setting of previous surgery, severe scarring, radiation, and preexisting comorbidities. The jejunum retains anatomic and physiologic characteristics that make it an excellent alternative conduit for esophageal reconstruction.[1–3] The jejunum has comparable luminal size, intrinsic peristaltic activity, relative abundance, low risk of intrinsic disease, and may not undergo senescent lengthening compared with the colon and obviates the need for a preoperative bowel prep. The jejunum has a reliable blood supply. The segmental nature has been a previous limitation to partial esophageal reconstruction. However, with advances in microsurgical techniques to assist in augmenting the blood supply in the proximal aspect of long segment interposition, these flaps can be reliably used for total esophageal reconstruction. Jejunal flaps can be mobilized as a pedicled, augmented ("supercharged") pedicled, or transferred as free flaps for reconstruction.

HISTORY

Jejunal interposition for esophageal reconstruction has evolved through technical advances from its introduction in the early 1900s.[4] Alexis Carrel, a French surgeon who won the Nobel Prize in medicine for his work in vascular anastomosis and organ transplantation, was among the first to describe the use of jejunal conduits for esophageal reconstruction in animal models.[5] This was subsequently followed by Roux in 1907 who reported the successful use of the pedicled jejunum for esophageal reconstruction in humans.[6] Since its description and initial development, Yudin,[7]

[a] Department of Surgery, Division of Plastic and Reconstructive Surgery, 200 First Street Southwest, Rochester, MN 55905, USA; [b] Department of Surgery, Division of Thoracic Surgery, Mayo Clinic, 200 First Street Southwest, Rochester, MN 55905, USA
* Corresponding author.
E-mail address: Blackmon.Shanda@mayo.edu
Twitter: @anitatmohan (A.T.M.)

Thorac Surg Clin 32 (2022) 529–540
https://doi.org/10.1016/j.thorsurg.2022.07.007
1547-4127/22/© 2022 Elsevier Inc. All rights reserved.

Ochsner and Owens,[8] and Rienhoff[9] were among the surgeons who subsequently published their experience using these flaps for both benign strictures and carcinoma. However, there were notable concerns on reliability and technical difficulty for total esophageal reconstruction, high rates of flap necrosis, and associated morbidity that was largely attributable to blood supply. Longmire[10] further modified Roux's technique by incorporating microvascular techniques and augmenting the blood supply between the mesenteric vessels and internal mammary vessels. In a similar period, both Longmire (1951) and Androsov (1956) reported benefits of vascular augmentation or "supercharging" the distal segment of the pedicled jejunal flaps.

The concept of supercharging was a significant development in esophageal reconstruction. Over the next 50 years, we have made considerable advances in the reliability and applicability of microsurgical techniques, including free tissue transfer of jejunal flaps for high esophageal reconstruction. Modern advances in these techniques and outcomes have made the use of pedicled jejunal flaps more widely accepted, particularly for total esophageal reconstruction. Ascioti and colleagues from the MD Anderson Cancer Center (MDACC) (2005) reported the first large American series of long segment supercharged pedicled jejunal (SPJ) interposition in 26 patients for esophageal cancer, with a success rate of 92.3%.[11] Blackmon and colleagues (2012) reported their multi-institutional series (MDACC and Houston Methodist Hospital HMH) in 60 combined patients to evaluate technical outcomes[12] and this study cohort was included in a subsequent review by Mays and colleagues (2019) of 100 patients between these same 2 institutions.[13]

NATURE OF THE PROBLEM

The complexity of surgery, patient presentation, and need for microsurgical expertise is a limiting factor to the popularity of the SPJ. There are still limited data on the clinical and functional outcomes using this technique. Most of these surgeries are performed in the setting of oncologic disease. Surgery among this complex group of patients is associated with notable morbidity. SPJ reconstruction can offer patients an improvement in quality of life when few salvage procedures are available to them.[13,14] Patients who present for salvage or secondary reconstruction of the esophagus when no gastric conduit is available, may also have associated risk factors including suboptimal nutritional status, advanced age, significant medical comorbidities, scarring or complications

from previous surgeries. Staged reconstruction following esophageal resection and diversion, is our preferred approach. It allows time for delivery of radiation therapy, assessment for metastatic disease, and patient optimization. The staged approach can be considered as reconstruction is not considered an emergency surgery.

ANATOMY

The jejunum is intraperitoneal and easily recognized at the ligament of Treitz. The jejunum and ileum are attached to the posterior wall by the mesentery. The motility of the jejunum consists of circumferential segmental contraction and peristalsis, which can become variable following transplantation.[15] The blood supply is segmental and arises from the superior mesenteric artery (SMA) and jejunal arteries arising from the left side of the artery. There are usually 4 to 5 jejunal arteries or "pedicles" to the jejunum. The jejunal arteries contribute to a branching network of tiered arcades that are usually supplied by a single arteriovenous origin and have a distinct pattern, then branching to create marginal arteries and finally terminating as the vasa recta of the bowel (**Fig. 1**). Anatomic variation of the classic patterns may also exist. Jejunal veins accompany the arterial branches.

PREOPERATIVE PLANNING

As previously noted, the complexity and heterogeneity of this patient population highlight the need for a multi-disciplinary approach to management and future monitoring. **Fig. 2** provides an overview of our systematic approach to the management of complex esophageal reconstruction. Oncologic, previous operative, medical, psychological, and planning of future surgical care are all elements that are integrated within the pathway with dedicated teams and support centered around patient care. It is important to ensure that there is the absence of active metastatic disease, improved malnutritional status (prealbumin >17, albumin >3), and an absence of infection, neutropenia, and deconditioning.[16] In complex cases whereby patients may have had multiple previous abdominal surgeries or reconstructive failure, the use of three-dimensional vascular mapping of the mesenteric vasculature can provide a valuable source of information for surgical planning and decision-making (**Fig. 3**).

The reconstruction is more typically performed after an esophageal diversion to optimize surgical circumstances. The optimal timing for reconstruction following diversion is also unknown, but is

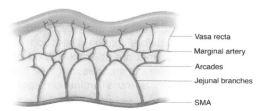

Fig. 1. Arrangement of vascular arcades and blood supply to the jejunum. (Used with permission of Mayo Foundation for Medical Education and Research.)

typically 6 months for patients with cancer and 3 months for noncancer etiology. Patients with benign disease may benefit from earlier reconstruction, compared with those with a malignant disease whereby adjuvant therapy may be completed, and patients can be optimized in terms of nutrition and comorbidities before undergoing a major reconstruction. Further benefits of planned staged reconstruction include a reduction in surgical operative time, reduced patient stress response, less edema, and enhanced hemodynamic instability.

Careful planning, optimization, and experienced cross-disciplinary team approach to surgery is an essential part of the success of the procedure and improve recovery and outcomes.

CHECKLIST PREPARATION AND PATIENT POSITIONING

- Stop all anticoagulants before surgery
- No bowel preparation required
- No thoracic epidural needed.

- Right-sided central venous access line, arterial line and urinary catheter, sequential compression devices, temperature probe, single endotracheal tube
- Supine positioning, arms tucked, pressure points padded and an inflatable shoulder roll placed to extend the neck
- Sterilize the J-tube site as much as possible as it can be a source of infection at the time of moving the J-tube. Nonalcoholic skin preparation is used around the esophagostomy and J-tube or G-tube site (fire risk).
- Patient is prepped from jawline, neck, chest, abdomen, groins, and bilateral legs (for possible saphenous vein grafts)
- Nerve monitoring system to provide recurrent laryngeal nerve alert during diversion procedures but not for reconstruction
- Avoid hypovolemia. Avoid vasopressors when possible
- Proactive transfusion as needed
- Hold heparin on induction and bilateral lower extremity sequential compressive devices placed
- Antibiotics on induction. Our primary choice is Cefazolin IV.

PROCEDURAL CHECKLIST
Exploratory Laparotomy

- In the second stage operation whereby the SPJ procedure is performed starting with exploratory laparotomy
- A completion gastrectomy if there is residual antrum only versus using for g-tube access

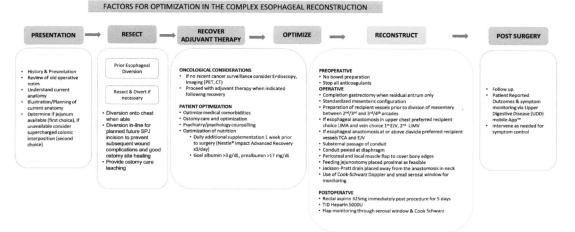

Fig. 2. Overview of our complex esophageal reconstruction pathway. CT, computed tomography; EJV, external jugular vein; LIMA, left internal mammary artery; LIMV, left internal mammary vein; NPO, nothing by mouth; SPJ, supercharged pedicled jejunal flap; SQ, subcutaneous; TCA, transverse cervical artery; TID, three times a day; PET, positive emission tomography; POD, postoperative day.

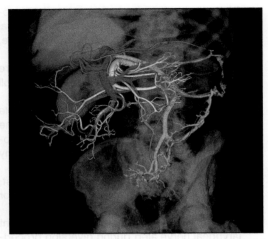

Fig. 3. Three-dimensional Computed Tomographic Angiography mapping of superior mesenteric artery and venous vasculature and assessment of available arcades.

- If an unexpected pathologic process is encountered early during exploratory laparotomy, do not proceed with the SPJ interposition operation[16]
- The entire length of the small bowel and mesenteric jejunal branches are identified
- If there is a presence of scar tissue or adhesions, perform lysis of adhesions
- Previous feeding jejunostomy tube site is taken down and oversewn. This site is considered a potential infection risk due to colonization and typically not included in the jejunal interposition.

Evaluation and Dissection of Mesentery

Selection of the jejunal arcades is based on the patient's anatomy, the length needed, previous jejunum surgery, previous placement of jejunal feeding tubes, and arterial anatomy including congenital variations in mesenteric vascular patterns. This can be complicated in patients with a history of previous Roux-en-Y procedures. The thoracic surgeon and plastic surgeon work closely to isolate the proper segments, with back lighting to dissect the vessels and prepare the flap for transposition.

- The goal is to preserve more than 20 cm of bowel from the ligament of Treitz and the first arcade
- The first mesenteric jejunal branch of the SMA is preserved on the planned arterial division of the mesentery between the first and second arcades (**Fig. 4**)
- Flap harvest and division of the arcades are performed by the thoracic surgeon and plastic surgery

- Inspect the entire arcade pattern to ensure the downstream branches are intact and favorable for use before ligation/dissection
- Jejunal segments are selected based on the arrangement of the arcades and their feeding vessels using a transillumination approach (**Fig. 5**)
- Prepare the second mesenteric branch of the SMA for microvascular anastomosis as the proximal segment of the jejunum that will reach into the neck (see **Fig. 5**)
- Division of the third arcade allowing use as a pedicle and to unfurl the bowel in a way it could also be used as a backup to connect as a supercharge if there is a complication to the second arcade
- Maintain the fourth or fifth jejunal arcade to be the primary blood supply to the distal segment of jejunum (the bowel that reaches into the chest), with the option to use the 4th as an additional pedicle like the 3rd, when length is an issue
- Transect the jejunum between the first and second jejunal arteries (**Fig. 6**)
- Do not perform the division of the mesentery between the second and third segments or between the third and fourth segments until the recipient vessels in the neck or chest are completed.
- Division of second jejunal arcade may start the clock for ischemic time.[16]

Preparation of Recipient Site in the Neck

- Esophageal diversion has been adapted to lie within the line of future incision for hemi-manubriectomy with SPJ cervical anastomosis (see **Fig. 6**)
- A left cervico-thoracic exploratory incision is made in a left-sided oblique orientation
- Takedown the diverting left esophagostomy with a wide vascular border to preserve collateral blood supply.
- Resection of a quarter of the superior left manubrium, the head of the clavicle, the head of the left first rib, and medial aspect of the second rib as needed (if further length for the IMA Is required). Leave periosteum on the left proximal 1st rib to cover bony edges
- A Midas Rex diamond tipped burr can assist to soften the bony edges to prevent erosion into the vessels.
- Perichondrium of the ribs is preserved to facilitate the dissection and preparation of the mammary vessels.

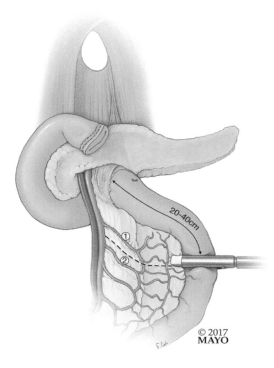

- Explore sites for recipient vessel selection for microanastomosis. Most of the recipient arteries and veins included the left internal mammary artery (LIMA), transverse cervical artery (TCA), left internal mammary vein (LIMV), and left external jugular vein (LEJV). The choice of recipient's vessels depends on the anticipated location of the pedicle of the jejunum after transposition and vessel size match (**Fig. 7**). Standardization includes the mesenteric artery to the LIMA and mesenteric vein to the EJV or LIMV.
- The external jugular vein is larger, a closer match to the jejunal pedicle, and can be dissected to provide length even for a lower esophageal anastomosis whereby the pedicle is below the clavicle.
- In cases whereby the esophagus stump is higher (mid-neck or higher, the pedicle of the jejunum ends up at the level of the clavicle or higher, the TCA and the LEJV are selected as recipient's vessels.
- If the patient has had a LIMA bypass, the right-sided vessels or transverse cervical vessels are typically selected as a second-choice recipient option. In these cases, an incision with esophageal diversion to the right neck is conducted in preparation for these less common cases.

Fig. 4. Illustration to show planned division of the jejunum between the first and second jejunal branches. (Used with permission of Mayo Foundation for Medical Education and Research.)

- Periosteal and perichondrial flaps from the medial aspect of the ribs and clavicle allow coverage of bony edges.
- Local muscle flaps can be raised using the superior aspect of the left pectoralis major muscle, dividing the medial fibers from its insertion, to allow the transposition of the medial portion to provide further coverage of the bone

Retrosternal Tunnel Creation and Flap Transposition

- A retrosternal tunnel is created, four–five finger breaths, with blunt dissection in front of the pericardium in the anterior mediastinal space, starting with an incision in the anterior midline of the diaphragm. This allows direct visualization of the flap on transposition and good orientation of the vessels for supercharging to nearby recipient's vessels.

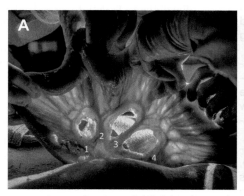
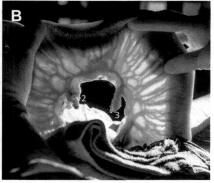

Fig. 5. Intraoperative evaluation of (*A*) jejunal vascular patterns using intraoperative transillumination and pedicle selection, (*B*) division and division of the mesentery to allow unfurling and adequate transposition of the flap.

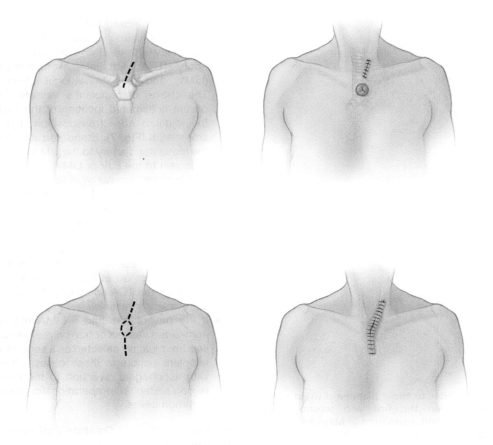

Fig. 6. Esophagostomy and cervical incision planning for SPJ interposition. (Used with permission of Mayo Foundation for Medical Education and Research.)

Jejunum is delivered antecolic if Roux previously performed. If jejunum is going to be connected to the antrum, then a retrocolic route is recommended.

- Jejunal branches and the mesentery is divided between either the second and third arcade or the third and fourth arcade. The bowel has a 3:1 radio of bowel length to mesentery, and such mesentery division allows straightening of the jejunum as it unfurls (**Fig. 8**)
- Adequate length achieved when the flap is unfurled before flap transposition. This often requires division of mesentery to the level of the bowel to straighten the conduit, with a few exceptional cases based on the arcade anatomy (**Fig. 9**).
- The bowel is then passed through the retrosternal tunnel using an ultrasound probe, cover to protect and ensuring that it remains straight and under no tension or twisting through the delivery. The bowel is sutured to the bag and the bowel is pushed into the

tunnel led by the bag. It is important to avoid pulling and always ensure the surgeon feels resistance
- Mesentery is placed to the left during transposition.
- A double-layered handsewn end-to-end anastomosis is performed between the cervical esophagus and proximal jejunum (inner layer 3–0 Vicryl and outer 3–0 Silk)
- Redundant bowel is discarded but mesentery leading up to that bowel is kept to lay on top of the anastomosis.

Microvascular Anastomosis: Supercharging

- The operating microscope is used to perform the anastomosis of the arteries and the veins
- The anastomosis is completed between typically the second jejunal pedicle and the selected recipient vessels
- Arterial microanastomosis is performed using 10/0 nylon sutures in an interrupted fashion

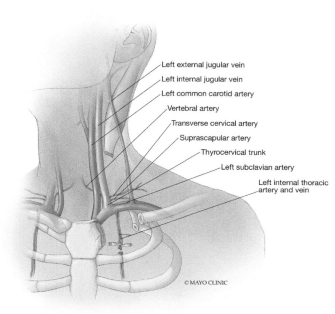

Fig. 7. Recipient site vessel selection and exposure in the neck for supercharged pedicled jejunal interposition. (Used with permission of Mayo Foundation for Medical Education and Research.)

Left external jugular vein
Left internal jugular vein
Left common carotid artery
Vertebral artery
Transverse cervical artery
Suprascapular artery
Thyrocervical trunk
Left subclavian artery
Left internal thoracic artery and vein

© MAYO CLINIC

- Venous anastomosis is performed using a microvascular anastomotic coupler (Synovis, Birmingham, AL)
- An internal Cook-Swartz Doppler probe (Cook Medical, Bloomington, IN) is placed on the vein for flap monitoring.
- Aim to keep ischemia time to less than 1 hour.
- A small 2 × 2cm serosal window of the jejunum or mesentery is left exposed for monitoring. We no longer use an external segment of jejunum as a sentinel flap for monitoring.

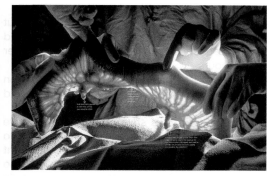

Fig. 8. Intraoperative example of unfurled jejunal flap as a straight conduit for esophageal reconstruction following division of the jejunal arteries and division of mesentery.

Feeding Tube Placement

- The feeding gastrostomy tube may be left in place if the jejunum is not used with a feeding tube.
- A new jejunal feeding tube may be fashioned and placed as proximal as possible, and at least 4 to 5 cm in length, and pexied to the abdominal wall to avoid bowel torsion

Closure and Dressings

- The serosal window is covered with Adaptic nonadherent dressing and is treated with regular wet to wet dressings (every 2 hours) until it granulates (**Fig. 10**)
- Once the serosal window has granulated it is dressed in impregnated petroleum gauze dressing daily until it heals by secondary intention (3–4 weeks).
- Two flat channel Jackson–Pratt drains are placed in the neck away from the site of the vascular and esophageal anastomosis.
- Neck incision is closed in 2 layers.
- The abdominal closure is performed during the neck microanastomosis.
- Mesenteric defects are closed to prevent internal herniation and the defect of the diaphragm is closed along the bowel, taking care to not damage the pedicle of the flap.

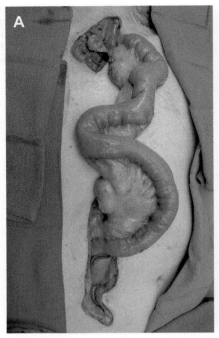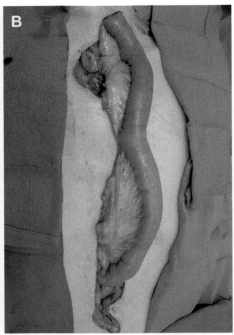

Fig. 9. Intraoperative example of furled and unfurled jejunal flap and length acquired for delivery of super-charged pedicled jejunal interposition. Furled (to the left) and unfurled with mesentery fully divided (to the right)

- The conduit is also pexied to the diaphragm at this level to prevent para-conduit herniation.
- No drains are placed in the peritoneal cavity.
- No nasogastric tube is inserted

POSTPROCEDURE CARE

- Maintaining a higher intravascular volume will reduce the need for intraoperative or postoperative vasopressors.
- Postoperative transfusion is rarely required; however, since large and rapid blood loss could be encountered a proactive transfusion protocol should be in place. Maintain Hemoglobin above 8.0 g/dL is preferred.
- The patient is transferred from the operating room bed directly to the ICU bed after surgery.
- Avoid transfer to a temporary bed for transport, with subsequent additional transfer to the ICU bed. Every transfer has a potential impact on perfusion to the flap.
- The patient is kept in the intensive care unit whereby close hemodynamic and flap monitoring for the first 24 hours is performed.
- The patient is typically extubated on the first postoperative day.
- Rectal aspirin is administered immediately at the end of the procedure and for 5 days postoperatively, and subcutaneous heparin is given the night of surgery and throughout the hospital stay.
- If there are any intraoperative concerns during microanastomosis, intravenous heparin bolus may be administrated intraoperatively and the patient may be placed on a heparin infusion for 24 to 48 hours
- Flap monitoring is performed hourly for the first 24 hours, every 2 hours between 24 and 48 hours and then every 4 hours until discharge
- Patient is provided with IV patient-controlled analgesia (PCA) and maintained for several days to ensure adequate pain control
- Bed rest is encouraged for 24 hours, then out to chair on the second postoperative day and subsequent ambulation with assistance after 48 hours
- The head is maintained in a neutral position and very gentle slight turning allowed, and no pressure over the neck or upper chest
- Enteral feeding is started after postoperative day 3 or when bowel activity beings, to advance slowly and suspended if the patient complains of abdominal pain. This will also help to avoid nonobstructive mesenteric ischemia (NOMI)
- Target discharge from hospital on postoperative day 7

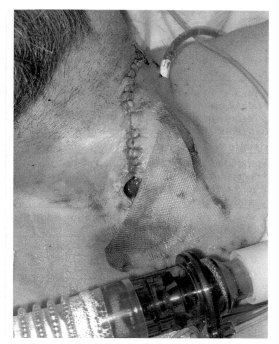

Fig. 10. Serosal window for flap monitoring following SPJ interposition covered with nonadherent dressing and kept moist with wet to wet gauze dressings every 2 hours.

Outcomes

Esophageal reconstruction in patients without a viable gastric conduit due to pathology or previous surgery creates a potentially hostile environment associated with a notable degree of morbidity. The use of supercharged pedicled jejunal flaps requires an experienced cross-disciplinary team that includes expertise in esophageal reconstruction and reconstructive microsurgery and is performed at specialized tertiary centers. Microsurgical techniques have expanded the utilization of the jejunum for proximal, distal, and total esophageal reconstruction to establish continuity, and are the preferred reconstructive option among many surgeons.[12,13,17–19]

Doki and colleagues (2008) reported jejunum reconstruction was superior to the colon due to lower anastomotic leak rates, shorter hospital stay, and lower postoperative loss of body-weight.[20] There are limited direct comparative studies between the use of the colon or jejunum, and therefore superiority of either approach is still debated. The following characteristics of the jejunum make it suitable as an alternative conduit:[1,2,12,13]

- A lumen size similar to that of the esophagus
- Relatively abundant length

- No requirement for formal preoperative preparation
- Lower incidence of intrinsic diseases
- Retains some segmental antegrade contraction that can assist in the clearance of swallowed food bolus through the conduit,
- Lower rates of senescent lengthening compared with the colon.

Most of the patients undergoing SPJ reconstruction are performed in the setting of oncologic disease.[12,13,21] Since the early reports of flap harvest and utility, there have been considerable advances in the adoption of microvascular techniques that have made a substantial change in the rates of flap survival (90%–100%) and ensuring a robust blood supply. Success in establishing a solid or oral diet following SPJ reconstruction has been reported between 86% and 92%. Despite advances in techniques and perioperative care, the reported rates of surgical complications and medical complications are still significant. In a multi-institutional series of 100 patients surgical complications have been reported at 42% with nearly half representing major inpatient complications, and an anastomotic leak rate of 13%.[13] In the same series of 28% medical complications, pneumonia was the most common at 18%. Potential risk factors for this include prior recurrent laryngeal nerve injury and propensity to aspirate when the jejunum is filled with food or liquids, distends, and then begins to contract which causes the regurgitation of fluid back into the throat. Patients are counseled to swallow three times more frequently than before the reconstructive surgery. In our institution, we have implemented targeted modifications to improve recovery and reduce complications through analysis of our own data and prior experience (**Table 1**).

An area of patient care that continues to grow in this patient population includes patient-reported outcomes (PROs) measures. The use of PROs can be used to acquire baseline functional data and symptoms and be used to evaluate interventions and postoperative symptom monitoring. There are limited published data in quality-of-life outcomes research and limited tools specific to esophageal reconstructive surgery. A variety of PRO tools have been established for patients with esophageal cancer and esophagectomies including quality of life scoring using Functional Assessment of Cancer Therapy Esophageal Cancer (FACT-E), European Organization for Research and Treatment of Cancer (EORTC) QLQ-OES18 questionnaires.[22,23] There are several published PROs have been developed for benign disease

Table 1
Intraoperative complications and associated targeted modifications in SPJ esophageal reconstruction

Type of Intraoperative Problem/Complication	Targeted Modification to Intraoperative Algorithm
Adjuvant therapy was delayed due to complication in single staged reconstruction,	2 stage approach with esophageal diversion to allow optimization and delayed reconstruction. Can reduce fluid sequestration and bowel edema
Intraoperative hypotension	Limit the use of epidurals
Ischemia of skin edges or delayed healing at the site of previous end esophagostomy	Esophageal diversion is designed to be incorporated within the line of future incision for hemi-manubriectomy with SPJ cervical anastomosis
Variation in mesenteric configurations	Standardized mesenteric configuration and dissection approach
Mesenteric bleeding	Careful Ligation of the largest vessels with 3–0 silk and reinforce with clips and LigaSure during flap harvest
Paraconduit hernia	Perform suspension of conduit as it passes through diaphragm
Jejunal scarring from feeding jejunostomy	Place feeding jejunostomy as proximal as possible
Abdominal wall adhesions	Use of Seprafilm® to reduce abdominal adhesions
Ulceration secondary to retained antrum	Perform completion gastrectomy when only residual antrum remains
Arterial postoperative bleeding	Prevent erosion by raising a periosteal flap covering over bony edges and smooth edges with diamond tipped burr
Cervical anastomosis recipient vein mismatch	Use external jugular vein or internal jugular vein due to better size match compared with the internal mammary vein and allows better inset of the flap following anastomosis
Complications from Monitoring loop of jejunum flap (including bleeding)	Flap monitoring provided by the use of internal Cook-Schwarz Doppler in addition to a small serosal window in the line of incision that heals by secondary intention, and avoiding the use of exteriorized bowel
Anastomotic Leak	Jackson Pratt drain placed away from the anastomosis site
Wound infections	Decontamination of J-tube sites before surgery, culture and treat sites as needed preoperatively.

conditions including the Gastrointestinal Symptom Rating Scale (GSRS), Quality of Life in Reflux and Dyspepsia (QOLRAD) questionnaire among others that have been validated to assess symptoms. Most studies evaluating health-related quality of life questionnaires were developed for patients undergoing a variety of treatment modalities, including nonsurgical management, or addressing concerns during active cancer management.[24] Treatment-specific postesophagectomy questionnaires have been developed such as the Dysfunction After Upper Gastrointestinal Surgery (DAUGS20) and the Upper Digestive Disease mobile application (UDD App), that was previously known as the CONDUIT tool.[23–25]

PROs can be used to monitor patient symptoms, guide therapeutic interventions, and assess the effectiveness of interventions or techniques. They can be used to better understand commonly experienced symptoms following reconstruction in this patient population and potential for prognostication in malignant disease.[26] Functional outcomes of SPJ interpositions have been shown to be comparable to that of the gastric conduits by using a comprehensive conduit assessment questionnaire too.[27] However, pain is more severe by comparison, likely due to hemi-manubriectomy, first rib resection, and additional scarring.

SUMMARY

Esophageal reconstruction with supercharged jejunum can be challenging and include high morbidity. A systematic approach, dedicated pathway, and a multidisciplinary approach can assist in optimizing outcomes and continue to monitor patients following surgery. Microsurgical techniques and cross-disciplinary approach to the execution have improved clinical outcomes and flap survival. Patient-reported outcomes are essential ways to compare groups of patients, techniques, and detect and manage problems.

CLINICS CARE POINTS

- The jejunum is relatively abundant, often free of disease, has intrinsic peristalsis, offers a good size match, and has a reliable blood supply for esophageal reconstruction.
- Success of the supercharged pedicled jejunal flaps interposition for esophageal reconstruction has been developed with advances in microvascular techniques to augment the blood supply of the proximal segment.
- A multidisciplinary and systematic approach, with standardization, is needed to assist in perioperative optimization, execution of the procedure, and reduction of errors.
- A delayed reconstruction can provide time for surgical and medical optimization, decrease the risk of prolonged anesthesia and hemodynamic instability, and enhance the delivery of adjuvant therapy.
- In spite of improving outcomes, the incidence of surgical and medical complications is still significant in this complex SPJ patient group.
- Patient-reported outcome data may provide an avenue to compare interventions and monitor symptoms following surgery, enhancing understanding of the long-term postoperative course, assisting in targeting persistent symptoms, and improving the overall quality of life.

DISCLOSURE

Dr S.H. Blackmon: esophageal anastomotic device patent, funded clinical trials by Medtronic and Steris.

REFERENCES

1. Gaur P, Blackmon SH. Jejunal graft conduits after esophagectomy. J Thorac Dis 2014;6(SUPPL.3): S333.
2. Bakshi A, Sugarbaker DJ, Burt BM. Alternative conduits for esophageal replacement. Ann Cardiothorac Surg 2017;6(2):137–43.
3. Chen HC, Rampazzo A, Gharb BB, et al. Motility differences in free colon and free jejunum flaps for reconstruction of the cervical esophagus. Plast Reconstr Surg 2008;122(5):1410–6.
4. Yasuda T, Shiozaki H. Esophageal Reconstruction Using a Pedicled Jejunum with Microvascular Augmentation. Ann Thorac Cardiovasc Surg 2011; 17(2):103–9.
5. Carrel A. The surgery of blood vessels etc. Johns Hopkins Hosp Bull 1907;18(190).
6. Roux C. A new operation for intractable obstruction of the esophagus (L'oesophago-jejuno-gastrosiose, nouvelle operation pour retrecissement infranchissable del'oesophage). Sem Med 1907;27:34–40.
7. Yudin SS. The surgical construction of 80 cases of artificial esophagus. Surg Gynecol Obs 1944;78: 561–83.
8. Ochsner A, Owens N. Anterothoracic Oesophagoplasty for Impermeable Stricture of the Oesophagus. Ann Surg 1934;100(6):1055.
9. Rienhoff WF. Intrathoracic esophagojejunostomy for lesions of the upper third of the esophagus. South Med J 1946;39(12):928–40.
10. LONGMIRE WP, RAVITCH MM. A new method for constructing an artificial esophagus. Ann Surg 1946;123:819–35.
11. Ascioti AJ, Hofstetter WL, Miller MJ, et al. Long-segment, supercharged, pedicled jejunal flap for total esophageal reconstruction. J Thorac Cardiovasc Surg 2005;130(5):1391–8.
12. Blackmon SH, Correa AM, Skoracki R, et al. Supercharged pedicled jejunal interposition for esophageal replacement: A 10-year experience. Ann Thorac Surg 2012;94:1104–13.
13. Mays AC, Yu P, Hofstetter W, et al. The Supercharged Pedicled Jejunal Flap for Total Esophageal Reconstruction: A Retrospective Review of 100 Cases. Plast Reconstr Surg 2019;144(5):1171–80.
14. Swisher SG, Hofstetter WL, Miller MJ. The Supercharged Microvascular Jejunal Interposition. Semin Thorac Cardiovasc Surg 2007;19(1):56–65.

15. Chen H-C, Spanio di Spilimbergo S, Evans KF, et al. In: Wei F-C, Mardini S, editors. Jejunum flap. 1st edition. Elsevier; 2009.

16. Blackmon SH. Long-Segment, Supercharged Pedicled Jejunal Interposition for Esophageal Replacement: How I Teach It. Ann Thorac Surg 2018; 105(2):345–50.

17. Sekido M, Yamamoto Y, Minakawa H, et al. Use of the "supercharge" technique in esophageal and pharyngeal reconstruction to augment microvascular blood flow. Surgery 2003;134(3):420–4.

18. Barzin A, Norton JA, Whyte R, et al. Supercharged jejunum flap for total esophageal reconstruction: Single-surgeon 3-year experience and outcomes analysis. Plast Reconstr Surg 2011;127(1):173–80.

19. Poh M, Selber JC, Skoracki R, et al. Technical challenges of total esophageal reconstruction using a supercharged jejunal flap. Ann Surg 2011;253(6): 1122–9.

20. Doki Y, Okada K, Miyata H, et al. Long-term and short-term evaluation of esophageal reconstruction using the colon or the jejunum in esophageal cancer patients after gastrectomy. Dis Esophagus 2008; 21(2):132–8.

21. Mohan AT, Mahajan NN, Mardini S, et al. Outcomes of Standardized Protocols in Supercharged Pedicled Jejunal Esophageal Reconstruction. Ann Thorac Surg 2022. In press.

22. Baker CR, Forshaw MJ, Gossage JA, et al. Long-term outcome and quality of life after supercharged jejunal interposition for oesophageal replacement. Surgeon 2015;13(4):187–93.

23. Straatman J, Joosten PJM, Terwee CB, et al. Systematic review of patient-reported outcome measures in the surgical treatment of patients with esophageal cancer. Dis Esophagus 2016;29(7): 760–72.

24. Mahajan NN, Lee MK, Yost KJ, et al. Preliminary Normative Standards of the Mayo Clinic Esophagectomy CONDUIT Tool. Mayo Clin Proc Innov Qual Outcomes 2019;3(4):429–37.

25. Lee MK, Yost KJ, Pierson KE, et al. Patient-reported outcome domains for the esophageal CONDUIT report card: A prospective trial to establish domains. Health Qual Life Outcomes 2018;16(1):197.

26. Ahmed M, Lau A, Hirpara DH, et al. Choosing the right survey—patient reported outcomes in esophageal surgery. J Thorac Dis 2020;12(11):6902.

27. Stephens EH, Gaur P, Hotze KO, et al. Super-Charged Pedicled Jejunal Interposition Performance Compares Favorably With a Gastric Conduit After Esophagectomy. Ann Thorac Surg 2015;100(2): 407–13.

Ongoing Controversies in Esophageal Cancer I
Feeding Tubes, Pyloroplasty, Thoracic Duct Clipping

Sidra N. Bonner, MD, MPH, MSc[a], Ryan Rebernick, BA[b],
Elliot Wakeam, MD, MPH[c],*

KEYWORDS

- Esophageal cancer • Jejunostomy tube • Pyloroplasty • Thoracic duct • Chyle leak

KEY POINTS

- If feeding tube placement is required, the ideal timing for placement is intraoperative—ideally as part of a minimally invasive procedure.
- Pyloric drainage procedures, depending on a surgeon's preference, can be performed safely and routinely with a nonsignificant reduction in delayed gastric conduit emptying and no clear benefit for reduced postoperative pulmonary complications or mortality.
- For surgeons who do not perform routine pyloric drainage, endoscopic interventions are a safe treatment for patients who develop clinically significant delayed gastric conduit emptying.
- Currently, there is no strong evidence to support prophylactic thoracic duct ligation.

INTRODUCTION

Esophagectomy remains a core component of treatment for patients with early-stage and locally advanced esophageal cancer.[1] Given the prevalence of perioperative complications, including anastomotic leaks, pneumonia, poor nutrition, reintubation, and mortality, some surgeons have advocated for routine placement of feeding tubes, pyloroplasty, and prophylactic thoracic duct clipping at the time of operation to reduce postoperative complications. Whether or not these procedures should be routinely done during esophagectomy remains controversial, and the data on whether these interventions reduce complications or paradoxically worsen outcomes are conflicting. This article outlines the rationale, current evidence, and new advances related to feeding tubes, pyloroplasty, and prophylactic thoracic duct clipping during esophagectomy.

Feeding Tubes

Patient evaluation and considerations of clinical appropriateness

Feeding tube placement is often deemed necessary when a patient is or is anticipated to experience malnutrition secondary to insufficient oral intake. Patients with esophageal cancer are at increased risk of malnutrition relative to other cancers due to the associated progressive dysphagia which is experienced by nearly 75% of patients at diagnosis.[2–4] Prolonged malnutrition can lead to a decline in body mass index (BMI), physical function, and increased mortality during neoadjuvant therapy or after surgery.[3,5] Patients whose BMI falls below 18.5 benefits from feeding tube placement are almost always indicated for nutritional access (Fenton and colleagues 2011, Alvarez-Serrado et al 2018). Further, nutritional access can be increasingly important if the patient

[a] Department of Surgery, University of Michigan, 1500 East Medical Center Drive, Ann Arbor, MI 48109, USA;
[b] University of Michigan Medical School, 1500 East Medical Center Drive, Ann Arbor, MI 48109, USA; [c] Section of Thoracic Surgery, Department of Surgery, University of Michigan, 1500 East Medical Center Drive, Ann Arbor, MI 48109, USA
* Corresponding author.
E-mail address: ewakeam@med.umich.edu

Thorac Surg Clin 32 (2022) 541–551
https://doi.org/10.1016/j.thorsurg.2022.07.003
1547-4127/22/© 2022 Published by Elsevier Inc.

experiences complications, such as an anastomotic leak. However, feeding tube placement is not without risks. Surgical placement of feeding tubes can result in damage to the gastroepiploic artery, bowel obstruction, tube dislodgement or blockage, and other issues which can occasionally require emergency treatment.[6] Routine placement of feeding tubes at the time of surgery, while classically considered part and parcel of esophagectomy, is increasingly being abandoned in favor of selective placement, however, institutional practices vary in this regard.

Rationale for usage in intraoperative settings

Although dysphagia affects the majority of esophageal cancer patients, the extent to which it affects patient nutritional status is highly variable and requires the care team to decide on the utility and timing of nutritional supplementation. Severe dysphagia preventing oral intake of liquids requires preoperative feeding tube placement, whereas less severe dysphagia may prompt intraoperative placement or be forgone entirely. However, intermediate or rapidly progressive dysphagia is a "gray area" where a feeding tube may be required but is dependent on the degree of nutritional depletion and rate of progression. In this scenario, failure to preoperatively place a feeding tube may lead to significant weight loss, complete obstruction, and the delay of definitive treatment. However, placement of the tube may expose the patient to unnecessary risks, such as surgical complications. To address whether feeding tubes should be placed when dysphagia is intermediate/rapidly progressive, a 2017 study of 156 patients with esophageal cancer examined outcomes in the context of nutrition intervention timing and found no perioperative benefit for enteral access before neoadjuvant chemoradiation.[7] Another study of 234 esophageal cancer patients who underwent esophagectomy showed no nutritional benefit for patients who received enteral feeding access.[8] The lack of benefit for preoperative feeding tube placement is thought to be due to reductions in dysphagia with the initiation of neoadjuvant therapy. Rapid initiation of neoadjuvant therapy is another strategy that can help obviate the need for preoperative feeding tube placement. Initiation of neoadjuvant therapy can in some cases reduce dysphagia by the completion of the first cycle of chemotherapy, and this reduction is independent of the degree of histologic response.[9,10] Thus, by rapidly initiating neoadjuvant therapy, preoperative feeding tube placement can often be postponed to intraoperative placement or avoided entirely.

Technique of placement

Preoperative Several methods exist for preoperative jejunostomy: open surgical, laparoscopic, and percutaneous techniques. Laparoscopic approaches are rapidly becoming standard due to their reduced complication rates in limited comparisons.[11] Briefly, in laparoscopic placement, 2 to 3 5 mm midline ports are placed linearly to allow for feeding tube placement in the left upper quadrant (LUQ). The upper port is used to retract the colon, the middle for the camera, and the lower for small bowel exposition. Once the ligament of Treitz is identified, the small bowel should be traced ~20 to 30 cm distally to identify the feeding tube site—ideally 2 cm below the costal margin. A fine needle is used to mark the site on the abdominal wall and tube fasteners are then placed through the abdominal cavity in a diamond configuration. These are used to secure the bowel to the abdominal wall where an 18-gauge needle is then passed in the center of the diamond through the abdominal cavity and into the bowel. The needle is followed by a wire, a dilator, and eventually a J tube which is assessed for patency with air/saline. The tube is then secured and patency is confirmed. A comprehensive overview of steps in laparoscopic placement and placement through other methods is available.[12]

Intraoperative An intra-operative jejunostomy is a straightforward procedure when paired with the high degree of visualization afforded by esophagectomy. The jejunum is mobilized and a segment of the intestine approximately 30 cm from the ligament of Treitz is selected. The chosen segment is examined downstream until the ileocecal valve to ensure an absence of torsion/adhesions and a 4 mm purse-string suture in box formation is placed on the antimesenteric side. From there, a small enterotomy is made within the purse string suture and the desired feeding tube is fed through approximately 10 cm (or more) distally. A Witzel tunnel is created and the intestine is imbricated over the feeding tube for a short segment. The jejunal segment is secured to the parietal peritoneum such that the intestinal loop is adherent to the LUQ abdominal wall. Finally, the external portion of the tube is secured to the skin and the abdomen is closed. A more detailed overview is available.[12]

Anatomy Key anatomic landmarks for jejunostomy placement center on identifying an appropriate segment of the small intestine. Notable landmarks include the ligament of Trietz and the ileocecal valve. The ligament of Treitz is a thin band of tissue that supports the small intestine and demarcates the transition from the duodenum to the jejunum. Understanding where the ligament of Treitz is in relation to the selected jejunal segment is critical to ensure that the tube is fed in the correct direction.

Prep and patient positioning For both open and laparoscopic jejunostomies, a patient should be placed in a supine position to facilitate access to the small intestine and the ligament of Treitz. For laparoscopic procedures, the patient's right arm can be tucked to facilitate increased standing room for personnel.

Recovery and rehabilitation Tube feeding can be initiated on the evening of the procedure. An initial rate of ~10 mL/h can be attempted and if tolerated advanced by 10 mL/h every 4 hours until the nutritional goal is met. This goal should be set in conjunction with a trained nutritionist familiar with the patient's nutritional status.

Management Following placement, the area surrounding the tube should be kept clean and monitored for signs of infection. An abdominal binder may be used to secure the tube and prevent unintentional removal.

Current evidence of outcomes: complications, survival, Length of Stay, utilization postoperatively

Although jejunostomy was once performed in all patients undergoing surgical treatment for esophageal cancer, these practices are changing. Even though jejunostomies facilitate obtaining nutritional goals in the postoperative period, most patients without complications do not require tube feedings and they are associated with significant complications which may offset their benefit. One study of 76 esophageal cancer patients showed that there was no difference in readmission rates or length of stay in patients who underwent jejunostomy versus those that did not.[13] Additionally, about 30% of patients who undergo esophagectomy visit the emergency department in the year following esophagectomy and feeding tube-related issues make up the majority of these visits.[14] In conjunction with the analyses highlighting the lack of benefit with preoperative jejunostomy placement, these studies collectively suggest that selective jejunostomy placement may minimize risks for patients who are unlikely to require tube feeding.

New developments

For malnourished patients with esophageal cancer, it is becoming increasingly important to facilitate refeeding through both (1) early neoadjuvant

therapy and (2) early oral intake after esophagectomy. As discussed earlier, significant reductions in dysphagia often occur within the first cycle of neoadjuvant therapy and facilitate improved nutritional status. Additionally, early oral intake after esophagectomy has been linked with improved outcomes. The Enhanced Recovery After Surgery program involved the resumption of a clear liquid diet by postoperative day #3 and advancement to a soft diet by day #4 and was associated with lower complication rates compared with the standard refeeding approach.[6,15] While this study was limited to 39 patients, it highlights a likely area of future study focused on less procedurally focused routes to optimizing nutritional status.

Recommendations

The majority of guidance on feeding tube placement in esophageal cancer is based on small, often retrospective studies that are limited to single institutions. However, these studies highlight some common themes. Collectively, the evidence suggests:

1. Avoid placing feeding tubes preoperatively unless a patient has severe malnutrition based on BMI and albumin. We strongly recommend placement for patients with BMI <18.5 and if the patient is unable to consume calories orally. It is likely that the patient's dysphagia and subsequently their weight gain will improve following the first cycle of neoadjuvant therapy.[16–18]
2. Consider forgoing intraoperative feeding tube placement in favor of early refeeding measures. Complication rates associated with tube placement are non-negligible and several studies have shown comparable outcomes ± placement.
3. If feeding tube placement is required, the ideal timing for placement is intraoperative—ideally as part of a minimally invasive procedure (**Table 1**).

Pyloroplasty

Introduction

One of the ongoing controversies in operative technique during esophagectomy are whether drainage procedures of the gastric conduit is associated with improved emptying and reduction in adverse postoperative outcomes.[19] Proponents of pyloric drainage procedures suggest that vagal damage during operation causes gastric dysmotility and denervation of the pylorus necessitating drainage procedures.[20–22] Postoperative dysfunction in gastric emptying has been proposed as a potential cause of nausea, vomiting, and

Table 1
Summary of important studies evaluating indications and outcomes for jejunostomy tube placement

Studies	Study Questions/ Objectives	Study Populations	Study Findings
Fenton et al[16]	What is the absolute indication for feeding tube placement in patients undergoing esophagectomy?	151 patients undergoing esophagectomy for esophageal malignancy	• The only absolute indication for feeding tube placement after esophagectomy was a BMI < 18.5. Patients above this threshold should have a feeding tube placed at the surgeon's discretion.
Álvarez-Sarrado et al[17]	Analyze the nutritional benefits of feeding jejunostomy for early postoperative enteral nutrition and directly related complications.	100 patients undergoing esophagectomy for esophageal malignancy	• Select patients with severe aphagia or BMI < 18.5 may benefit from feeding tube placement
Jenkins et al[7]	Does enteral access before neoadjuvant chemoradiation for esophageal cancer provides benefit compared with placement during definitive esophagectomy?	156 patients undergoing esophagectomy for esophageal malignancy	• No nutritional or perioperative benefit for enteral access before neoadjuvant chemoradiation for esophageal malignancy as measured by weight loss, serum albumin, dysphagia, and complication rates
Cools-Lartigue et al[10]	Determine if dietary counseling and neoadjuvant chemotherapy could obviate the need for invasive tube feeding.	130 patients with cT3 or N+ esophageal and esophagogastric junction adenocarcinoma undergoing neoadjuvant chemotherapy	• Dysphagia scores improved in 96% of patients, primarily after the first therapy cycle.
Giacopuzzi et al[14]	Is an Enhanced Recovery After Surgery protocol safe and feasible for esophagectomy (including both the Ivor Lewis and McKeown procedures) compared with standard perioperative protocol?	39 patients undergoing esophagectomy for esophageal malignancy	• Enhanced Recovery After Surgery protocol displayed earlier extubation, earlier intensive care unit discharge, earlier thoracic drain/urinary catheter/nasogastric tube removal, earlier mobilization, and earlier resumption of oral feeding.

(continued on next page)

Table 1
(continued)

Studies	Study Questions/ Objectives	Study Populations	Study Findings
Berkelmans et al[18]	This study investigates the effect of direct start of oral feeding following minimally invasive esophagectomy compared with standard of care.	132 patients undergoing minimally invasive esophagectomy randomized to either direct oral feeding resumption ($n = 65$) or nil by mouth and tube feeding for 5 d post-op ($n = 67$)	• Direct oral feeding after esophagectomy does not affect functional recovery or increase severity of postoperative complications.

aspiration leading proponents to suggest that pyloric drainage can reduce postoperative adverse events.[19–22] However, surgeons who do not routinely perform pyloric drainage during esophagectomies argue that the clinical incidence of delayed gastric conduit emptying (DGCE) postoperatively is low and that dysfunction in gastric motility may be reversible over time.[19–22] In this section, we discuss the clinical epidemiology and physiology of delayed gastric conduit drainage, different techniques for pyloric drainage, current literature about the association to outcomes as well as new procedural approaches.

Clinical epidemiology and pathophysiology of delayed gastric conduit emptying

Earlier research has demonstrated that following esophagectomy the incidence of DGCE with relevant clinical features is 10% to 20%.[23–25] However, there remains a wide range of definitions of DGCE with investigations using varied clinical and/or radiological methods to assess the incidence. For instance, using water-soluble contrast swallow studies postoperatively has demonstrated DGCE in up to 96% of patients.[26] However, a meta-analysis, including studies with clinical and radiologic diagnostic measures found incidence ranging from 2% to 47%.[19] The collection of these studies highlights that radiologic findings do not fully correlate to symptomology and that clinically significant DGCE affects a minority of patients undergoing esophagectomy.[25] To date the pathophysiology of DGCE remains complex. Given the oncologic principles necessary during esophagectomy, the vagal nerves are divided, and the sympathetic components of the celiac and mesenteric axis may be disrupted during lymphadenectomy.[23] Dysfunction in the motility of the conduit is complex with abnormal pyloric functioning, coordination, anastomosis location, peristalsis, or pressure gradients all found to be

potential contributors.[23] However, earlier studies have found that return to normal motor activity begins at 12 months postoperatively.[27]

Operative techniques for pyloric drainage

Historically, pyloroplasty and pyloromyotomy have been the two most common procedures used for pyloric drainage. Earlier systematic reviews have demonstrated that when pyloric drainage is performed during esophagectomy, pyloroplasty and pyloromyotomy represent the majority of operative methods used for drainage, however, techniques, such as finger fracture and pylorus stretching have been reported as well.[19] Pyloroplasty is performed to widen the pylorus with the most common approach being the Heineke–Mikulicz technique.[28] This involves a longitudinal incision through the pylorus starting at the distal antrum and continuing through the proximal duodenum typically traveling 5 to 7 cm. This incision is then closed transversely with either single-layer or two-layer closure with appropriate attention to approximate serosal and mucosal layers. This transverse closure allows for an increased diameter in the pylorus.[28] Pyloromyotomy includes an anterior incision involving the serosal and muscular layers until the submucosa is visualized. This nontransmural incision is then buttressed with an omental flap.

Outcomes

The effect of pyloric drainage procedures on short- and long-term outcomes remains central to the ongoing debate about whether it should be standard practice for patients undergoing esophagectomy. The key outcomes of reduced DGCE, pulmonary complications (related to aspiration), leak, and mortality are discussed here.

Delayed gastric conduit emptying and gastric outlet obstruction The association between pyloromyotomy and reduced DGCE and gastric outlet obstruction remains unclear. Pooled meta-analysis of randomized trials and single-center retrospective studies have demonstrated a nonsignificant reduced incidence of DGCE for patients receiving pyloric drainage procedures, including pyloromyotomy compared with no procedures [pooled odds ratio (OR) = 0.54; 95% confidence interval (CI) = 0.2–1.44; $P = 0.22$]. Notably, the 24 studies included in this pooled analysis included varying methods of measuring DGCE with questionnaires, swallow studies, radionuclide scintigraphy, and direct gastroscopic visualization.[19] A single-center study comparing pyloromyotomy to no pyloromyotomy found no differences in gastric outlet obstruction (9.6% versus 18.2%; $P = 0.078$).[24] Other studies have demonstrated a similar nonsignificant reduction in DGCE when pyloromyotomy is performed compared with other pyloric drainage procedures or no pyloric drainage.[29,30]

Pulmonary complications Advocates for the routine performance of pyloric drainage procedures have often cited that DGCE can increase the risk of aspiration and pulmonary complications. An earlier meta-analysis has demonstrated that pulmonary complications were nonsignificantly less among patients receiving any pyloric drainage procedure (pooled OR = 0.77; 95% CI = 0.46–1.28; $P = 0.31$).[25] Another meta-analysis demonstrated no difference in pulmonary complications (OR = 2.5, 95% CI = 0.34–18.98; $P = 0.36$) or fatal pulmonary aspiration on subanalysis (OR = 0.25, 95% CI = 0.04–1.60; $P = 0.14$).[30] An earlier prospective randomized trial by Law and colleagues, demonstrated no difference in pulmonary complications either.[22]

Anastomotic leak To date, there is no clear evidence that pyloromyotomy is associated with reduced anastomotic complications. Single-center studies have demonstrated no difference in anastomotic leaks between pyloromyotomy, pyloroplasty, and nonpyloric drainage groups.[31] For instance, in an analysis of 211 patients undergoing Ivor Lewis esophagectomy, there was no difference in the rate of anastomotic leak between no drainage, pyloroplasty, or pyloromyotomy (1.9% versus 0% versus 0%). A pooled analysis of five studies demonstrated no significant difference in anastomotic leak with pyloric drainage with pyloroplasty, and pyloromyotomy of finger fracture compared with no pyloric drainage procedure (OR = 0.65; 95% CI = 0.38–1.11; $P = 0.12$).[19]

Mortality In-hospital mortality following pyloric drainage procedures has not been found to have

a significant difference in postoperative mortality in meta-analyses.[16,27,29] Single-centers studies have additionally demonstrated no difference in mortality when comparing no drainage, pyloromyotomy, and pyloroplasty.[22,24,31]

New developments
Given the overall low clinical incidence of DGCE and mixed evidence on its effect on postsurgical outcomes, there has been increased interest in the use of intrapyloric Botulinum toxin (Botox) injections and endoscopic interventions for symptomatic patients and intra-op compared to routine prophylactic surgical pyloric drainage. A single-center retrospective study of 283 patients undergoing minimally invasive esophagectomy comparing no drainage, surgical drainage, and intrapyloric Botox injection demonstrated no difference in postoperative outcomes, pneumonia, or anastomotic leak. However, patients receiving Botox injection had significantly more symptoms at 6 and 12 months than no drainage and required more endoscopic dilation by 12 months postoperatively.[32] Additional studies have demonstrated that the use of intrapyloric Botox injection is associated with increased postoperative reflux and utility of prokinetic agents compared with pyloric drainage procedures.[33] The use of endoscopic pneumatic pyloric dilation has been demonstrated to be a safe and effective treatment for early DGCE.[34–36] For instance, in patients undergoing endoscopic dilation for postsurgical acquired pyloric stenosis it has been found that approximately 35% require more than one endoscopic dilation.[35] A single-center retrospective review of 25 patients receiving preoperative endoscopic pyloric balloon dilation before esophagectomy found that no patients needed a second operation for pyloric drainage and that only one patient required postoperative endoscopic dilation. Given the increased availability of advanced endoscopic techniques in addition to overall low incidence rates of DGCE, postoperative endoscopic pneumatic dilation is a reasonable alternative approach for surgeons who do not routinely perform pyloric drainage. Lastly, the role of per oral endoscopic myotomy of the pylorus (POP), for delayed conduit emptying following esophagectomy is an additional option for patients. To date, no randomized studies comparing POP to standard operative techniques have been performed. However, small case studies have demonstrated that POP is safe and associated with reduced symptoms.[37,38]

Recommendations
At this time, there is evidence suggesting a nonsignificant reduction in DGCE for patients receiving

Table 2
Summary of important studies evaluating outcomes following pyloric drainage procedures for gastric conduit

Studies	Study Questions/ Objectives	Study Populations	Study Findings
Lanuti et al[24]	What is the incidence of gastric outlet obstruction after esophagectomy with or without pyloromyotomy?	242 patients undergoing esophagectomy with gastric conduit formation. Two groups: no pyloromyotomy (*n* = 83) and pyloromyotomy (*n* = 159)	• Pyloromyotomy did not significantly reduce the incidence of gastric outlet obstruction
Arya et al[19]	Is pyloric drainage associated with improved clinical outcomes?	Pooled analysis of 25 studies with 3172 patients undergoing esophagectomy	• Pyloric drainage procedures were associated with a nonsignificant reduction in the incidence in anastomotic leaks and pulmonary complications and no significant difference in mortality
Palmes et al[31]	What is the effect of pyloric drainage on gastric outlet obstruction, mortality, and anastomotic leak?	198 patients with esophageal carcinoma treated with transthoracic esophagectomy with gastric conduit reconstruction with pyloromyotomy (*n* = 118), pyloroplasty (34) or no drainage procedure (46)	• No difference between the three groups in hospital mortality, anastomotic leak rate, or gastric outlet obstruction
Nobel et al[33]	What is the difference in postoperative outcomes following minimally invasive esophagectomy between different pyloric drainage methods?	283 patients undergoing esophagectomy with surgical pyloric drainage (*n* = 73), intrapyloric Botulinum injection (*n* = 53), no procedure (*n* = 157)	• Pyloric drainage was not associated with lower rate of postoperative complications, pneumonia, or anastomotic leak between groups. Botox injection was associatied with higher gastric outlet obstructive symptoms at 6 and 12 mo compared to surgical drainage.

pyloroplasty. There is no clear evidence that pyloric drainage reduces pulmonary complications or postoperative mortality. Additionally, pyloroplasty has not been found to have higher adverse events compared with no drainage procedure. Taken together, we recommend:

(1) Pyloric drainage procedures can be performed safely and routinely depending on a surgeon's preference.
(2) For surgeons who do not perform routine pyloric drainage, endoscopic interventions are a

safe treatment for patients who develop clinically significant DGCE (**Table 2**).

Thoracic Duct Ligation

Introduction
The complication of chylothorax following esophagectomy occurs in up to 4% of cases.[39,40] The sequelae of chylothorax, including immunosuppression, malnutrition, and respiratory complications, make it a dreaded complication with significant implications for postoperative morbidity

and mortality. In this section, we detail the clinical features of a thoracic duct leak, the role of prophylactic duct clipping, and outcomes and new developments.

Anatomy of the thoracic duct

The anatomy of the thoracic duct is central to understanding the development of chylothorax and operative management. The thoracic duct is typically 36 to 45 cm in length with a 2–3 mm diameter. The thoracic duct originates at the cisterna chyli, which is a dilated lymphatic sac located posterior to the abdominal aorta on the body of the first and second lumbar vertebral bodies (L1 and L2). It travels superiorly within the posterior mediastinum on the right side between the aorta and azygous vein until the level of the fifth thoracic vertebra (T5). At this level, it crosses to the left side and ascends posterior to the aortic arch and anterior to the subclavian vein until it reaches the apex of the chest. At that location, the thoracic duct forms an arch and terminates at the junction of the left internal jugular vein and left subclavian vein.[40,41] This anatomy occurs in approximately 65% of patients with a wide variation in anatomy contributing to the possible development of this complication.

Clinical features and medical management of chyle leak

The presence of a chyle leak typically becomes clinically relevant when the patients begin oral or enteral feeding. It is typically identified as a milky fluid in the thoracostomy tubes and confirmed with fluid analysis demonstrating high levels of lymphocytes. An earlier analysis has found that high chest tube exceeding greater than 400 mL per day within the first 6 postoperative days is associated with higher odds of chylothorax (OR = 36; 95% CI = 8.2–157.8).[42] Medical management remains fundamental to the initial treatment of chylothorax. The combination of dietary restrictions of no oral intake with total parental nutrition or a diet with low fat and medium chain fatty acid along with medical management with somatostatin or octreotide infusions has been found to be effective for many postoperative chylothoraxes. Despite conservative nonoperative management being the first line in treatment, it is important to not prolong conservative management. The timing of definitive intervention remains controversial but many advocate limiting conservative management to 2 weeks.[41,43] Early postoperative surgical intervention has been found to be effective for individuals with persistent chest tube drainage typically greater than 10 to 12 mL/kg after conservative management to reduce serious

complications and mortality.[42,44] The seriousness of chylothorax on postoperative outcomes has led some surgeons to advocate for prophylactic ligation to reduce the clinical incidence of these devastating complications.

Operative technique to prophylactic thoracic duct ligation

To date, there are multiple techniques used for prophylactic thoracic duct ligation. Guo and colleagues found that ligation of the thoracic duct with double ligation with two 10 mm clips encircling the lympho-fatty tissue between the aorta and azygous vein was demonstrated to be safe in a case series of video-assisted thoracoscopic esophagectomy.[45] Lin and colleagues have also demonstrated that prophylactic ligation of lymphatic tissue between the azygous vein and aorta with 0.0 silk suture is affected.[46] Other studies have detailed the use of absorbable polyglactin sutures or other nonabsorbable sutures for mass ligation as an effective approach as well.[47,48] Notably, each of these investigations represents single-center trials and therefore are limited in generalizability to all operating surgeons.

Outcomes

The evidence supporting prophylactic thoracic duct ligation during esophagectomy on the incidence of postoperative chylothorax and short-term outcomes remains mixed. The outcomes of postoperative chylothorax incidence, serious complications, and mortality are discussed here.

Postoperative chylothorax incidence The association between prophylactic thoracic duct ligation and decreased incidence of postoperative chylothorax has demonstrated mixed results. For instance, Crucitti and colleagues found in a meta-analysis of seven studies comparing prophylactic duct ligation to no prophylactic ligation found a significantly lower difference in the incidence rate of postoperative chylothorax (RR = 0.47; 95% CI = 0.27–1.002; P = 0.08). Notably of the seven studies included in this analysis, only one was a prospective randomized trial.[49] However, a meta-analysis of 15 studies, including 1 randomized trial demonstrated no significant difference in postesophagectomy chylothorax between prophylactic ligation and nonligation groups (OR = 0.73; 95% CI = 0.50–1.07; P = 0.11).[50] Similarly, Lei and colleagues found in a meta-analysis that prophylactic thoracic duct ligation had no significant reduction in postoperative chylothorax incidence (RR = 0.431; 95% CI = 0.186–1.002; P = 0.050).[51] Taken together, these studies demonstrate that there is no clear evidence supporting routine prophylactic

Table 3
Summary of important studies evaluating outcomes following prophylactic thoracic duct ligation

Studies	Study Questions/Objectives	Study Populations	Study Findings
Bao et al[52]	What is the association of prophylactic thoracic duct ligation on short- and long-term outcomes?	Patients undergoing esophagectomy with prophylactic thoracic duct ligation ($n = 559$) and no ligation ($n = 41$)	• Prophylactic ligation group had significantly lower postoperative chylothorax with no difference in median survival or 5 y survival.
Lai et al[48]	Is prophylactic mass ligation of the thoracic duct associated with reduced postoperative chylothorax rates?	Patients undergoing transthoracic esophagectomy randomly assigned to preservation group ($n = 328$) and prevention ligation ($n = 325$).	• Prophylactic ligation was associated with a significant reduction in chylothorax rates between groups
Liu et al[51]	Is prophylactic mass ligation of the thoracic duct associated with reduced postoperative chylothorax rates and survival?	Meta-analysis of 15 studies, including 1 randomized controlled study. Included 3658 patients undergoing thoracic duct ligation and 4638 preserved thoracic duct.	• There was no difference in chylothorax between the two groups and patients with preserved thoracic duct had significantly better 5 y overall survival.

ligation as a method to significantly reduce the development of postoperative chylothorax.

Mortality and survival The impact of prophylactic ductal ligation and short- and long-term surgical outcomes has been limited. Prospective single-center studies have not detected a difference in hospital mortality between patients receiving and not receiving prophylactic ligation.[52] In a meta-analysis of thoracic duct ligation prophylactically or postoperatively for chylothorax demonstrated that patients with preserved thoracic duct have improved 5-year survival (OR = 1.25; 95% CI = 1.08–1.44, $P = 0.002$).

New developments
Thoracic duct embolization (TDE) has become an alternative to surgical management of postoperative chyle leaks. In 1 analysis of 50 patients with persistent chylous leak following traditional surgical thoracic duct ligation, TDE was associated with resolution of the leak in 90% of patients.[53] The mechanisms of embolization used included coils and glue with higher success when both are used.[54] Earlier assessment of long-term complications has found that abdominal swelling, lower extremity swelling, and diarrhea are the most common complications. Despite the promise of TDE as a safe minimally invasive approach to managing chyle leaks, it is not uniformly available at all

sites and requires unique interventional radiology expertise.

Recommendations
There is no strong evidence to support prophylactic thoracic duct ligation at this time. Given this, we recommend that:

(1) Postoperative chyle leaks are managed with nonoperative management first with a maximum duration of 5 to 7 days.
(2) If nonoperative management is unsuccessful, we recommend surgical ligation if interventional radiology is unavailable. However, if expert interventional radiology is available, then TDE can be performed first (**Table 3**).

DISCLOSURE

Dr. Sidra Bonner is funded by an NIH T32 grant (T32HL007749).

REFERENCES

1. National Comprehensive Cancer Network. Esophageal Cancer (Version 1.2022). Available at: https://www.nccn.org/professionals/physician_gls/pdf/esophageal.pdf. Accessed January 20, 2021.
2. Daly JM, et al. Esophageal cancer: results of an American College of surgeons patient care evaluation study. J Am Coll Surg 2000;190:562–72.

3. Anandavadivelan P, Lagergren P. Cachexia in patients with oesophageal cancer. Nat Rev Clin Oncol 2016;13:185–98.

4. Bozzetti F, SCRINIO Working Group. Screening the nutritional status in oncology: a preliminary report on 1,000 outpatients. Support Care Cancer 2009; 17:279–84.

5. Tuca A, Jimenez-Fonseca P, Gascón P. Clinical evaluation and optimal management of cancer cachexia. Crit Rev Oncol Hematol 2013;88: 625–36.

6. Kidane B, et al. Emergency department use is high after esophagectomy and feeding tube problems are the biggest culprit. J Thorac Cardiovasc Surg 2018;156:2340–8.

7. Jenkins TK, Lopez AN, Sarosi GA, et al. Preoperative enteral access is not necessary prior to multimodality treatment of esophageal cancer. Surgery 2018;163:770–6.

8. Huerter ME, et al. Enteral access is not required for esophageal cancer patients undergoing neoadjuvant therapy. Ann Thorac Surg 2016;102:948–54.

9. Sunde B, et al. Relief of dysphagia during neoadjuvant treatment for cancer of the esophagus or gastroesophageal junction. Dis Esophagus 2016; 29:442–7.

10. Cools-Lartigue J, et al. Management of dysphagia in esophageal adenocarcinoma patients undergoing neoadjuvant chemotherapy: can invasive tube feeding be avoided? Ann Surg Oncol 2015;22: 1858–65.

11. Mastoridis S, et al. Laparoscopic vs. open feeding jejunostomy insertion in oesophagogastric cancer. BMC Surg 2021;21:367.

12. Hawn MT, Mulholland MW. Operative techniques in colon and rectal surgery. Philadelphia: Wolters Kluwer; 2015.

13. Akiyama Y, et al. Evaluation of the need for routine feeding jejunostomy for enteral nutrition after esophagectomy. J Thorac Dis 2018;10:6854–62.

14. Giacopuzzi S, et al. Enhanced recovery after surgery protocol in patients undergoing esophagectomy for cancer: a single center experience. Dis Esophagus 2017;30:1–6.

15. Bakhos C, Patel S, Petrov R, et al. Jejunostomy-technique and controversies. J Visc Surg 2019;5:33.

16. Fenton JR, Bergeron EJ, Coello M, et al. Feeding jejunostomy tubes placed during esophagectomy: are they necessary? Ann Thorac Surg 2011;92(2): 504–12.

17. Alvarez-Sarrado E, Mingol Navarro F, Rosellon J, et al. Feeding Jejunosotmy after esophagectomy cannot be routinely recommended. Analysis of nutritional benefits and catheter-related complications. Am J Surg 2019;217(1):114–20.

18. Berkelmans GHK, Fransen LFC, Dolmans-Zwartjes ACP, et al. Direct oral feeding following minimally invasive esophagectomy (nutrient ii trial): an international, multicenter, open-label randomized controlled trial. Ann Aurg 2020;271(1):41–7.

19. Arya S, Markar SR, Karthikesalingam A, et al. The impact of pyloric drainage on clinical outcome following esophagectomy: a systematic review. Dis Esophagus 2015;28:326–35.

20. Cheung HC, Siu KF, Wong J. Is pyloroplasty necessary in esophageal replacement by stomach? a prospective, randomized controlled trial. Surgery 1987; 102:19–24.

21. Gupta S, Chattopadhyay TK, Gopinath PG, et al. Emptying of the intrathoracic stomach with and without pyloroplasty. Am J Gastroenterol 1989;84: 921–3.

22. Law S, Cheung MC, Fok M, et al. Pyloroplasty and pyloromyotomy in gastric replacement of the esophagus after esophagectomy: a randomized controlled trial. J Am Coll Surg 1997;184:630–6.

23. Konradsson M, Nilsson M. Delayed emptying of the gastric conduit after esophagectomy. J Thorac Dis 2019;11(Suppl 5):S835–44.

24. Michael L, E. de Delva P, Wright CD, et al. Post-esophagectomy gastric outlet obstruction: role of pyloromyotomy and management with endoscopic pyloric dilatation. Eur J Cardio-Thoracic Surg 2007; 31(Issue 2):149–53.

25. Zhang L, Hou SC, Miao JB, et al. Risk factors for delayed gastric emptying in patients undergoing esophagectomy without pyloric drainage. J Surg Res 2017;213:46–50.

26. Cerfolio RJ, Bryant AS, Canon CL, et al. Is botulinum toxin injection of the pylorus during Ivor Lewis [corrected] esophagogastrectomy the optimal drainage strategy? J Thorac Cardiovasc Surg 2009;137(3):565–72. published correction appears in J Thorac Cardiovasc Surg. 2009 Jun;137(6): 1581.

27. Nakabayashi T, Mochiki E, Garcia M, et al. Gastropyloric motor activity and the effects of erythromycin given orally after esophagectomy. Am J Surg 2002; 183(3):317–23.

28. Søreide K, Sarr MG, Søreide JA. Pyloroplasty for benign gastric outlet obstruction–indications and techniques. Scand J Surg 2006;95(1):11–6.

29. Nguyen NT, Dholakia C, Nguyen XM, et al. Outcomes of minimally invasive esophagectomy without pyloroplasty: analysis of 109 cases. Am Surg 2010; 76(10):1135–8.

30. Urschel JD, Blewett CJ, Young JE, et al. Pyloric drainage (pyloroplasty) or no drainage in gastric reconstruction after esophagectomy: a meta-analysis of randomized controlled trials. Dig Surg 2002;19(3):160–4.

31. Palmes D, Weilinghoff M, Colombo-Benkmann M, et al. Effect of pyloric drainage procedures on gastric passage and bile reflux after

esophagectomy with gastric conduit reconstruction. Langenbecks Arch Surg 2007;392(2):135–41.

32. Nobel T, Tan KS, Barbetta A, et al. Does pyloric drainage have a role in the era of minimally invasive esophagectomy? Surg Endosc 2019;33(10): 3218–27.

33. Eldaif SM, Lee R, Adams KN, et al. Intrapyloric botulinum injection increases postoperative esophagectomy complications. Ann Thorac Surg 2014; 97(6):1959–65.

34. Mertens A, Gooszen J, Fockens P, et al. Treating early delayed gastric tube emptying after esophagectomy with pneumatic pyloric dilation. Dig Surg 2021;38(5–6):337–42.

35. Maus MK, Leers J, Herbold T, et al. Gastric outlet obstruction after esophagectomy: retrospective analysis of the effectiveness and safety of postoperative endoscopic pyloric dilatation. World J Surg 2016;40(10):2405–11.

36. Swanson EW, Swanson SJ, Swanson RS. Endoscopic pyloric balloon dilatation obviates the need for pyloroplasty at esophagectomy. Surg Endosc 2012;26(7):2023–8.

37. Anderson MJ, Sippey M, Marks J. Gastric per oral pyloromyotomy for post-vagotomy-induced gastroparesis following esophagectomy. J Gastrointest Surg 2020;24:715–9.

38. Malik Z, Kataria R, Modayil R, et al. Gastric Per Oral Endoscopic Myotomy (G-POEM) for the Treatment of Refractory Gastroparesis: Early Experience. Dig Dis Sci 2018;63:2405–12.

39. Worrell SG, Chang AC. Silencing the bird: Should surgical thoracic duct ligation shuffle off this mortal coil? J Thorac Cardiovasc Surg 2018;156(2):844.

40. Martucci N, Tracey M, Rocco G. Postoperative Chylothorax. Thorac Surg Clin 2015;25(4):523–8.

41. Nair Sukumaran K, Petko Matus, Hayward Martin P. Aetiology and management of chylothorax in adults. Eur J Cardio-Thoracic Surg 2007;32(2):362–9.

42. Shah RD, Luketich JD, Schuchert MJ, et al. Postesophagectomy chylothorax: incidence, risk factors, and outcomes. Ann Thorac Surg 2012;93(3): 897–904. https://doi.org/10.1016/j.athoracsur.2011. 10.060.

43. Marts BC, Naunheim KS, Fiore AC, et al. Conservative versus surgical management of chylothorax. Am J Surg 1992;164(5):532–5. https://doi.org/10.1016/ s0002-9610(05)81195-x.

44. Merigliano S, Molena D, Ruol A, et al. Chylothorax complicating esophagectomy for cancer: a plea for early thoracic duct ligation. J Thorac Cardiovasc Surg 2000;119(3):453–7. https://doi.org/10.1016/ s0022-5223(00)70123-1.

45. Guo W, Zhao YP, Jiang YG, et al. Prevention of postoperative chylothorax with thoracic duct ligation during video-assisted thoracoscopic esophagectomy for cancer. Surg Endosc 2012;26(5):1332–6. https://doi.org/10.1007/s00464-011-2032-3.

46. Lin Y, Li Z, Li G, et al. Selective en masse ligation of the thoracic duct to prevent chyle leak after esophagectomy. Ann Thorac Surg 2017;103(6):1802–7.

47. Lai FC, Chen L, Tu YR, et al. Prevention of chylothorax complicating extensive esophageal resection by mass ligation of thoracic duct: a random control study. Ann Thorac Surg 2011;91(6):1770–4.

48. Cagol M, Ruol A, Castoro C, et al. Prophylactic thoracic duct mass ligation prevents chylothorax after transthoracic esophagectomy for cancer. World J Surg 2009;33:1684–6.

49. Crucitti P, Mangiameli G, Petitti T, et al. Does prophylactic ligation of the thoracic duct reduce chylothorax rates in patients undergoing oesophagectomy? A systematic review and meta-analysis. Eur J Cardiothorac Surg 2016;50(6): 1019–24.

50. Liu L, Gong L, Zhang M, et al. The effect of prophylactic thoracic duct ligation during esophagectomy on the incidence of chylothorax and survival of the patients: an updated review. Postgrad Med 2021; 133(3):265–71.

51. Lei Y, Feng Y, Zeng B, et al. Effect of prophylactic thoracic duct ligation in reducing the incidence of postoperative chylothorax during esophagectomy: a systematic review and meta-analysis. Thorac Cardiovasc Surg 2018;66(5):370–5.

52. Bao T, Wang YJ, Li KK, et al. Short- and long-term outcomes of prophylactic thoracic duct ligation during thoracoscopic-laparoscopic McKeown esophagectomy for cancer: a propensity score matching analysis. Surg Endosc 2020;34(11):5023–9.

53. Nadolski GJ, Itkin M. Lymphangiography and thoracic duct embolization following unsuccessful thoracic duct ligation: Imaging findings and outcomes. JTCVS 2018;15692:838–43.

54. Chen E, Itkin M. Thoracic duct embolization for chylous leaks. Semin Intervent Radiol 2011;28(1): 63–74.

Ongoing Controversies in Esophageal Cancer II

Gastrectomy versus Esophagectomy for Siewert Type II Esophageal Adenocarcinoma

Nicolas Devaud, MD[a,b], Paul Carroll, MB, BCh, MD, FRCSI[c],*

KEYWORDS

- Esophageal cancer • Siewert classification type 2 • Esophagectomy • Gastrectomy

KEY POINTS

- Type II junction cancers are a challenging disease.
- Gastrectomy or Esophagectomy are viable options without a clear demonstrable superior option.
- Accurate staging is vital to determine junctional cancer type.
- Lymph node metastasis pathway is bidirectional-abdominal/mediastinal.

INTRODUCTION

Adenocarcinoma arising from the distal esophagus and the esophagogastric junction (GEJ) is increasing in Western populations (**Fig. 1**).[1–4] The incidence of gastric adenocarcinoma, on the contrary, has been steadily decreasing, but remains the 4th commonest cause of cancer death worldwide.[4] The diminishing incidence of gastric cancer may be explained by an epidemiologic drift based on decreasing intestinal type tumors of the distal stomach (predominant Eastern population subtype) with a reflected rise in the incidence of proximal diffuse type/signet cell gastric adenocarcinomas.[5]

The incremental impact of distal esophageal cancer and the emerging preponderance of proximal, poorly differentiated gastric adenocarcinoma defines an emerging debate around the optimal management of cancers of the gastroesophageal junction (GEJ). Siewert first described the division of cancers of the GEJ (AEG I–III) into 3 types depending on their endoscopic location using the center of the tumor as the marker and nominal measurements of 2–5 cm to define the junctional subtype.[6] Since 2010, the American Joint Committee on Cancer (AJCC) has considered cancers of the GEJ as a distinctive subtype. This staging system was intended to harmonize esophageal and gastric cancers using pathologic data derived from an international collection of 4627 patients (60% adenocarcinoma) gathered under the direction of a consortium of experts, the Worldwide Esophageal Cancer Collaboration (WECC).[7] The 7th edition of the staging system incorporated cancers of the esophagus and GEJ within the first 5 cm of the stomach that extends into the esophageal junction or distal esophagus, that is, the Siewert I–III classification.[8] This has been most lately refined within the 8th edition of AJCC TNM for esophageal cancer, using the epicenter of the tumor and a cutoff of 2 cm to define its subtype. Importantly, if the epicenter is greater than 2 cm from the EGJ it is now defined as a gastric cancer.[9]

This new consensus has driven an agreement as to how best to approach those more clearly defined esophageal and gastric cancers, that is, Siewert I and III lesions. However, disease with a tumor epicenter within 1 cm above and 2 cm below the GEJ (AEG II), still causes debate as to what is the optimal surgical approach. The

[a] Instituto Oncológico Fundación Arturo López Pérez (FALP), Santiago, Chile; [b] Universidad de Los Andes, Santiago, Chile; [c] Galway University Hospital, School of Medicine, University of Galway, Galway
* Corresponding author.
E-mail address: Paul.carroll@hse.ie

Thorac Surg Clin 32 (2022) 553–563
https://doi.org/10.1016/j.thorsurg.2022.07.004
1547-4127/22/© 2022 Elsevier Inc. All rights reserved.

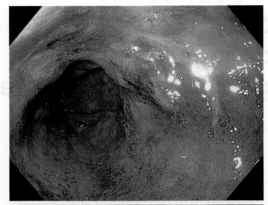
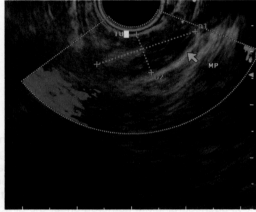

Fig. 1. Endoscopic and EUS evaluation of Siewert II, GEJ adenocarcinoma.

argument is driven perhaps by historical surgical expertise and the background training of Upper GI surgeons and Thoracic surgeons rather than by a clear biological definition. Interestingly, a recent survey among surgeons involved in the care of GEJ cancers highlighted that 66% preferred an extended total gastrectomy for the management of type 2 AEG cancers.[10]

GASTROESOPHAGEAL JUNCTIONAL ADENOCARCINOMA-DEFINITIONS AND CLASSIFICATIONS

The GEJ is the anatomic transition from the tubular intra-abdominal esophagus to the proximal stomach. This transition is determined by the histologic change in the esophageal squamous mucosa to the gastric columnar mucosa. The squamocolumnar junction, also known as the Z-line, is normally identified endoscopically at a distance between 38 and 40 cm from the incisors.[11] This transitional segment includes a narrow segment of mucus-secreting columnar mucosa, distal to the squamous esophageal mucosa but proximal to the

acid-secreting gastric oxyntic mucosa referred as the "gastric cardia". The cardia is characterized histologically by glands, coiled and loosely packed in abundant lamina propria. These glands are lined by tall, neutral mucin-producing columnar cells and endocrine cells.[12]

The squamocolumnar histologic transition line may vary and not coincide with the anatomic transition from the esophagus to the proximal stomach. This is particularly evident among patients with hiatal hernia and/or Barrett's esophagus. The increasing incidence of distal esophageal adenocarcinoma secondary to Barrett's disease together with the anatomic ambiguity to differentiate from proximal gastric adenocarcinomas gave way to a tumor epicenter definition.[13]

Siewert and colleagues described GEJ adenocarcinoma as tumors that have their center within 5 cm proximal or distal to the anatomic cardia, defining three distinct tumor entities[13–15]:

- *Type I:* Adenocarcinoma arising at a distance between 1 and 5 cm proximal to the cardia. They are considered tumors of the distal esophagus that develop from an area with intestinal metaplasia (Barrett's esophagus) and may infiltrate the GEJ from above.
- *Type II:* Adenocarcinoma with an epicenter within 1 cm proximal to 2 cm distal of the GEJ. Considered true carcinomas of the cardia that develop from the cardiac epithelium or short segments with intestinal metaplasia at the GEJ.
- *Type III:* Adenocarcinoma with epicenter at a distance between 2 and 5 cm distal to the cardias. Considered subcardial gastric carcinomas that can infiltrate the GEJ and distal esophagus from below.

The classification of GEJ adenocarcinoma into 3 subtypes has been based mainly on epidemiologic differences. Specialized intestinal epithelial metaplasia in the distal esophagus with subsequent development of severe dysplastic changes has been clearly proven as the main precursor lesion for adenocarcinoma in Type I tumors.[16] Therefore, there is a recognized preponderance among male patients with severe GERD and secondary Barrett's disease who develop these tumors.[16,17] On the contrary, Siewert's type II and III tumors show a high incidence of poorly differentiated/diffuse type tumors which is rarely seen among type I tumors, with no identified gender-related difference.[18] This tumor histology resembles the Western pattern for gastric cancer.[4,19,20]

The definition of a true junctional cancer from its epicenter is somewhat more complex considering the understanding of the genomic and molecular landscape of gastric and esophageal cancers. A number of studies have also suggested gene expression differences within GEJ tumor types[21,22] as well as different patterns of lymphatic spread. These discoveries will likely guide oncologic therapeutic modalities (chemotherapy/immunotherapy/radiation) in the future. In current practice, accurate identification of the location and staging of these lesions is critical for treatment planning.

DIAGNOSIS AND STAGING ASSESSMENT OF ESOPHAGOGASTRIC JUNCTION TUMORS
Diagnosis

Clinical presentation of GEJ tumors may be characterized by GERD symptoms including heartburn, regurgitation, retrosternal pain, and progressive dysphagia. Symptoms can correlate with endoscopic findings of erosive inflammatory changes and proximal displacement of the squamocolumnar junction to the distal esophagus, suggesting Barrett's esophagus. Diagnosis of adenocarcinoma will be confirmed with the endoscopic biopsy in the context of intestinal metaplasia and early/high-grade dysplasia at the GEJ.

This sequential presentation is probably more evident for proper Siewert Type I tumors in patients being followed endoscopically as part of a Barrett's esophagus multidisciplinary program at the time of diagnosis of adenocarcinoma. Routine follow-up of these patients may secure earlier cancer stage diagnosis,[23] considering the annual risk of esophageal adenocarcinoma of 0.12% (95% CI, 0.09–0.15) among patients with Barrett's esophagus.[24] Patients with low-grade dysplasia on the index endoscopy in the context of Barrett's esophagus have an incidence rate for adenocarcinoma of 5.1 cases per 1000 person-years.[24] However, these surveillance programs have not proven to substantially reduce the risk of death from esophageal adenocarcinoma.[25] 95% of esophageal adenocarcinomas arise without a prior diagnosis of Barrett's esophagus and nearly 80% of esophageal adenocarcinoma arise without a prior diagnosis of GERD.[26]

The most common presentation among patients with GEJ tumors is dysphagia to solid food with secondary weight loss with no previous GERD-related symptoms described. Endoscopic diagnosis is most frequently conducted at more advanced tumor stages, defining a bulky tumor mass at the GEJ extending from or to the distal esophagus or proximal stomach.

The Siewert tumor type is a clinical definition of the tumor epicenter at the time of pretreatment endoscopy and CT staging. The assignment to each of these tumor types is purely morphologic/topographic, based originally on the findings from contrast radiography, but mainly after endoscopy with orthograde and retroflexed views of the GEJ [14] in the modern era. The accuracy of this classification will be determined by tumor cT stage at the time of index endoscopy; therefore, the ability to view the GEJ through to the proximal stomach with the endoscope is important, and can sometimes be difficult from the bulk of the tumor. The yield to accurately define endoscopically the tumor subtype may be higher for early Siewert I & III tumors and not so straightforward for Siewert II tumors, particularly in more advanced cTNM lesions. (pure 1, Endoscopic and Pathology picture)

Endosonography

Endosonography (EUS) is the most sensitive test for locoregional staging in esophageal cancer. EUS can determine the depth of tumor invasion (cT), as well as confirm the nodal involvement of suspicious paraesophageal or perigastric lymph nodes through fine-needle aspiration (cN). The accuracy of EUS for evaluating primary tumor and nodal status has been reported to be 85% and 75%, respectively, while the sensitivity has been reported to be in the range of 85% to 95% for primary tumor evaluation and 70% to 80% for nodal evaluation.[27]

EUS has been suggested to impact the evaluation in early-stage tumors and spare the need for neoadjuvant treatment and radical surgery with the benefit of endoscopic or surgical resection solely. Intramucosal cancers (T1a) have a 6%-10% risk of nodal metastasis, while invasion into the submucosa (T1b) increases the risk of lymph node metastasis to 19%–23%.[28] **(Fig. 2**, EUS

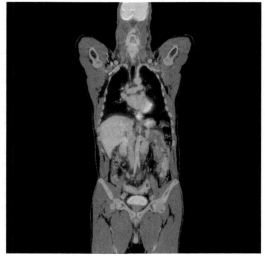

Fig. 2. FDG-PET CT staging of Siewert II GEJ adenocarcinoma.

picture). T1a lesions may benefit then from the endoscopic resection of the mucosa, with clear margins, whereas T1b will require radical surgery considering the higher risk of nodal involvement. The accuracy though of EUS to discriminate between T1a and T1b superficial lesions has been a matter of debate. A retrospective cohort of 131 patients with early-stage esophageal cancer undergoing EUS, compared endosonographic to pathologic staging of specimens removed with endoscopic mucosal resection. In 80% of cases, EUS did not demonstrate any submucosal involvement. Evaluation of the endoscopically resected specimens, however, revealed either submucosal invasion, positive resection margin for cancer, or lymphovascular invasion in 24% of these patients. In the remaining 20% of subjects whereby EUS defined signs of submucosal invasion or lymph node metastasis, the pathology specimen after diagnostic endoscopic resection also showed major discrepancies.[29] Meta-analyses on this matter have also been contradictory proving a concordance rate between EUS and pathology staging as low as 65% while others show a sensitivity and specificity for superficial lesions ranging from 86% to 87% and no differences between T1a and T1b.

EUS is a costly and operator-dependent procedure. For GEJ tumors, the staging benefit of EUS has not been clearly defined. Retrospective studies have found that EUS accuracy at the GEJ is inferior to that of other regions of the esophagus when compared with resected specimens; with 23% under-staged and 29% over-staged by EUS. The negative effect is particularly pronounced with early GEJ tumors being more frequently overstaged.[30]

Positron Emission Tomography-Computed Tomography

Considering the lymphatic spread of GEJ adenocarcinomas to the mediastinum, pericardial, celiac axis, and paraaortic nodes, [18F]Fluorodeoxyglucose-PET-CT has proven to be useful for locoregional and metastatic staging in advanced esophageal and GEJ tumors.[31]

FDG-PET-CT can determine the baseline FDG uptake of the primary tumor before neoadjuvant therapy, the presence of locoregional disease, the presence of distant metastatic disease, and the response to therapy. FDG-PET is superior to contrast-enhanced CT for the detection of metastatic nodes. The sensitivity, specificity, and accuracy of PET-CT are 52%, 94%, and 84%, respectively, compared with 15%, 97%, and 77%, respectively, for CT.[32] PET has also shown

a higher accuracy (82% vs 64%) and sensitivity (74% vs 47%) compared with CT and EUS for the detection of distant metastatic disease.[32] (Fig. 3, PET CT picture). However, within GEJ adenocarcinomas, diffuse/nonintestinal growth type and mucus-containing tumor type (signet ring variant) may have a reduced FDG uptake. Therefore, in advanced poorly differentiated tumors, clinical staging may rely better on the CT images. For early-stage disease (cTis, cT1), FDG-PET-CT has also proven to be of limited accuracy. FDG uptake increases with increasing pT stage. In a study by Betancourt Cuellar and colleagues on superficial esophageal cancer, comparing FDG uptake with final pathologic staging after resection, median FDG uptake values for early-stage disease were low, with 3.7 for pTis, 3.8 for pT1a and 4.2 for T1b. Sensitivity and positive predictive value for pN disease were 0% and accuracy was 82%.[33]

Surgical Approaches

With respect to surgical oncologic options, the debate continues as to what is the best modality for true junctional or type 2 EGJ cancers as they straddle the boundaries of true gastric and esophageal adenocarcinomas. The surgical options for Type 2 cancers include gastrectomy/extended gastrectomy, transhiatal esophagectomy, and transthoracic (intrathoracic or cervical anastomosis) esophagectomy. Clearly, the approaches have significant similarities; abdominal lymphadenectomy, resection of the proximal stomach/cardia, and clearance around the hiatus. There is, however, discord with respect to the extent of proximal resection within the thorax and the requirement for a mediastinal lymphadenectomy.

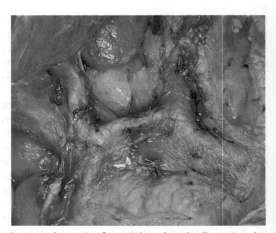

Fig. 3. Celiac axis after D2 lymphnode dissection during total gastrectomy with distal esophagectomy for Siewert II GEJ adenocarcinoma.

Irrespective of approach, the principles of any resection of AEG II lesions are the same:

a. Complete resection of the tumor with negative proximal, distal, and circumferential margins (R0 resection)
b. Thorough lymphadenectomy
c. Acceptable surgical morbidity/mortality
d. Reasonable quality of life (QOL)
e. Oncologic outcomes (disease free/overall survival)

To date, the evidence supporting a superior option for the treatment of these cancers has not been forthcoming due to somewhat heterogenous and limited data. There has not been a randomized trial to compare both approaches specifically for AEG II tumors, with conclusions inferred from other studies. A Japan Clinical Oncology Group (JCOG) trial examined the difference between a transhiatal (n = 82) and the left thoracoabdominal approach (n = 85). No significant difference was seen in 5-year survival (52% vs 38%).[34] The thoracoabdominal group did accumulate a higher morbidity (41% vs 22%, $P = .008$). Limited subgroup analysis showed no survival advantage in Type 2 cancers with advisement that a thoracic approach should not be conducted for tumors involving <3 cm of the esophagus.[35] A further study examining 220 people with mid to distal esophageal cancers incorporating tumors of the cardia, examined differences between a transthoracic and transhiatal esophagectomy. 5-year survival was equivalent (36% vs 34%, $P = .71$). A subgroup study highlighted that a transthoracic approach in Type I AEG may provide a long-term advantage (51% vs 37%, $P = .33$). This was not seen with Type 2 tumors.[36,37] A retrospective study by Blank and colleagues, examined an institutional experience of 242 AEG II lesions, 56 (23.1%) undergoing a right thoracoabdominal esophagectomy (transthoracic/Ivor Lewis) compared with an extended total gastrectomy. Morbidity and mortality were equivalent. Resection margins and nodal yield were also similar. Overall survival was significantly better in those who had an esophagectomy (33.6 months vs not reached, $P = .02$). Multivariate analysis demonstrated that pN status ($P = .0017$) and surgery type in locally advanced cancers (cT3/4 or cN1) ($P = .0017$) as independent prognostic factors. One must be cognizant that there was a selection bias in this study toward gastrectomy in the more elderly, potentially more frail population which may influence the data somewhat.[38] Finally, most recently, Kamarajah and colleagues, in a registry analysis of 9594 cases in the US National Cancer Database (NCDB) show clear prognostic superiority for esophagectomy over gastrectomy for Type 2 junctional tumors. With propensity matching, esophagectomy cases had a better median survival (68 vs 51 months, $P < .001$), 5-year Survival (53 vs 47 months, $P < .001$) and R0 rates (94 vs 91%, $P = .001$). Length of stay, readmission rates, and 30/90 day mortality were similar.[39] Of note, there is some concern that there were more advanced cancers in the gastrectomy cohort, with more T3/4 lesions (38% vs 25%, $P < .001$) and N2/3 tumors (18% vs 10%, $P < .001$). Stage-specific survival was not examined in this article. This most recent data provides some evidence that esophagectomy is superior to gastrectomy for these cancers; however, it is still not fully apparent.

Lymphadenectomy

Clearly, a universal question regarding GEJ tumors is the extent of the lymphadenectomy to deliver the best oncological outcome. Summarily, whether a 2 field (abdominal and mediastinal) lymphadenectomy is required. Given the location of AEG II tumors, between true gastric and esophageal cancers, the pathway for lymph node metastasis can be intrathoracic, intraabdominal, or both. Understanding the metastatic nodal spread from cancers of the junction and cardia would help to guide lymphadenectomy. Importantly, not every positive node carries the same impact on survival. Proximal mediastinal lymph nodes-Paratracheal nodes 2 and 4, Station 5 Aorto-pulmonary window, Station 7 subcarinal node, Station 10 R/L paraesophageal nodes, carry a poorer prognosis compared with locoregional nodes (15.4 vs 35.3 months, $P < .001$).[40] Siewert reported the lymphatic distribution in 1002 type I-III AEG lesions with a combination of extended total gastrectomy for AEG II/III and a transthoracic esophagectomy for AEG I lesions. Spread to lower mediastinal nodes was 12% in AEG II cancers. Interestingly, only 2% of AEG II lesions were found to have positive lymph nodes in the distal stomach, station 5 suprapyloric, station 4 greater curve, and at station 6 at the infrapyloric region. Most notably in this study was that AEG I-III cancers had a preponderance to spread to the same stations-paracardial, left gastric, and lower mediastinum.[14] An elegant study from Newcastle, performed a simulation analysis looking at the impact of obviating an extended lymphadenectomy in the thorax (ie, via a transhiatal esophagectomy) or performing a minimal abdominal resection based on a cohort of patients with positive nodes. 61% were AEG I or II tumors. They demonstrated hypothetically that omitting a

2-field lymphadenectomy would result in a 23% reduction in predicted 5-year survival of patient with N1 or N2 disease.[41] Mitchell *and colleagues* examined the mediastinal nodal involvement post chemoradiation in 204 AEG II and III junctional tumors (151%–47% AEG II lesions). Recurrences within the mediastinum at 2 years were also included. 15% (n = 31/204) met the criteria for mediastinal involvement. 24 (11.8%) had pathologic involvement with the majority involving paraesophageal nodes (20/24). 4.9% (10/24) recurred within 2 years, 3 patients had both ypN + ve disease and subsequent recurrence.

Gastrectomy or Esophagectomy

Locally advanced GEJ adenocarcinoma can be treated with radical surgery by a completely abdominal approach (D2 Total Gastrectomy + Distal Esophagectomy vs Transhiatal Esophagectomy), or a combined abdominal/transthoracic approach (Left Lateral Thoracoabdominal Esophagogastrectomy vs Transthoracic Esophagectomy). The benefits and issues with each approach are delineated in **Table 1**. Studies comparing oncologic and perioperative outcomes for different esophagectomy approaches have shown a higher number of lymph nodes dissected after a transthoracic surgical approach[42] with superior 5-year survival,[43] but increased morbidity particularly after left thoracoabdominal esophagectomy.[35] A transthoracic esophagectomy has traditionally been associated

with higher thoracic and pulmonary complications; therefore, favoring abdominal resections in frail/elderly patients with pulmonary comorbidities.[14,44] A single-center experience demonstrated equal morbidity between the 2 approaches, with respiratory complications occurring in 28.2% of esophagectomies as compared with 33.3% of gastrectomies.[38] The development of minimally invasive approaches to esophagectomy (thoracoscopic/laparoscopic and Robotic) have now challenged this perception with demonstrable improvement in pulmonary complications.[45–47]

Data on proximal free margin length,[44] tumor grade, tumor growth pattern, and lymphatic spread based on Siewert tumor classification,[14] has led to a mostly accepted consensus regarding Transthoracic Esophagectomy (TTE) as the best approach for Siewert Type I tumors and D2 Total Gastrectomy + Distal Esophagectomy for Siewert Type III tumors (TG).

Finally, studies comparing the quality of life on surgical approach for GEJ tumors, have usually favored a Total Gastrectomy. These studies were based on previously validated general health and cancer-specific questionnaires,[48–50] and proved that after short (6 months) and long-term follow-up (1–2 years postsurgery), patients who undergo a Total Gastrectomy for GEJ adenocarcinoma report better quality of life than those with transthoracic esophagectomy.[51–53] Patients postesophagectomy describe a reduced physical function, increased reflux symptoms and

Table 1
Comparison of transthoracic esophagectomy versus extended total gastrectomy for AEG II cancers

	Esophagectomy with Gastric Conduit	Extended Gastrectomy with Roux-en Y Esophagojejunostomy
Organ Space	Thorax + Abdomen	Abdomen
Oncologic factors		
Margin threat	Gastric	Esophagus
Lymphadenectomy	D1+/mediastinal	D2-lower mediastinum
Reconstruction factors		
Organ preservation	2/3 stomach	Loss of stomach
Capacity	Large reservoir	Minimal reservoir
Conduit length	Proximal thorax	Jejunal restriction
Hiatal Herniation	Moderate risk	Low risk
Conduit issues		
Emptying	Delayed gastric emptying + pylorospasm	Minimal issues with jejunal emptying
Reflux	Gastroesophageal reflux++	Rare alkaline reflux
Dumping	Low	Low-moderate
Medications	PPI	Vit B12 supplementation

dyspnea.[53] In a recent study, Jezerskyte *and colleagues*, documented quality of life scores in 30 patients with gastrectomy and 71 after esophagectomy. Most of these surgeries were completed in a minimally invasive approach. No significant differences were seen in global health or functioning domains. Similar reflux and fatigue scores were equivalent. The only separation in the groups in favor of gastrectomy was in the less clinically relevant health-related quality of life (HR-QoL) domain of choking when swallowing" and "coughing". These QoL studies may aid in shared decision-making when a choice between the surgical options is available.[52]

Reflux symptoms secondary to an esophagectomy may be defined by the negative intrathoracic pressure over a tubular gastric conduit, in continuity to the proximal esophagus that has no esophagogastric sphincter to protect from the positive abdominal pressure. Total Gastrectomy, on the contrary, is reconstructed following a Roux-en-Y jejunal loop with an alimentary limb that is mostly intraabdominal and a biliary limb distant from the esophago-jejunal anastomosis and therefore reducing the risk of bile reflux to the esophagus **(Fig. 4)**. One must be aware that biliary reflux is also a symptom postgastrectomy.

A nuanced stratagem for the approach to these cancers is recommended. Consideration for the stage of the malignancy must be included in the approach. With earlier stage cancers (cT1/2), with a likely low yield for metastatic lymphadenectomy, an extended gastrectomy might be the best option. For advanced lesions, the length of esophageal infiltration is a key consideration in the approach for resection and reconstruction. Tumor extent ≥1.5 cm into esophagus, irrespective of Siewert classification, was the single most important factor in determining mediastinal lymph node involvement in the absence of clinical evidence of intrathoracic concerning nodes.[54] This is further reinforced by Mine *and colleagues,* highlighting a poorer outcome with margins <2 cm in transhiatal gastrectomy.[55] One must factor in whether an R0 resection can be obtained via an abdominal approach in the presence of individual patient factors, such as a large hiatal hernia, a short esophagus, and body habitus. These factors may also compromise the surgeon's ability to fashion an anastomosis at the hiatus/low mediastinum.

Future Directions

In the current era of multimodal and personalized treatment of cancer, the question of which should be the best approach for Siewert type II tumors includes confronting perspectives over neoadjuvant chemoradiation versus perioperative chemotherapy for locally advanced disease.

Multimodal treatment has proven a significantly better survival compared with surgery alone, regardless of the surgical approach. The CROSS randomized controlled trial analyzed the benefit of neoadjuvant carboplatin + paclitaxel and 41.4 Gy chemoradiation therapy.[56] This trial

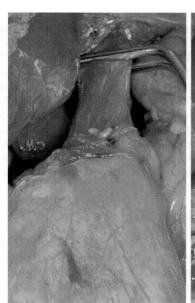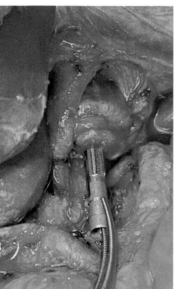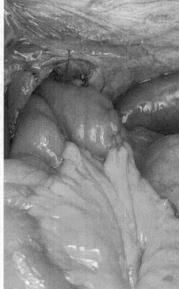

Fig. 4. Total gastrectomy with distal esophagectomy and intra-mediastinal esophago-jejunal anastomosis for Siewert II GEJ adenocarcinoma.

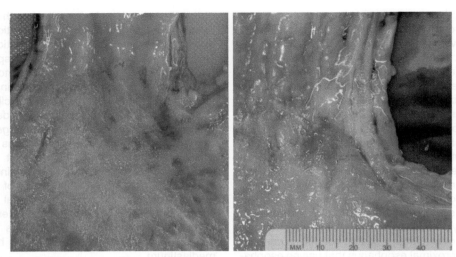

Fig. 5. Siewert II GEJ tumors with complete macroscopic and histologic response after FLOT neoadjuvant treatment.

proved an OS benefit of neoadjuvant chemoradiation among patients with esophageal and GEJ tumors including Siewert type II tumors, even after long-term follow-up.[57] The survival benefit was stronger though, within patients with squamous cell carcinoma compared with those with adenocarcinoma (81.6 vs 43.2 months).

Perioperative chemotherapy without radiation has also proven a survival benefit for patients with GEJ adenocarcinoma compared with surgery alone. Trials have included patients with locally advanced adenocarcinoma of the stomach, GEJ, and distal esophagus (MAGIC, FLOT-4).[58,59] The complete disease response proven by neoadjuvant chemoradiation and perioperative chemotherapy (**Fig. 5**) versus the distant metastatic progression among patients with residual disease, highlights the question over the need of systemic treatment after surgery. This question has not been answered over a head-to-head study, though is currently being tested in two phase III RCT comparing CROSS versus FLOT for distal esophageal and GEJ adenocarcinoma; ESOPEC and Neo-AEGIS, with Neo-AEGIS, suggesting equipoise between the 2 options.[60,61]

Moreover, survival results with perioperative chemotherapy on GEJ adenocarcinoma have promoted a more ambitious analysis among patients with limited metastatic disease in a phase II study which proved favorable results for responders or stable metastatic disease after 4 cycles of pseudoneoadjuvant chemotherapy(AIO-FLOT3).[62]

The recent development in targeted therapies for gastric and GEJ adenocarcinoma have also highlighted this question about adjuvant systemic treatment in high-risk tumors, proving the benefit of postoperative treatment in patients with residual disease after neoadjuvant chemoradiation. CheckMate-577 is a phase III RCT that proved a disease-free survival benefit of 11.4 months with adjuvant Immune Checkpoint Inhibitors in patients with locally advanced esophageal/GEJ cancer and pathologic residual disease after neoadjuvant chemoradiation followed by surgery.[63] The median disease-free survival was 22.4 months among patients who received nivolumab and 11.0 months among those who received placebo (hazard ratio for disease recurrence or death, 0.69; 96.4% CI: 0.56–0.86; $P < .001$). The median distant metastasis-free survival was 28.3 in the nivolumab group and 17.6 months in the placebo group. The risk of distant recurrence or death was, therefore, 26% lower with nivolumab than with placebo.[63] This study proved again the role of adjuvant systemic treatment in preventing the high incidence of distant metastatic progression in patients with stage II-III disease, as well as a promising future of targeted therapies in esophageal and GEJ adenocarcinoma. Other trials are currently under recruitment to define the benefit of immune-targeted therapies in esophageal and GEJ metastatic disease.[64]

SUMMARY

Siewert Type II tumors represent a gray area of debate whereby various questions have not yet been answered. Both TTE and TG achieve a complete oncologic tumor resection, though with an ongoing controversy about the best surgical approach in terms of quality of life, oncological outcome, and survival. Recent evidence suggests a better oncological outcome after TTE,[65] whereas others show no survival differences and better postoperative quality of life after TG.[51–53,66] The ongoing CARDIA-trial is a multinational, multi-center, randomized, clinical superiority trial, designed to solve this question.[42]

Overall, current data indicate that both approaches are acceptable. Individual patient/tumor factors must be incorporated into the decision-making and the capability of the surgeon to adapt to intraoperative findings is vital to provide the patient with a satisfactory outcome both in relation to oncological and morbidity considerations.

CLINICS CARE POINTS

- Operative approach remains the choice of the surgeon. The capability to operate on both sides of the diaphragm is an important component of the surgeon's armamentarium in treating junctional adenocarcinoma.
- Accurate staging of junctional cancer is key. This includes assessing lymphadenopathy in the mediastinum and abdomen with multiple modalities (EUS, CT. PET-CT).

DISCLOSURE

The authors have nothing to disclose.

REFERENCES

1. Al-Kaabi A, Baranov NS, van der Post RS, et al. Age-specific incidence, treatment, and survival trends in esophageal cancer: a Dutch population-based cohort study. Acta Oncol 2022;1–8.
2. Coupland VH, Allum W, Blazeby JM, et al. Incidence and survival of oesophageal and gastric cancer in England between 1998 and 2007, a population-based study. BMC Cancer 2012;12:11.
3. Dubecz A, Solymosi N, Stadlhuber RJ, et al. Does the Incidence of Adenocarcinoma of the Esophagus and Gastric Cardia Continue to Rise in the Twenty-First Century?-a SEER Database Analysis. J Gastrointest Surg 2013;18(1):124–9.
4. Bray F, Ferlay J, Soerjomataram I, et al. Global cancer statistics 2018: GLOBOCAN estimates of incidence and mortality worldwide for 36 cancers in 185 countries. CA Cancer J Clin 2018;68(6): 394–424.
5. Collaborators GBDSC. The global, regional, and national burden of stomach cancer in 195 countries, 1990-2017: a systematic analysis for the Global

Burden of Disease study 2017. Lancet Gastroenterol Hepatol 2020;5(1):42–54.
6. Siewert JR, Holscher AH, Becker K, et al. [Cardia cancer: attempt at a therapeutically relevant classification]. Chirurg 1987;58(1):25–32.
7. Rice TW, Rusch VW, Apperson-Hansen C, et al. Worldwide esophageal cancer collaboration. Dis Esophagus 2009;22(1):1–8.
8. AJCC cancer staging Manual, TNM classification of malignant tumours. 7th Edition. New York: Springer-Verlag; 2010.
9. TNM classification of malignant tumours, 8th Edition. Wiley-Blackwell 2016. James D. Brierley CW, editor: Wiley-Blackwell; 2016.
10. Haverkamp L, Seesing MF, Ruurda JP, et al. Worldwide trends in surgical techniques in the treatment of esophageal and gastroesophageal junction cancer. Dis Esophagus 2017;30(1):1–7.
11. Delattre J-F, Avisse C, Marcus C, et al. Functional Anatomy of the Gastroesophageal Junction. Surg Clin North Am 2000;80(1):241–60.
12. Greenson JKLG, Owens SR, Montgomery EA. Diagnostic pathology: Gastrointestinal. 2nd edition. Elsevier; 2016.
13. Siewert SH JR. Adenocarcinoma of the gastroesophageal junction: classifcation, pathology and extent of resection. Dis Esophagus 1996;9: 173–82.
14. Rudiger Siewert J, Feith M, Werner M, et al. Adenocarcinoma of the esophagogastric junction: results of surgical therapy based on anatomical/topographic classification in 1,002 consecutive patients. Ann Surg 2000;232(3):353–61.
15. Stein HJ, Feith M, Siewert JR. Cancer of the esophagogastric junction. Surg Oncol 2000;9(1):35–41.
16. Cameron AJLC, Pera M, Carpenter HA. Adenocarcinoma of the esophagogastric junction and Barrett's esophagus. Gastroenterology 1995;109:1541–6.
17. Chalasani N, Wo JM, Hunter JG, et al. Significance of intestinal metaplasia in different areas of esophagus including esophagogastric junction. Dig Dis Sci 1997;42(3):603–7.
18. Siewert JR, Stein HJ. Classification of adenocarcinoma of the oesophagogastric junction. Br J Surg 1998;85(11):1457–9.
19. Sitarz R, Skierucha M, Mielko J, et al. Gastric cancer: epidemiology, prevention, classification, and treatment. Cancer Manag Res 2018;10:239–48.
20. Etemadi A, Safiri S, Sepanlou SG, et al. The global, regional, and national burden of stomach cancer in 195 countries, 1990–2017: a systematic analysis for the Global Burden of Disease study 2017. Lancet Gastroenterol Hepatol 2020;5(1):42–54.
21. van Dekken HGE, Dinjens WN, Winjnhoven BP, et al. Comparative genomic hybridization of cancer of the gastroesophageal junction: deletion of 14Q31-32.1 discriminates between esophageal (Barrett's) and

gastric cardia adenocarcinomas. Cancer Res 1999; 59:748–52.

22. van Dekken H, Alers JC, Riegman PHJ, et al. Molecular Cytogenetic Evaluation of Gastric Cardia Adenocarcinoma and Precursor Lesions. Am J Pathol 2001;158(6):1961–7.

23. Codipilly DC, Chandar AK, Singh S, et al. The Effect of Endoscopic Surveillance in Patients With Barrett's Esophagus: A Systematic Review and Meta-analysis. Gastroenterology 2018;154(8):2068–20686 e5.

24. Hvid-Jensen F, Pedersen L, Drewes AM, et al. Incidence of adenocarcinoma among patients with Barrett's esophagus. N Engl J Med 2011;365(15): 1375–83.

25. Corley DA, Mehtani K, Quesenberry C, et al. Impact of endoscopic surveillance on mortality from Barrett's esophagus-associated esophageal adenocarcinomas. Gastroenterology 2013;145(2):312–319 e1.

26. Reid BJ, Li X, Galipeau PC, et al. Barrett's oesophagus and oesophageal adenocarcinoma: time for a new synthesis. Nat Rev Cancer 2010;10(2):87–101.

27. Romagnuolo JSJ, Hawes RH, Hoffman BJ, et al. Helical CT versus EUS with fine needle aspiration for celiac nodal assessment in patients with esophageal cancer. Gastrointest Endosc 2002;55:648–54.

28. Dubecz A, Kern M, Solymosi N, et al. Predictors of Lymph Node Metastasis in Surgically Resected T1 Esophageal Cancer. Ann Thorac Surg 2015;99(6): 1879–85 [discussion: 86].

29. Pouw RE, Heldoorn N, Alvarez Herrero L, et al. Do we still need EUS in the workup of patients with early esophageal neoplasia? A retrospective analysis of 131 cases. Gastrointest Endosc 2011;73(4):662–8.

30. Dhupar R, Rice RD, Correa AM, et al. Endoscopic Ultrasound Estimates for Tumor Depth at the Gastroesophageal Junction Are Inaccurate: Implications for the Liberal Use of Endoscopic Resection. Ann Thorac Surg 2015;100(5):1812–6.

31. Yang GYWT, Jobe BA, Thomas CR. The role of positron emission tomography in esophageal cancer. Gastrointest Cancer Res 2008;1(2):3–9.

32. Flamen P, Lerut A, Van Cutsem E, et al. Utility of positron emission tomography for the staging of patients with potentially operable esophageal carcinoma. J Clin Oncol 2000;18(18):3202–10.

33. Cuellar SL, Carter BW, Macapinlac HA, et al. Clinical staging of patients with early esophageal adenocarcinoma: does FDG-PET/CT have a role? J Thorac Oncol 2014;9(8):1202–6.

34. Sasako M, Sano T, Yamamoto S, et al. Left thoracoabdominal approach versus abdominal-transhiatal approach for gastric cancer of the cardia or subcardia: a randomised controlled trial. Lancet Oncol 2006;7(8):644–51.

35. Kurokawa Y, Sasako M, Sano T, et al. Ten-year follow-up results of a randomized clinical trial comparing left thoracoabdominal and abdominal

36. Hulscher JB, van Sandick JW, de Boer AG, et al. Extended transthoracic resection compared with limited transhiatal resection for adenocarcinoma of the esophagus. N Engl J Med 2002;347(21):1662–9.

37. Omloo JM, Lagarde SM, Hulscher JB, et al. Extended transthoracic resection compared with limited transhiatal resection for adenocarcinoma of the mid/distal esophagus: five-year survival of a randomized clinical trial. Ann Surg 2007;246(6): 992–1000 [discussion -1].

38. Blank S, Schmidt T, Heger P, et al. Surgical strategies in true adenocarcinoma of the esophagogastric junction (AEG II): thoracoabdominal or abdominal approach? Gastric Cancer 2018;21(2):303–14.

39. Kamarajah SK, Markar SR. Esophagectomy or Total Gastrectomy for Siewert 2 Gastroesophageal Junction (GEJ) Adenocarcinoma: An Ongoing Debate. Ann Surg Oncol 2022;29(1):750.

40. Anderegg MC, Lagarde SM, Jagadesham VP, et al. Prognostic Significance of the Location of Lymph Node Metastases in Patients With Adenocarcinoma of the Distal Esophagus or Gastroesophageal Junction. Ann Surg 2016;264(5):847–53.

41. Phillips AW, Lagarde SM, Navidi M, et al. Impact of Extent of Lymphadenectomy on Survival, Post Neoadjuvant Chemotherapy and Transthoracic Esophagectomy. Ann Surg 2017;265(4):750–6.

42. Mertens AC, Kalff MC, Eshuis WJ, et al. Transthoracic Versus Transhiatal Esophagectomy for Esophageal Cancer: A Nationwide Propensity Score-Matched Cohort Analysis. Ann Surg Oncol 2021;28(1):175–83.

43. Colvin H, Dunning J, Khan OA. Transthoracic versus transhiatal esophagectomy for distal esophageal cancer: which is superior? Interact Cardiovasc Thorac Surg 2011;12(2):265–9.

44. Barbour AP, Rizk NP, Gonen M, et al. Adenocarcinoma of the gastroesophageal junction: influence of esophageal resection margin and operative approach on outcome. Ann Surg 2007;246(1):1–8.

45. Biere SS, van Berge Henegouwen MI, Maas KW, et al. Minimally invasive versus open oesophagectomy for patients with oesophageal cancer: a multicentre, open-label, randomised controlled trial. Lancet 2012;379(9829):1887–92.

46. van der Sluis PC, van der Horst S, May AM, et al. Robot-assisted Minimally Invasive Thoracolaparoscopic Esophagectomy Versus Open Transthoracic Esophagectomy for Resectable Esophageal Cancer: A Randomized Controlled Trial. Ann Surg 2019;269(4):621–30.

47. Mariette C, Markar SR, Dabakuyo-Yonli TS, et al. Hybrid Minimally Invasive Esophagectomy for Esophageal Cancer. N Engl J Med 2019;380(2): 152–62.

48. Aaronson NK, Ahmedzai S, Bergman B, et al. The European Organization for Research and Treatment of Cancer QLQ-C30: a quality-of-life instrument for use in international clinical trials in oncology. J Natl Cancer Inst 1993;85(5):365–76.

49. Blazeby JM, Alderson D, Winstone K, et al. Development of an EORTC questionnaire module to be used in quality of life assessment for patients with oesophageal cancer. Eur J Cancer 1996;32(11):1912–7.

50. van der Schaaf M, Derogar M, Lagergren P. Reference values of oesophago-gastric symptoms (EORTC QLQ-OG25) in a population-based setting. Eur J Cancer 2012;48(11):1602–7.

51. Barbour AP, Lagergren P, Hughes R, et al. Health-related quality of life among patients with adenocarcinoma of the gastro-oesophageal junction treated by gastrectomy or oesophagectomy. Br J Surg 2008;95(1):80–4.

52. Jezerskyte E, Saadeh LM, Hagens ERC, et al. Long-Term Quality of Life After Total Gastrectomy Versus Ivor Lewis Esophagectomy. World J Surg 2020; 44(3):838–48.

53. Fuchs H, Holscher AH, Leers J, et al. Long-term quality of life after surgery for adenocarcinoma of the esophagogastric junction: extended gastrectomy or transthoracic esophagectomy? Gastric Cancer 2016;19(1):312–7.

54. Mitchell KG, Ikoma N, Nelson DB, et al. Mediastinal Nodal Involvement After Neoadjuvant Chemoradiation for Siewert II/III Adenocarcinoma. Ann Thorac Surg 2019;108(3):845–51.

55. Mine S, Sano T, Hiki N, et al. Proximal margin length with transhiatal gastrectomy for Siewert type II and III adenocarcinomas of the oesophagogastric junction. Br J Surg 2013;100(8):1050–4.

56. van Hagen P, Hulshof MC, van Lanschot JJ, et al. Preoperative chemoradiotherapy for esophageal or junctional cancer. N Engl J Med 2012;366(22): 2074–84.

57. Shapiro J, van Lanschot JJB, Hulshof MCCM, et al. Neoadjuvant chemoradiotherapy plus surgery versus surgery alone for oesophageal or junctional cancer (CROSS): long-term results of a randomised controlled trial. Lancet Oncol 2015;16(9):1090–8.

58. Cunningham D, Allum WH, Stenning SP, et al. Perioperative chemotherapy versus surgery alone for resectable gastroesophageal cancer. N Engl J Med 2006;355(1):11–20.

59. Al-Batran S-E, Homann N, Pauligk C, et al. Perioperative chemotherapy with fluorouracil plus leucovorin, oxaliplatin, and docetaxel versus fluorouracil or capecitabine plus cisplatin and epirubicin for locally advanced, resectable gastric or gastro-oesophageal junction adenocarcinoma (FLOT4): a randomised, phase 2/3 trial. Lancet 2019; 393(10184):1948–57.

60. Reynolds JV, Preston SR, O'Neill B, et al. Neo-AEGIS (Neoadjuvant trial in Adenocarcinoma of the Esophagus and Esophago-Gastric Junction International Study): Preliminary results of phase III RCT of CROSS versus perioperative chemotherapy (Modified MAGIC or FLOT protocol). (NCT01726452). J Clin Oncol 2021;39(15_suppl):4004.

61. Hoeppner J, Lordick F, Brunner T, et al. ESOPEC: prospective randomized controlled multicenter phase III trial comparing perioperative chemotherapy (FLOT protocol) to neoadjuvant chemoradiation (CROSS protocol) in patients with adenocarcinoma of the esophagus (NCT02509286). BMC Cancer 2016;16:503.

62. Al-Batran SE, Homann N, Pauligk C, et al. Effect of Neoadjuvant Chemotherapy Followed by Surgical Resection on Survival in Patients With Limited Metastatic Gastric or Gastroesophageal Junction Cancer: The AIO-FLOT3 Trial. JAMA Oncol 2017;3(9): 1237–44.

63. Kelly RJ, Ajani JA, Kuzdzal J, et al. Adjuvant Nivolumab in Resected Esophageal or Gastroesophageal Junction Cancer. N Engl J Med 2021;384(13): 1191–203.

64. Puhr HC, Preusser M, Ilhan-Mutlu A. Immunotherapy for Esophageal Cancers: What Is Practice Changing in 2021? Cancers (Basel) 2021;13(18).

65. Kamarajah SK, Phillips AW, Griffiths EA, et al. Esophagectomy or Total Gastrectomy for Siewert 2 Gastroesophageal Junction (GEJ) Adenocarcinoma? A Registry-Based Analysis. Ann Surg Oncol 2021; 28(13):8485–94.

66. Haverkamp L, Ruurda JP, van Leeuwen MS, et al. Systematic review of the surgical strategies of adenocarcinomas of the gastroesophageal junction. Surg Oncol 2014;23(4):222–8.